Praise for *Energetic Herbalism*

"This amazing book almost leaves me speechless. *Energ....* .. many different sources that flow into moder.... tion and practice. This is the type of book th.... been practicing for decades, yet it also repres.... the plants themselves, expressing themselves.... book touches upon everything that I hold dea......, ...unded upon the real experience of Nature as a living, intelligent, spiritual being."

—Matthew Wood, MS (Herbal Medicine), founder, Matthew Wood Institute of Herbalism; author of *The Book of Herbal Wisdom*

"Although I have been an herbalist for forty years, I was never able to understand the concepts of Chinese or Ayurvedic energetics as applied to healing with plants. Kat Maier is the first person to make the connection clear, and I am grateful— I get it! Just getting started as an herbalist? Want to be a better herbalist? A better steward of the planet? This is the wisdom book for you."

—Dr. Rosita Arvigo, DN, founder, The Abdominal Therapy Collective; author of *The Urban Herbalist*

"A wonderfully practical and accessible guide to energetic herbalism, filled with the wisdom and Viriditas of a Real Herbalist. Thank you, Kat!"

—David Hoffmann, RH (AHG), fellow, National Institute of Medical Herbalists; principal scientist, Traditional Medicinals

"I always ask my students: Do you want to be a good herbalist or a great herbalist? One of the essentials necessary to achieve a high level of herbal practice is the study of herbal energetics. In *Energetic Herbalism*, Kat Maier has distilled the teachings of the world's great herbal traditions into a concise, easy to learn guide that will allow any herbalist to begin to treat each person as an individual rather than generically treating diseases, and in so doing, to truly achieve excellence."

—David Winston, RH(AHG), DSc(hc), author of *Adaptogens: Herbs for Strength, Stamina, and Stress Relief*

"Beginning with her story of how she got into herbalism—a journey that became her life's work—Kat Maier takes on the hard task of making complex herbal systems easily understandable. She also does something that is even harder. She leads her readers to understand that plant medicine is a relationship that needs to be approached from the heart."

—Karyn Sanders, cofounder, Blue Otter School of Herbal Medicine; cohost, *The Herbal Highway*

"A beautifully written, all-encompassing guide to understanding the major healing traditions from around the world. Lest you think that this is all Kat Maier offers, let me dispel that thought. Diving deep into sacred healing traditions, Kat leads us to the plants. She enlightens with the uses, indications, and preparations of the plants she has chosen for the apothecary. *Energetic Herbalism* is a book you'll return to again and again."

—Phyllis Light, author of *Southern Folk Medicine*

"That Kat Maier's book so wonderfully conveys the essence and importance of energetic herbalism is a blessing. That the book also frames our use of herbs within the larger relationships we hold with the land, the seasons, and the sacred is essential. In *Energetic Herbalism*, Kat doesn't share mere uses of herbs but keen insights into establishing a deeper understanding of the patterns of health and nature."

—jim mcdonald, herbalist and founder, herbcraft.org

"In this beautifully written resource, Kat Maier has distilled her immense understanding of plant medicine into a captivating and comprehensive guidebook. Her extensive trainings in both the herbal energetic arts and the world of conventional medicine make her a trustworthy guide. . As an herbal teacher, this is a book I would recommend. As a practicing herbalist, this is a book I will reference. And as a reader, this is a book that offers me inspiration and hope."

—Lorna Mauney-Brodek, founder and director, Herbalista

"Kat Maier has crafted a very necessary book for these times and the era ahead. We all come from an herbalism tradition somewhere in our lineage. Kat weaves together many of these global practices, paying attention to giving credit where it is due and honoring the sources of the wisdom she shares. Ultimately, this book delves into the sometimes subtle yet significant ways seasonality and energetics aid in healing, filling a niche greatly needed in the herbal community."

—Marc Williams, ethnobiologist; facilitator, Botany Every Day; executive director, Plants and Healers International

"*Energetic Herbalism* nurtures an awareness of partnership between people and plants—it is a reverent call to sustainability. Kat's profound teachings always leave me awestruck and entice me further into my love affair with herbs. In her book, her impassioned voice penetrates the healer's heart."

—Mimi Hernandez, executive director, American Herbalists Guild

Energetic Herbalism

A Guide to Sacred Plant Traditions
Integrating Elements of
Vitalism, Ayurveda,
and Chinese Medicine

Kat Maier

Foreword by Rosemary Gladstar

Chelsea Green Publishing
White River Junction, Vermont
London, UK

Project Manager: Patricia Stone
Editor: Fern Marshall Bradley
Copy Editor: Deborah Heimann
Proofreader: Angela Boyle
Indexer: Shana Milkie
Designer: Melissa Jacobson

Printed in the United States of America.
First printing October 2021.
10 9 8 7 6 5 4   24 25 26 27 28

Library of Congress Cataloging-in-Publication Data
Names: Maier, Kat, 1955– author.
Title: Energetic herbalism : a guide to sacred plant traditions integrating
   elements of vitalism, ayurveda, and Chinese medicine / Kat Maier.
Description: White River Junction : Chelsea Green Publishing, 2021.
   | Includes bibliographical references and index.
Identifiers: LCCN 2021036531 (print) | LCCN 2021036532 (ebook)
   | ISBN 9781645020820 (paperback) | ISBN 9781645020837 (ebook)
Subjects: LCSH: Herbs—Therapeutic use.
Classification: LCC RM666.H33 M34 2021 (print) | LCC RM666.H33 (ebook)
   | DDC 615.3/21—dc23
LC record available at https://lccn.loc.gov/2021036531
LC ebook record available at https://lccn.loc.gov/2021036532

Chelsea Green Publishing
White River Junction, Vermont, USA
London, UK
www.chelseagreen.com

To my loving parents, Loretta and Hank,
and the light they birthed in me.

And to my son, Ian, who carries the flame forward.

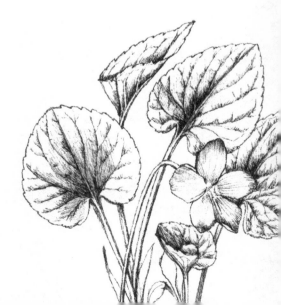

Contents

PART 2

The Apothecary

Foreword

How wise you are to be holding this brilliant book in your hands, getting ready to open the first pages, to plunge into the very heart of energetic herbalism. A magnificent world awaits you, and what better guide than renowned herbalist Kat Maier. As a teacher, practitioner, and steward of healing herbs, Kat brings decades of herbal experience to her writing, but also the curiosity and open mind of someone who is forever enchanted by the green world around them. Like so many herbalists I know, Kat fell into the world of herbs when she was quite young, and she has been on a heartful journey with the plants ever since. Lucky for us she's also found it part of her path to share with others what she's learned along the way.

I had the good fortune to meet Kat over thirty years ago at an herbal conference. We quickly became herbal sisters and best friends. I've had plenty of opportunities to witness Kat's passion and brilliance as we worked together on herbal projects over the years. Kat doesn't look at things simply, and she seldom takes the "normal" route. Her path is eclectic, deepened and enriched by her desire to explore life deeply, to get to the root of things, and to understand with her heart as well as her mind. That depth, wisdom, and experience is woven into the very core of *Energetic Herbalism*.

The world has been enriched by many excellent herb books written in the past few decades, but few contemporary herbalist authors explore the ideas of energetic herbalism, plant stewardship, and the spiritual relationship between plants and humans with such depth and insight as Kat. I do not know of any book that attempts to synthesize the teachings of several of the great traditions of herbalism into a cohesive body of knowledge. But that's precisely what Kat does, and does so magnificently, in this book. Her primary focus is on Traditional Chinese Medicine, Ayurvedic herbalism, and Vitalism, or what is sometimes called Western Herbalism. Each is unique and different in many aspects, but all are based on the universal principles of energetics, or the elemental life forces of Nature.

If we observe and reflect Nature, then we begin to understand our own nature, and also begin to understand how herbs, a force of Nature, affect our health and well-being.

As Kat readily admits, it can take a lifetime to understand and master the concepts underlying even one of these ancient traditions of healing. Thus, she does not propose that *Energetic Herbalism* will make anyone a master of any of the systems she explores. Rather, she clearly establishes that by understanding the underlying concepts described by each of these systems, we can begin to understand the energetics of how herbs work in the body. In turn, this knowledge leads us to a deeper, more personal relationship with the plants, as well as our own personal healing and our healing work with others.

Kat is not only a skilled herbalist but also an excellent storyteller and writer. She weaves in her own personal stories and experience, as well as insights and quotes from the many herbal teachers, shamans, and healers she has known and worked with. *Energetic Herbalism* is certainly not lacking in the practical, hands-on, easy-to-digest information that one finds in many popular herbal books but, in her usual style, Kat leads us farther afield, deeper into the world of plants. She invites us to explore the spiritual and energetic or elemental relationship between people and plants and gives us the necessary tools to do so. As she states in the introduction, the core essence of this book is ". . . to reveal the depth of relations that exist within ourselves and therefore with our external environment." Plants, as we come to understand them, are some of our greatest teachers on this path. Kat's intent is always to show us the path to greater knowledge and understanding, yes, but also to heartful connection with plants as living beings and spiritual teachers. As she so simply states, ". . . plants teach us how to be fully human."

I believe you'll find this book, as I did, not only insightful and instructional, but also inspiring and a joy to read. I've made a habit of collecting favorite quotes from my herbal friends over the years. I have quite the collection of "Kat Quotes" because what she says is so often quotable. This is one of my favorites:

What amazing dinner hosts plants are as they gather the best of folks together and, always, a good time is had. Rarely does anyone leave wanting, for these medicines and foods nourish us in places we never knew were hungry.

That's precisely what *Energetic Herbalism* does—it's a book that nourishes and feeds us in places we might never have known we were hungry. Kat offers us a feast for the senses and the soul. Enjoy!

Rosemary Gladstar
Misty Bay, Vermont

BEGINNINGS

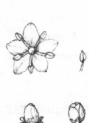

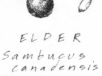

ELDER
*Sambucus
canadensis*

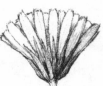

CALENDULA
*Calendula
officinalis*

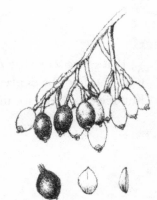

BLACK HAW
Viburnum prunifolium

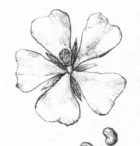

MARSHMALLOW
Althaea officinalis

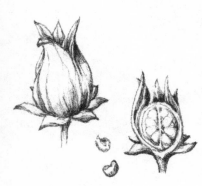

ROSELLE
Hibiscus sabdariffa

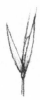

OATS
Avena sativa

BLACK COHOSH
Actaea racemosa

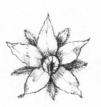

BORAGE
Borago officinalis

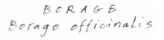

Honoring the Sacred

In the late 1980s, I had the honor and pleasure of living with the Shenandoah National Park as my neighbor. I would often end my day with a hike into the mountains to deepen my relationship with the medicinal plants I was learning about. One hot July day, I was particularly excited to head into the woods as I knew the white plume flowers of black cohosh would be in full glory. As I rounded a bend in the trail, I caught sight of the cohosh I had been visiting on my walks. Then, quite unexpectedly, energy leapt from the plant and penetrated my being. I stood there, breathless and in shock. As I gasped for air, I concentrated on calming myself. I began to realize that breath was flowing between this plant and myself. This has been described as "aisthesis—an exchange of soul essence accompanied by a gasp of recognition."[1] My breath was literally taken away—but then returned only to be accompanied by a multitude of sensations that culminated in a wash of profound peace. I could taste the sweet soil that held minerals and biota, life itself. I could smell the sophisticated yet fetid perfume of the cohosh's flowers. All my senses were heightened as I received an invitation to enter a sacred union. I slowly knelt, weeping in disbelief and awe, knowing that this black cohosh had communed with my being in a way that would change my life forever.

My experience with black cohosh was magical, cosmic, and spiritual, but the most vivid quality of the encounter was an exchange of information that I *sensed* rather than *thought*. Through my sense of smell, cohosh informed me who pollinates her blossoms. Through my taste buds, I learned what soil conditions are needed to nourish the plant's medicine. Through my heart, I was moved to understand that this plant would be a significant ally.

I learned all of this even though I did not have any direct physical contact with the plant that day; some other form of communication had taken place. I felt initiated into a world of service, reverence, and awe.

This extraordinary event of aisthesis was not unique to me—this transcendent experience has been described by others who study and work with plants as well. It did not descend on me as a novice herbalist—my encounter with cohosh happened more than ten years after my first yearning to understand the experience of the sacred world of plants. I had been devouring books about medicine people from across the globe who experienced deep healing through plant medicine. Their stories would often arise from the curing of a personal malady, and most beguiling to me were the relationships these elders, shamans, midwives, and herbalists had with the mysterious and potent world of plant spirit energy.

I had no illusions of becoming a shaman myself—I feel that the shaman's calling rises from a clear invitation from the spirit world. I am descended from Irish and German ancestry, and my path to becoming an herbalist was uniquely my own and oftentimes involved being confronted with more questions than answers. I have come to realize that herbalism as we know it today can allow anyone to richly explore their personal journey. Whether you engage with herbs through parenting, farming, wildcrafting, or deep clinical studies, your path is enriched by the relationships you cultivate, one by one, with the plants who are your teachers. The pleasure and power of plant medicine is a lifetime study.

Origin Stories

Holding a meaningful relationship with plants may be a new concept for some, but it is very familiar among First Nation peoples who grow up in cultures that name planets, bodies of water, and nonhuman species as relatives. Grandmother Moon, Father Sky, and Mother Earth are authentic and essential relationships. Indigenous creation stories are of cooperation and interdependence with Nature—rocks, animals, wind, and rain—as their primary relationship. This creates a sense of belonging, purpose, and an identity that inextricably links one to the whole of creation. In referring to Indigenous people in this book, I am speaking of original peoples all around the globe; first peoples of Europe, India, South America, Africa, and everywhere.

How is it that so many people have lost their sense of connectedness? What sets people on a path of falsely thinking they are separate from the rest of creation and superior to other creatures? The reasons are complex and deep seated, entwined with religious and cultural beliefs and prejudices that date back more than a thousand years. They are also inextricably bound to the worldwide history of colonization—of people invading lands and brutally exploiting their natural resources and Indigenous peoples. In the United States, this is prominent in the historical record of colonization and cultural appropriation by white European immigrants.

In the Old Testament creation story of Adam and Eve, danger arose from Nature herself in the form of an apple, a snake, and a woman. In Indigenous creation stories, however, interdependence with Nature is the primary relationship. When we shift our view and regard aspects of the natural world as beings rather than objects, it dramatically alters how we engage with them. Ecotheologian Thomas Berry says, "We are talking only to ourselves. We are not talking to the rivers, we are not listening to the wind and stars. We have broken the great conversation. By breaking that conversation, we have shattered the universe."[2]

The work now is to join the efforts historically led by BIPOC (Black, Indigenous, People of Color) groups to deconstruct and transform the colonizers' influence that has shaped the structures of the current world we live in. The natural world is not a grouping of resources to be consumed and exploited, but rather a gathering of beings to honor and respect. Objectification of the sentient beings who inhabit our landscapes creates a hierarchy where only humans are considered alive and conscious; Nature is referred to as "it." Often when I lead a plant walk, people ask me whether this plant or that one is "good for anything." In that context, it seems like an acceptable question. But imagine if someone introduced me to you and, after greeting you, I wondered aloud whether you were good for anything, or how I could use you. I am confident that our relationship would not evolve much further from that initial meeting.

I am not suggesting that our role is to anthropomorphize or attribute human personality to plants. Instead, let us learn to receive with gratitude the gifts plants offer us. Environmental scientist and Potawatomi elder Robin Wall Kimmerer has helped clarify the language that is embedded in Indigenous practices of reciprocity. This is the exchange of gifts and gratitude for all that these creative beings give us. Kimmerer calls the restoration of these relations the "grammar of animacy." As we engage inhabitants of the natural world as kin, elders, and teachers, there is a ripe opportunity for a paradigmatic shift to take hold.

Journey to the Plants

I was not born into a family, tribe, or culture that sang songs honoring ancestors or the spirits of the trees. For me, the sacred was held in a church where we weren't allowed to dance. It was held in the Eucharist wafer I was forbidden to touch. And only through the intercession of another human could I attain a union with my creator. Even so, I loved the rituals and ceremonies of coming together and singing. I owe the birth of my dream to this seed of love.

My childhood cosmology of Catholicism presented Jesus as the ultimate healer. At age six, I was enthralled by stories of Jesus walking on water and raising the dead, and the instantaneous healings that would occur. This was my introduction to energetic healing, in which mysterious forces are gathered to create a miraculous outcome. I did not know how to name it at that time, but I was seeking the sacred, and these stories nourished my dream to become a healer.

When I was twelve, I saw a movie about the Peace Corps, and I immediately knew I had found my calling—a resounding sense of connection seeded in the desire to serve. It wasn't until I arrived in another land seven years later that I understood that the drive to serve was coupled with a desire to live with diverse cultures of color and learn their ancestral ways.

The year was 1978, the country was Chile, and I was a Peace Corps health educator working in a rural town. Rich in natural resources, Chile is a culturally sophisticated South American treasure. The health care system was well developed, and modern medicine (in simple form) was available in even the remotest towns.

With the transition to contemporary medicine, traditional ways were perceived as backward. There was a common phrase, "*no sea bruja*," which means "don't be a witch" (i.e., a traditional healer). The year prior to my arrival, there had been a horrific coup seeded in part by US interests. For a twenty-year-old US woman to choose to live in a remote area was difficult for the Chileans to fathom. It wasn't until I had spent a few months traveling to satellite clinics, sharing many meals with hospital staff and their families, that a group of women elders took me into the fields with them to harvest plants. One of the first times I drank their healing tea, I felt a stirring, a reverie, a deep sense of peace enveloping me. As I listened to their stories of healing, I was transported to a place ancient yet familiar. This feeling was fleeting but impactful; it showed me that plants were a portal to the energetic world of healing I was determined to find.

Sadly, I also witnessed these traditions disappearing into the shadow of the emerging structures of a dominant culture where only the white man's medicine was to be trusted. This rejection and scorn of a magnificent people and their traditions provoked a deep grief in me.

The time I spent in Chile was the beginning of the "golden thread" that William Stafford describes in his poem, "The Way It Is." He writes there is a thread we follow that never changes. It is our heart's journey, and it is hard to explain to others because they cannot see it: The thread is ours alone. Life proceeds, circumstances change, tragedies occur, yet all through life we never let go of the thread. We know as long as we hold onto it, we will never get lost.

I returned home from Chile to a graduate school program in Washington, DC, with a grand vision of working with international groups to save traditional plant medicines. As a student I soon came to realize that the international programs offered to developing countries were a Western template for improvement that did not originate with invitations or requests of the nation or culture that was receiving aid.

For me, one disquieting question spiraled to another. How could I save a tradition that I had no experience with? Who was I to tell other cultures that plant medicine is superior when millions were suffering from lack of basic human needs and rights? Who was I actually saving traditions for? In that era (late 1970s), the articulation of the white savior complex—whites helping non-whites as a self-serving gesture—was not well articulated, not among white people, that is. As Nigerian American art historian and Harvard professor Teju Cole writes about well-intentioned US efforts, "His good heart does not always allow him to think constellationally. He does not connect the dots or see the patterns of power behind the isolated 'disasters.' . . . He is putting food in those mouths as fast as he can. All he sees is need, and he sees no need to reason out the need for the need."[3]

The issues of deep systemic injustices stemming from colonization and cultural appropriation have come to the forefront of my heart and personal work. The more I learn, the humbler I become as I see how deeply the colonizers' mind has influenced my lens of the world. The herbal community as well is coming to terms with the ways in which descendants of white European immigrants stole Indigenous American and enslaved African wisdom and practices and then sold them as their own. It is a process that requires humility, introspection, and painful discussion of how to decolonize herbalism.

In the midst of this foundational reckoning, I believe that there is a way forward in understanding how energetics are shared by diverse cultures of the world and how to honor the teachings of the ancestors. Thus, I am beginning this book with my own story, but not as a template for anyone else to follow. It is simply to say that each person's search for their way to work with plant medicine is unique. Your path will reveal the place in yourself that resonates with authenticity and what your special relationship with the sacred will hold.

Returning to my story, much to the chagrin of family and my favorite academic advisor, I left graduate school before completion. The choice to leave was the thread guiding me on my search to understand healing from direct experience. I left Washington, DC, to work in a wilderness school in the Appalachian Mountains near Shenandoah National Park. My motivation was a deep-seated need to steep myself in Nature, live among the plants, and learn about them through the seasons. The two years I spent in the mountains were possibly the most intense of my life. This school was a brilliant model of working with resilient young women of all races who were deeply struggling with challenges arising from their family and school experiences and the trauma of social injustices.

I naively assumed there would be lots of staff support, but many staff members left due to the high demands of the physical environment and the nature of the work. Eventually, only a handful of us remained to fend for the students and ourselves. It was a peer-run program, and learning came through immediate consequences. If the group did not chop firewood, it would be a long, cold night. We felled trees to build buildings, used draw blades to clear bark, lashed and notched critical joints of the structures we built. There were so many skills needed—for counseling, for construction, and for group work.

The thread I followed in order to live in intimate connection with plants led me into the hearts and souls of these beautiful young women who were far braver than I would ever have to be. When they left this program, they would be on their own, which is why the school focused on daily life skills. From balancing checkbooks to learning math through measuring, to learning cooperation so we would be warm at night. These women taught me how many privileges I had enjoyed in life, including to choose to live at the camp in order to study plants. Those that I stayed in contact with would sometimes ask if I was still as crazy about plants now as I had been during those memorable seasons. How could I tell them, yes—even more so!

Close to the end of my two-year commitment, a brochure for the California School of Herbal Studies showed up on the mountain. The literature literally just showed up at the school. It included a beautiful calendar of the curriculum, complete with field trips to enchanting California coastlines and inland forests. I called the phone number on the brochure, and Rosemary Gladstar, the founder of the school, answered. At that time, I had no idea how special that conversation was. Rosemary was so gracious and helpful, and she said she would call me back with the name of someone I could rent a room from.

My heart felt the pulse of the plants, yet the voice in my head said that I needed a medical license, some legitimation of my studies and hard work so I could work in rural clinics with underserved populations. I was torn between my elusive dreams of living and working with Nature and my rational beliefs. Very reluctantly, I decided to thank Rosemary, decline the rental room, and continue my search. Had I let go of the thread? Or was the declining of California dreaming helping me to define more clearly where my path lay?

Soon after, I met a British woman who owned a local health food store. She said if I was that interested in herbal medicine for the people, I needed to go to the British School of Phytotherapy at Tunbridge Wells in Southeastern England, a respected medical school that instructed in the use of medicinal plants as the pharmacopeia. It sounded like a dream come true. I decided to go to Tunbridge Wells and apply, but made Dublin my first stop, so I could visit friends and explore the island of my ancestors. Two weeks into that solo journey, I found myself on the west coast of Ireland, in love with many aspects of the wild and coastal lands. I found a job at a bed and breakfast with a view of the Aran Islands. This put a roof over my head and provided enough money to pay the penalty for canceling my flight home. The mythical lands of Ireland's west coast had enchanted me. I lived in County Clare in the tiny yet musically renowned town of Doolin, just south of the Burren, a lunar-like landscape, with arctic, Andalusian, and alpine wildflowers and portal dolmens—ancient, Megalithic tombs shrouded in mystery and magic.

After morning tasks, I would venture out on long walks with my field guides of plants of the Burren. I developed a side business taking international travelers on walking and botany tours of this landscape. We would hike for miles, and the wildness of this landscape was so raw and liminal that I felt I could easily enter another dimension. Getting lost was not uncommon, and the vast expanse and freedom was intoxicating. Ancient ceremonial treasures that had witnessed a thousand years of winds and storms sat free for all to experience.

For the first time in my life, I felt indigenous to a place. The dictionary definition of *indigenous* is "native to an area," but the Latin derivative *gignere* means "to bring into being." I had grown up hearing stories of the strong Irish American women in my mother's family, just one generation removed from those who had arrived at Ellis Island from Ireland, but most of them had passed before I was old enough to appreciate their wisdom and character. During my months in Ireland, it slowly dawned on me that although the school at Tunbridge Wells was the thread I had followed across the Atlantic, the real education awaiting me was to come into selfhood by experiencing the deep home ground of my ancestors. I had thought I needed a certificate, approval from a higher power to deem me worthy of pursuing my goals. But what higher education is there than to follow the thread to one's source, to encounter the lineage that makes you who you are? The enchantment of Ireland's west coast, the songs I heard in my wanderings, were hauntingly familiar and simply so right.

I returned to the United States with a deepened sense of identity, and I enrolled in the physician's assistant program at Hahnemann Medical College in Philadelphia. This may seem a strange choice after my experiences in Ireland, but I knew I wanted to learn clinical skills of emergency medicine and enough basic knowledge of allopathic medicine to help others navigate the complexities of that system. Not wanting to devote several years of study to medical school, I decided that the two-year, deeply intensive training as a physician's assistant fit perfectly with my dream of continuing plant studies.

After I completed the training, I assumed I would soon get a job in a medical practice, work for five or so years, gather lots of experience, then move on to working with the plants. In the meanwhile, I began exploring the Shenandoah mountains with an old friend named Clyde Perry. After retiring from a meaningful career at NASA, Clyde had moved to the farthest hollow one could find in the mountains, and there he served anyone and everyone as a deeply gifted healer. These mountains were a veritable living apothecary of wild native medicines. On one of our plant expeditions, Clyde took me to La Dama Maya Herb Farm in Luray, Virginia. At the farm, I was transported back to the liminal quality of Ireland. Maureen Messick and Lee McWhorter were the stewards and they introduced me to biodynamic farming, which views the farm as a whole, living organism just as a wild woodland creates its own ecosystem. The goal is to utilize and support the interrelatedness of resources that exist in a homestead landscape. Balancing elements and harmonizing relationships in this way was my first glimpse into the teachings of what I was to later learn in the practice of vitalism.

After a year of planting according to the stars and movements of the planets (biodynamic practices), it gradually dawned on me that the rejections I was receiving to my applications to work as a physician's assistant were actually affirmations that my education in plant medicine was now in full swing. I began in earnest my apprenticeship to the plants. It can take a while to see that rejection is an ally keeping us on the true path to self.

Like any back-to-the-lander in the 1980s working in an undefined profession, I hustled a number of jobs while living and studying plant medicine in the mountains. I gave free lectures, learned new skills in bodywork, and began offering people recommendations on how to use herbal medicines I was familiar with. After seven years of this, my community began referring to me as an herbalist. This is how it used to be: You were deemed an herbalist when your medicine worked and you had gained the requisite trust. I feel I was truly a community-created herbalist and define myself as such to this day.

My winding path to herbalism inspired me to create two schools so others could have a container for learning this amazing craft. The first, in Washington, Virginia, with wonderful co-founder Teresa Boardwine, was Dreamtime Center for Herbal Studies. After seven very successful years, the golden thread brought me to Charlottesville, where I opened my second school, Sacred Plant Traditions. Reflecting back to my early concern about obtaining licensure as a form of legitimization, it's important to acknowledge that standards of competency serve as a guide to making sound choices. However, I contend that the miraculous fact that herbalism in the United States is *unlicensed* offers untold benefits for those who seek the services of herbalists. This freedom to claim herbalism as medicine of the people is to be celebrated, treasured, and fiercely protected. It is a privilege to have access to so many forms of plant medicines as well as a diversity of traditional ways of working with the plants.

About This Book

This book is a culmination of my thirty years of study, travel, explorations, and, most importantly, practice of herbal medicine. These chapters represent what I feel is a strong foundation for individuals who wish to deeply engage with plants for care of themselves and of their communities. Remember, herbal medicine was the main health care system only one hundred years ago in the United States. The traditional healing cultures of Ayurveda and Chinese medicine I explore in this book have been developing sophisticated botanical medicine systems for the last five thousand years, and they have done so explicitly working with energetic medicine. The common denominator of all energetic systems, whether African, Caribbean, or Tibetan, are the elements of Nature that make us who we are. These are constant the world over. Fire, water, air, earth, wood, ether, and metal are representations of energy. Heat is transformative, earth is grounding, and air is movement. The ways in which these elements relate to each other in our health or in Nature create the patterns we work with. I am grateful that contemporary herbalism is now adopting the lens of these energetic systems. It makes so much sense, and it reflects a notion I have loved from the practice of permaculture—the edge effect. This effect arises when two or more systems merge and their coming together creates a diversity that would not exist otherwise. This happens in natural ecosystems as well as cultural ones.

This is the core of this book, to reveal the depth of relations that exist within ourselves and therefore with our external environment. Dry lands invite winds to blow and stir the air. Dry tissues bring winds or tremors and stir our energy. Earth and all her elements of fire, water, and air are in constant relationship, adjusting to forces that are adjusting to other forces with the intent of self-correction. Nothing lives in isolation. Like a pebble tossed into a pond, the ripples created affect life beyond the shore. Ever so gently, barely perceptible, energy constantly touches the world we live in.

It is my hope that through this book you will begin to develop a fluency with the language of energetics so you can help your family and friends enjoy better health, and if you are a practitioner, to work more deeply with your apothecary and community. Energetic herbalism not only has borne the test of time, it is the most ecological system of medicine in existence today. It teaches us that less is better, that we can improve health and vitality simply by shifting patterns in the body versus by administering medicines or undertaking procedures that produce drastic changes. I am deeply grateful for the sophisticated success of modern medicine, such as setting a broken bone, removing a tumor, or brilliantly imaging a nerve lesion. But for most of our day-to-day maladies, simpler, safer remedies often are all we need.

Unlike many herbal books today, the materia medica chapter in this book offers a limited palette of plants: twenty-five medicinal herbs. This is an intentional choice. When I studied herbalism in Mexico and Central America, most of the powerful women healers I encountered worked with an apothecary of only five to ten plants. Rosita Arvigo, who lives in Belize and has devoted her life to the preservation of traditional Mayan herbalism, talks often about using only her three favorite plants, marigold (*Tagetes erecta*), basil (*Ocimum basilicum*), and rue (*Ruta graveolens*). When we develop relationships with plants, their medicine extends far beyond the tidy definitions and categories we tend to place them in. In Chinese medicine, there is a concept of Fifty Fundamental Herbs. These are the plants that have the widest basic applications and thus are the foundation of an apothecary.

As I considered which plants to include in my materia medica for this book, I was keenly aware of the plight of many wild medicinal plants, whose populations are threatened by the booming herbal products industry that is growing exponentially with each passing year. In 2019, US consumers spent more than nine and a half billion dollars on herbal supplements, according to the American Botanical Council's herb market report.[4] According to a report published by Botanic Gardens Conservation International, "Plant extinctions are occurring at a rate unmatched in geological history, leaving ecosystems incomplete and impoverished. Current extinction rates are at least 100 to 1,000 times higher than natural background rates, with a quarter of the world's coniferous trees known to be in jeopardy and as many as 15,000 medicinal plants under threat."[5]

When I began my practice in the 1980s, I worked with only a small number of plants. I was a stubborn, radical bioregionalist who only used plants available on the farm where I lived or from surrounding fields and woodlands. While we think the "buying local" movement is a recent arrival, many have been living this solution for quite some time. Early on I was also influenced by the writings of author and herbalist Svevo Brooks, who said, "My idea of a good herbalist isn't someone who knows the uses of forty different herbs, but someone who knows how to use one herb in forty different ways."[6]

Over the years, though, my apothecary reflected my travels, both geographically and as an herbalist. As I began learning from other teachers, my shelves of medicines expanded to an apothecary full of exotic remedies sourced from around the world. Many of these plants are profound medicines and they taught me about their energetics of flavor, smell, and medicinal effects. Now in my wiser years, I have circled back, and my apothecary once again fits on fewer shelves. I have come to grips with the hard truth that to save healing plants, we need to commit to bioregionalism as best we can and engage in thoughtful conversations about these issues. Before today's popular books on herbal medicine become fables about extinct plants, we are challenged to find alternatives to endangered species. Just as these times are demanding that we restructure our institutions, so, too, does the herbal community need to have the courage to restructure their apothecaries and seek to work effectively with fewer plants or with those whose lives are not endangered.

Throughout my career, and also in this book, I honor the teachers I have been blessed with, but my deepest training came from the seven years I apprenticed to the plants, one on one, in my exploration of the rich apothecary of the Appalachian Mountains. The learning continues to this day.

Kat Maier
Charlottesville, Virginia
Unceded land of the Monacan Indian Nation

PART 1

Sacred Relationships and Healing Traditions

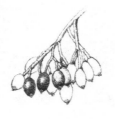

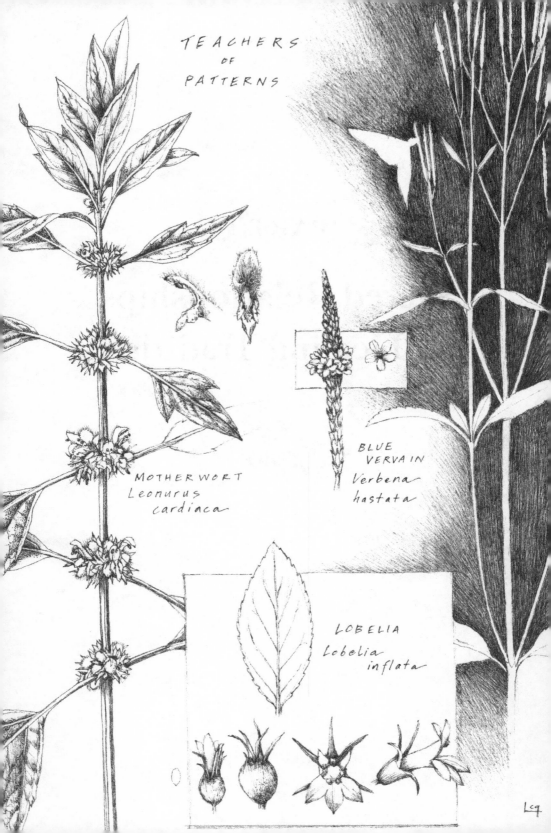

TEACHERS OF PATTERNS

MOTHERWORT
Leonurus
cardiaca

BLUE
VERVAIN
Verbena
hastata

LOBELIA
Lobelia
inflata

Lcg

CHAPTER 1

The Language of Energetics

I can still picture her. My client was hovering on the edge of her seat, face flushed and foot tapping incessantly. My efforts to calm this client had seemed only to aggravate her. I excused myself and went to my apothecary to recruit help. Returning, I asked my client, I'll call her Maria, if she felt comfortable taking an herb so we could better assess her needs. She agreed, and I gave her 10 drops of motherwort (*Leonurus cardiaca*) tincture. After a few minutes, Maria visibly relaxed. She sat back, loosening her jaw a bit, and made a joke about how anxious she was and asked, could she have another sip? After the second sip, she shifted position, planted both feet on the floor, and then tears welled up in her eyes. "I knew I had come to the right place," she said.

That magic elixir, motherwort, is a common garden plant. In fact, as a member of the mint family, it can be a bit intrusive in the garden. The profound effect Maria experienced was not elicited by some rare and exotic plant from the Amazon or Tibet. It was a common garden plant, motherwort, that allowed this client to experience profound changes. Maria presented with heat and tension that had been present for so long she was barely aware of her fidgeting and spastic movements. My client had recounted her many visits to practitioners, which brought her little to no relief. A few symptoms had improved at times, but truth be told, she was getting worse. Maria described her cracking joints and stiffness, cold hands and feet, sluggish bowels, and dry skin and eyes. Her most distressing symptom, she said, was the insomnia. And by the way, what was that herb that she had just taken, and could she have another sip?

The energy of motherwort directly affected the energy of Maria. As a bitter herb, motherwort is cooling, so it chilled the heat from her anxiety. As a bitter relaxant, motherwort allowed Maria to settle into herself with a little more ease. Cracking of the joints can signify dryness, and when tension relaxes for extended periods of time, fluids flow easier to lubricate tendons and bowels. Pretty magical that this wild and weedy plant could have such a profound effect on Maria's energy, physical being, and even state of mind! Maria's immediate ability to relax allowed her to self-correct and thereby better access her senses, emotions, and, ultimately, her true nature.

This is energetic herbalism. Its elegance lies in its simplicity and its sensuality: reading patterns of the person and matching the patterns to those found in plants. Maria's pattern of long-term tension led to a pattern of dryness, which in turn possibly led to a pattern that energetic practitioners call *wind*, or internal, changing patterns. Obviously, treating the needs of clients—and even ourselves—is not always so simple and clear-cut. Yet I can say I have journeyed with a multitude of "Marias" to reach greater health through the lens of energetics.

Generally, energetics in herbalism relates the energetics of the plant (cooling, moving motherwort) to a current imbalance or condition (anxiety, tension), then lastly to the energetics of the person or constitution (sensitive, dry). The underlying foundation is the energetics of the spirit (unconditional support) of the plant and the sacred relationship an herbalist develops with the land and these sentient beings, the plants.

Honoring Roots of Energetic Models

The word *energetic* may conjure images of New Age crystals, and the term is sometimes misapplied to any and all new healing modalities. In truth, though, energetic herbalism is as old as the Earth herself. This mode of healing is based on the truth that the vital force of nature and the vital force of an individual human are one and the same. Indigenous cultures the world over call this force *spirit* in their native language. Ancient Greeks called this force *vitality*, the Chinese call it *Qi* (chi), Iroquois nation calls it *Orenda*, Ayurveda calls it *Prana*, West Africans call it *Ashe*.

The goal of energetic herbalism is to enhance our terrain, which is our inner landscape—our tissues, organs, vessels, and all the forces that are engaged to maintain our health. The aim is to create an environment where we optimize nutrition from food, breath from air, and joy from our surroundings so our vitality flows with the least hindrance. To be in the flow is the goal of these traditions.

In the late 1960s, chemist James Lovelock and microbiologist Lynn Margulis proposed the theory that the Earth is endowed with an ability to communicate across species in effort to provide homeostasis. The well-known Gaia hypothesis or Gaia theory states that the biota communicates with organic as well as inorganic material to ensure evolution as well as feedback systems for an elegant self-regulating balance to occur. This theory is named after the Mother Earth goddess from Greek mythology. Margulis and Lovelock described planet Earth as a self-regulating being who automatically adjusts the temperature, salinity of the ocean, and atmospheric content in response to changes in the ecosystem. In this respect, the living system of Earth is identical to the workings of our bodies. We are constantly regulating temperature, fluids, and the tone of organs and tissues. *Vitalism* is a teaching that states there is an invisible force governing our health, lives, and planet that is unseen and unmeasurable. This force has the intelligence to be not only self-directing but brilliantly self-correcting.

Of course, this is what Indigenous teachings have been saying for millennia in describing the sacred connections of all forms of Nature. Amazonian tribes still work with plants according to the stories and dreams that have been sung through ancestral wisdom keepers, as do many First Nation peoples. Creation stories can seem incomprehensible to Westerners, yet they provide meaningful direction and patterns for peoples who experience Nature and time in a sacred and nonlinear fashion. Vitalist traditions, Ayurveda, Traditional Chinese Medicine, Unani Tibb, and North American Eclectic medicine represent the organization of elements of Nature. These systems describe the patterns of energy present in humans as well as in the plants themselves. Throughout history, there have been translations and modifications of energetic models, whether from within a culture or from outside it, in attempts to appeal to the politics of the day or to be more accessible to other cultures. For example, folkloric, Taoist, shamanic traditions in China were being practiced for centuries before the beginning of the beautiful cosmology of Classical Chinese Medicine. The Classical model then was adapted after the Cultural Revolution of the 1960s, which attempted to modernize and standardize this system, thus birthing Traditional Chinese Medicine, or TCM. This is the nature of systems; there is adaptation and conformity, but still, bodies of knowledge are preserved that can be shared through the ages.

Reading Patterns

Energetic herbalism is a framework that matches the pattern or spirit (warming, cooling, moving, sedating) of an herb to that of the imbalance (tension, stagnation, dryness) in the body in an effort to gently nudge the body back into balance via the path of least resistance. This is accomplished by removing impediments to the body's natural state of relaxation. A relaxed person is a highly functioning one because all systems are able to communicate and support each other with optimum efficiency and spirit. As mechanical as that may sound, the less resistance there is in our beings, whether mentally, physically, or spiritually, the brighter our life force and spirit will shine.

My training as a practitioner in allopathic medicine gave me an awe of the articulation of our bodies through the language of biomedicine. In practice, though, I was allotted only fifteen minutes per patient, and I realized that such a rigid system could not allow for the grandeur of medicine/healing to play out. It would be impossible to treat a person in a truly holistic sense in such a brief encounter. I also found myself wondering why preventable diseases such as diabetes and hypertension were on the rise at exponential rates. These diseases have become the dreaded comorbidity factors in this time of pandemics. In my training as a physician's assistant, I seemed to spend all my time chasing numbers and trying to control symptoms rather than restoring a person's healthy terrain or ecology so that the numbers would take care of themselves.

Wide-angle vision is a technique I use to teach the art of pattern recognition. It involves allowing the gaze to transition from a hard focus to a softer, more expansive contemplation of a scene with the full range of peripheral vision (I describe how to do this in "Sensory Noticing" on page 44). As you make this shift, your consciousness drops from sympathetic mode (fight or flight) and enters the parasympathetic world of sensing environs from a more holistic vantage point. The body relaxes and awareness is heightened because the analytical mind is put aside. Patterns emerge and sounds that were inaudible can be heard as you release the mental gyrations that were drowning out the present moment. Trackers, gardeners, hunters, wildcrafters, and those gifted with a natural acumen for high awareness live in this state of being in which many levels of the world can be perceived simultaneously.

This level of perceptiveness is critical in energetic medicine, where the goal is to treat the whole person and not just superficial symptoms. The mantra is to treat what you see, but this "seeing" must include all the senses, not just the eyes. We *listen* to the client's history, *feel* their pulse, *smell* their scent, and *observe* (with the heart as well as the eyes) their movements and spirit.

To skillfully observe patterns of disease, we first need to spend time observing patterns in Nature, to learn to grasp patterns of harmony and disharmony. Blowing winds that dry the land, flooding waters that swell rivers, excess heat that rises, and cold that depresses are all vital expressions of Nature that play out in our organs, joints, muscles, thoughts, and spirit. This is the practice of traditional folk herbalism: Through observation of Nature's patterns, the inherent self-regulating systems of the body are acknowledged and supported.

This practice is the heart of preventative medicine. According to Ayurvedic teachings, if you know the pattern of imbalance, you can successfully treat 80 percent of illnesses with foods and herbs to support self-healing mechanisms, especially when disruptions in patterns are observed early on. The challenge is to trust the inherent wisdom of the body and resist the inclination to take over for the vital force.

An exception is when an illness is left without remedy for too long, and an example of that is mononucleosis (mono). In my clinical practice, I frequently consult with clients who had mono during their young adult years. Although Western medicine considers mono a benign illness, it can seriously drain a person's vitality. The client recovers from acute symptoms, but modern medicine has nothing to offer in terms of the lost art of convalescence or *re-vitalization*. Thus, even after the patient "feels better," they may still experience fatigue. At an energetic level, their body is running colder due to loss of vital energy. They experience a need to add a layer of clothes more often or drink warming beverages. This shift is so subtle that many people don't register this change. But over time, even ordinary stress can exacerbate this energetic condition of cold or deficiency, leading to lowered immune function. Eventually, stress can push this condition into chronic fatigue syndrome, which results when the Epstein Barr virus (the same virus that causes mono) takes over the body due to low vitality. As stress continues to drain vitality, this person may progress to metabolic syndrome or hypothyroidism, the latter being a condition that is epidemic in women over age fifty.

In energetic medicine, the approach to helping someone fully recover from mono is to warm the person through use of appropriate tonics and herbs to support the immune system. It is vital to understand the energetics of the herbs you work with, however. For example, echinacea (*Echinacea* spp.) is specific for mono, but its energy is cold (which is why it excels at clearing toxic heat from snakebites). With mono, echinacea can be helpful, but it should be offered in combination with warming herbs to address deficient vitality. With this kind of simple, knowledgeable herbal support, the patient recovering from mono can potentially avoid years of suffering and loss.

I have found that naming patterns of imbalance for clients empowers them with a greater understanding of their nature and their health. Instead of overwhelming a client by telling them they might have four or five diseases, we can address one, or perhaps two, underlying conditions. That said, herbalists make use of many tools to help clients on their journey toward health, including blood work, bodywork, allopathic testing, and scans when appropriate. Yet time and again I have seen cases that involved a multitude of issues, and by working energetically, as I did with my client Maria, the path to healing unfolds with greater simplicity than might have been imagined.

Chapter 2 presents ways to begin the lifelong journey of deeply knowing plants and their spirits or personalities. In addition to their wonderful energetics, plants bring a unique level of compassion to our lives. Plants have an uncanny ability to get in between the spaces to remind our bodies that their self-healing mechanisms are still intact. They are the perfect teachers indeed.

Elements of Nature

The common denominator of all energetic systems is the elements of Nature. Fire, water, air, earth, wood and metal are representations of energy in many cultures. Fire transforms and moves, water nourishes and moistens, air cools and dries, and earth builds and grounds. The ways in which the elements relate to each other creates patterns in our terrain or state of health. When we have a red-hot infection, we work with the energy of temperature and apply cooling balms and medicine to clear the heat. As mentioned above, in the case of mononucleosis, the issue is not enough heat or vitality, so we want to warm and nourish. The magnificence of energetic herbalism is that elements are constant. Those suffering from the Spanish flu during the pandemic of 1918 were treated with many of the same herbs used to treat

COVID-19 one hundred years later, because those herbs address the same conditions. A fever is excess heat, and boggy lungs are excess water, and the energetic remedies for these imbalances are unchanged. Traditional medicine does not focus on destroying the virus (though we do have amazing plants for that purpose when we need them) but rather on strengthening the terrain in order to prevent the virus from spreading. This is one of the greatest gifts of energetic healing. The constancy of Nature (the elements) provides reassurance that we will be equipped to respond, even to seemingly novel health challenges in this era of changing climate. The Earth may become warmer, but heat is the same fundamental pattern today as it was seventy or seven hundred years ago—there will just be more of it. Now is the time to learn to navigate unpredictable changes by embracing the wisdom of the teachings of ancient healing systems. These teachings are becoming the language of twenty-first-century natural medicine. Whether the topic is Anthropocene extinction or pandemics, the way through the darkest of times is to engage with the wisdom and sanctity that is instilled in every breath, rock, leaf, or shooting star. Nature is guiding us more than we can imagine.

Global Healing Systems

Over the past thirty years, herbalists have gained vast experience with global energetic traditions, from Chinese medicine to Greek, Arabic, African, and Ayurvedic medicine. People are eager to learn and practice these ancient global healing traditions.

Over the years I have gotten lost, found my way, grown confused again, and ultimately emerged humbled by the challenge of how to honor these global healing traditions in my teaching. How to present complex systems that require years of study, quite honestly lifetimes of study, in the space of a month-long, or even three-year course? I persisted because I believe these systems fill a great need in our times, offering a deeply compassionate way of learning about who we are and how we can navigate an increasingly complex world. On my path, I was fortunate to find teachers who brought these systems and languages home to me in a way that deeply enriched my practice, teachings, and life. And now I have created this guide for working with self-care. I want to stress that this book is not intended to teach how to practice Five Phase Theory or Ayurveda—such training requires many years of dedication. It is also not an attempt to merge the distinct qualities of different energetic systems. Rather, it is intended as an honoring of the wisdom keepers who have walked this planet for millennia. It is a manual of the most useful tools I have found and stocked in my medicine bag during my decades as a community herbalist and teacher. For many readers, the chapters that follow will be a deep dive into unfamiliar concepts and vocabulary. For more experienced readers, I acknowledge that I have left out a substantial amount of theory that these thousand-year systems offer. My goal is to offer stories and teachings that will serve as a practical foundation for those who wish to care for the health needs of their family and community. And for serious students of herbalism, it is the introduction that I hope will inspire them to pursue more training.

The three models of energetics I particularly focus on are Five Phase Theory, Ayurveda, and Western energetics. These three traditions are the scaffolding, and the matrix that holds it all together is the truth from Indigenous teachings that the Earth and all her creations are imbued with a sacred spirit. I invite you to *experience* these complex systems through the *elements* of Nature. Each of these energetic models encompasses layer upon layer of nuanced, intricate studies of centuries of brilliant theories. This may sound intimidating, but remember, you are already using plant medicines from all over the world in your daily life—just take a look at your spice rack to see that this is so.

I offer my experience using these models as tools of healing, and for me, healing is an act of beauty. These systems are treasures that deserve deep appreciation. The artful expression of our relationship to the elements, seasons, and emotions deserves study and reverence. Energetic herbalism was born from the Earth after millennia of pattern observation by diviners, artists, healers, and physicians. The diversity of these systems is what gives depth to our healing journey.

Five Phase Theory

The introduction of Five Phase (Five Element) Theory into my practice was life-changing. While many refer to this system as Five Element, I prefer the original translation, Five Phase, because this system reveals relationships and patterns. Ted Kaptchuk writes, "The Chinese term that we translate as 'Five Phases' is *wu xing*. *Wu* is the number five, and *xing* means 'walk' or 'move,' and perhaps most pertinently, it implies a process."[1] Five Phase Theory is a guide to moving through the five seasons, or five phases, with a greater understanding of the functions and qualities of our physiology, both physically and emotionally. The fifth season is late summer and the five elements related to the seasons are Earth, Water, Wood, Metal, and Fire. Many acupuncturists and clinicians work with the yin/yang theory or the Eight Principal Theory of TCM because these theories are thought to be more pragmatic. Five Phase is seen as more metaphysical though many practitioners use a blend of theories for clinical diagnosis and treatment. For our purposes of studying patterns and elements, Five Phase Theory provides an elegant template for the contemplation of the phases of our lives and seasons as well as our daily rhythms.

Let's look at one simple example of relationships in Five Phase Theory. Spring relates to the Liver and Gallbladder, and this is the season we eat spring greens—bitter greens to cleanse the liver and clear the stagnancy of winter. The element connected to the season of spring is Wood, which is the element that relates to growth, change, and vision. As sap rises in the springtime, so too do we feel a stirring of energy. Projects dormant during the winter "spring" forth. How empowering to learn seasonal celebrations, remedies, and lifestyle choices to focus on liver health.

For me, one of the most profound teachings from this model is the emotions that are governed and processed by each element. For example, the emotion of anger is processed by the element Wood in the season of spring. Anger is a necessary energy to experience when there is danger or a threat. It can be lifesaving, and allowing this energy to move within the body is important for our physical and mental health. Suppression of anger, which is endemic in Western culture, can be damaging to the liver and causes excess heat. This is referred to as Liver heat rising—picture the classic image of a red-faced, overheated, angry person who suffers with high blood pressure and cholesterol issues, and too much heat.

In my teaching experience, students find learning the medicine of the seasons empowering because it affirms their intuitive sensibilities. And while beneficial to the individual, seasons also engage us with the ecology of community and the Earth. There are many new concepts to take in and assimilate when first learning Five Phase Theory, but once you begin to experience the seasons with a new perspective, so much of this information becomes second nature.

Ayurveda

Westerners have embraced Ayurvedic medicine, from yoga to diet advice to the brilliant system of working with *doshas*. Doshas are the patterns created in an individual at the moment of conception, and these patterns are also called our *prakruti*. We can draw an analogy to our astrological birth chart or expression of the positions of the planets in the sky at the time we were born.

In Ayurvedic philosophy, the elements of Nature are Ether, Air, Fire, Water, and Earth. Dosha means *humor* or *fault*, and thus while it represents our nature and personality, it also represents our challenges. Vata dosha is a blend of Air and Ether, pitta is Water and Fire, and kapha is Water and Earth. Our *constitution*, or temperament, is an expression of the two elements that were predominant at conception. To know your constitutional tendencies is to be empowered with the ultimate guide for a lifetime of self-care.

I have found the study and practice of these elemental doshas to be enormously useful for my self, clients, and community. To know our nature and grasp how deeply we share truths and traits of the planet we call home is profound. The greatest gift I have received through this study is compassion for self and others. Understanding, for example, that our fiery pitta selves are prone to jealousy and that there are practices and foods to temper this flame and redirect our light, fosters tolerance of one's nature. The substantial and earthy kapha dosha is often misunderstood as lazy and slow, yet they are the most loyal and loving of companions and allies, as is the solid earth below our feet. Balancing of the doshas is not simply a way to improve digestion, get a better night's sleep, or achieve more lustrous hair. Working with these elements is our divine act of manifesting our individual and collective evolutionary nature. Ayurveda teaches that through our doshas we have incarnated this time around with these elements in order to understand *Prema* (kapha), *Jyoti* (pitta), and *Prana* (vata), or love, light, and life. The Ayurvedic model also includes a detailed model for responding to current health challenges an individual faces. These challenges are called *vikruti*. In Western energetics, there is another lens for describing current health challenges in terms of energetic imbalances. This lens is the tissue states.

Vitalism and Western Herbalism
Herbalist and ethnobotanist David Winston has made a lifelong study of early North American herbalism, and he holds a wealth of knowledge regarding the vibrant storied past of herbalism on this continent. He wrote, "The core of American herbal medicine comes from the ethnobotanical traditions of Native Americans using plants indigenous to America."[2] It is important to pay respect to those cultures that have shaped American herbalism. The medicine lore of the Indigenous, enslaved, women and poor

in North America was an oral tradition. Without written records, it has been hard to follow the threads of all who carried the medicine of the plants to this time. Fortunately, there are amazing historians and herbalists of color telling these stories and uncomfortable truths, so as a nation we may heal. These authors are weaving the stories to bear witness to the vast contributions made by those of the oral traditions.

Two schools of medical practice were born from Thomsonianism, the practice of botanic medicine started by a root doctor (a lay practitioner who used plant medicines) named Samuel Thomson in the mid-1800s. Thomson was influenced by a village wise woman, Mrs. Benton who learned much of her craft from Indigenous healers, most likely the local Abenaki or Wabenaki Nations. Those schools of medicine, Eclecticism and Physiomedicalism, were comprised of physicians who wanted to create alternative treatments to the horrific medical practices of the day, such as use of mercury and excessive bloodletting to "balance the humors." These new physicians would use "eclectic" medicines to serve their community instead, including home-opathy, steam bathing, and botanical formulas. From botanical descriptions to complex dispensing formulas, the writings of the Eclectic physicians are the only written texts representing over a hundred years of herbal medi-cine practice in the United States. Fortunately, many of these texts are still accessible, and I have listed many in "Recommended Reading" on page 331. In an article on the history of Physiomedicalism, Canadian herbalist Todd Caldecott wrote, "Despite its relatively short history, the systems of healing that rose up in opposition to Regular medicine [the conventional medicine of the era] represent an important source of knowledge for modern clinical herbalists. Freed from the shackles of humoral medicine, these practitioners based their practices on nothing more than empirical observation, and in so doing, developed a system of practice, including diagnostic and assessment techniques, that are the basis of modern clinical herbal medicine."[3]

In 1900 Physiomedicalist physician J.M. Thurston published *The Phi-losophy of Physiomedicalism* wherein he articulated the six tissue states as a vocabulary to describe expressions of imbalance in the body. In *Principles and Practice of Phytotherapy*, herbalists Simon Mills and Kerry Bone stated, "JM Thurston produced the last authoritative physiomedical text, posing operational definitions of the vital force . . . and elaborating on the need to use only such remedies as supported vitality."[4] The terms Thurston used to describe the states seem a bit archaic today; they were derived from the theories of the time. The terminology that herbalist Matthew Wood has brought forward is more understandable in our present-day vernacular, and Wood's articulation of the tissue states forms the foundation of my discussion of them throughout this book, and particularly in chapter 6.

The six tissue states are patterns that describe our inner terrain when it is *out of balance*. The six states are hot/cold, dry/damp, and tense/lax. The art of energetic healing lies in appreciating the subtle, nuanced shifts in these states. They are not polar opposites; they delineate a continuum along the spectrum. In this way, they are a reflection of *homeodynamics*, a concept that is replacing the conventional concept of homeostasis. Homeodynamics more accurately describes the fluidity of the natural world, the constant movement that characterizes life. Stasis is defined as a period of inactivity or equilibrium. In regard to life-forms, though, long-term inactivity equals death. A living organism may pass through a point of equilibrium but as a living, self-correcting system, it is constantly adjusting its internal milieu with that of the environment. Tissue states reflect the dynamic quality all organisms employ in order to maintain internal coherence.

A Contemplative Practice

Admittedly, there is a lot of juicy material between the covers of this book. Reading it cover to cover may not be the best way for you to digest it. Energetic herbalism is not a linear subject, and there is no requirement to read chapters in order. I suggest that you begin with the chapters that are of most interest to you. You may find that with many of the chapters, you'll need to put the book down for a while after reading, contemplate the models presented, and then return and reread. As you visit and revisit energetic models of healing, the experience will clarify, enlighten, astound, and simply blow your mind that our world is so blessed with an intelligence that transcends all reason, a cosmology so generous, loving, and limitless that it is hard to comprehend. As fifteenth-century ecstatic poet Kabir wrote, "Those who hope to be reasonable about it fail. The arrogance of reason has separated us from that love. With the word reason you already feel miles away."[5]

Through the magnificence of Five Phase Theory, we will come to learn that we digest not only foods but thoughts, experiences, and far-reaching notions from Nature. At Sacred Plant Traditions school, there is a bitter bar, where we offer bitter elixirs all day, every day. Bitters, as you may know or are about to discover, facilitate digestion. These herbal offerings help students not only digest information but also transform a language of archetypes, mythology, plant spirits, and the beauty of Nature into a comprehensible template. Thank goodness we have plants to help us navigate these realms. Through their limitless love and ego-dissolving medicinal ways, the plants teach us how to be fully human.

At the root of the word *ecology* is the Greek word *oikos*, which means home. With energetic herbalism, as we tend our terrain, our ecology, and our spirit, we are, in essence, finding our way home. For me, the web that gathers together the multifaceted craft of herbalism is the equally ancient practice of honoring plant spirits. Herbalist and author Rosita Arvigo said, "It is folly to ignore the sacred in life or medicine. Skirting the spiritual has had a shattering effect on every dimension of contemporary existence."[6] With energetic herbalism, we gather the pieces and reweave integrity back into our lives. We work with not only patterns of Nature but also the world of the sacred, which contains the stories and songs that are our birthright. When we honor the intelligence and spirit of plants, we acknowledge our place in the scheme of life. Our humanness is defined by our ability to engage in our natural world, and we express this holy life through ceremony. Ceremony is an energetic language that transcends the physical realm, and all of our work with plants is a beautiful ceremony. This can be as simple as making a cup of nourishing tea.

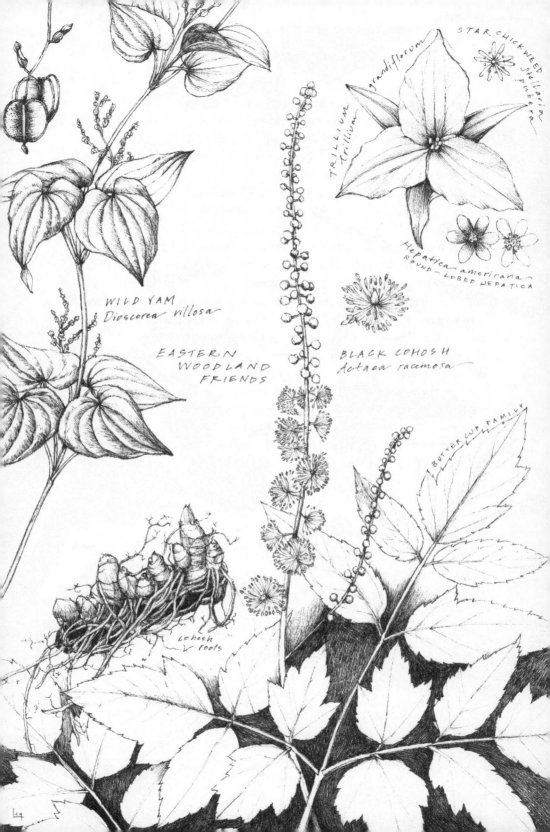

WILD YAM
Dioscorea villosa

TRILLIUM grandiflorum
Trillium

STAR CHICKWEED
Stellaria pubera

Hepatica americana
ROUND-LOBED HEPATICA

EASTERN
WOODLAND
FRIENDS

BLACK COHOSH
Actaea racemosa

BUTTERCUP FAMILY

cohosh
roots

Plant Relations with All the Senses

Our ancestors experienced the plants through their senses and their dreams, and above all, they listened. Imagine the sound-scape that blessed the Earth ten thousand years ago. Amid the cacophony of woodland or jungle sounds, the medicine songs were just coming into being. The composers were Spirit (of many names), Nature, and the new player, humans. Through creation songs and stories, people learned who their relations were and how the mountains, rivers, stones, and forces of weather were part of their family. The same, of course, happened with the plants.

Experiencing plants as kin is inherent to Indigenous cultures all over the world, from Celts in Ireland to the Quechua in Peru to the Taino people of Puerto Rico. Today we speak of plants as allies, partners to work with in creating optimal health. I credit the plants as *teachers* even more than as partners, because their healing abilities are like none I have witnessed before. Think of the spirit of motherwort (*Leonurus cardiaca*), which had such an immediate effect on my client Maria (see chapter 1). Yes, *Leonurus* has many beneficial qualities (cooling, relaxing), but the immediacy of the effect was through the *spirit* of motherwort's connection to Maria. Through my own relationship with this herb, I have come to feel that the spirit of motherwort is one of unconditional support. This is what enabled Maria to drop so quickly into herself and feel safe enough to allow tears to well up. The energy of motherwort created a pattern in Maria that allowed her to make necessary changes to become more herself.

Although I am an experienced practitioner, I did not have the capacity to comfort Maria and help her transform in such a short span of time. Motherwort initiated her healing. My role was to recognize the pattern of Maria and to know which plant might "teach" her how to relax. This is the beauty of energetic herbalism: A person continues taking doses of the plant until its pattern has had time to repattern their mind or spirit, allowing them to then hold that new way of being and make it their own.

The same phenomenon happens on a physical level. For example, the pattern that is created by the energetics of ginger (*Zingiber officinale*) is stimulating and warming. For someone who has run colder than normal all their life, drinking ginger tea for an extended period of time will eventually shift the cold pattern to a more healthful one, flush with vitality. The energetics of the herb marshmallow (*Althaea officinalis*) is moistening, cooling, and building. Through use of marshmallow, someone who has suffered from a chronic dry cough can change the pattern or terrain of their lungs to one that is nourished and less irritated.

Plant spirit medicine is a deeply personal journey. Working with the spirit aspect of the plant is often captured in what are called flower essences. (In chapter 8, I describe these and how to make them.) These are beautiful medicines that address emotional and spiritual health. I have found, however, that when I make teas and tinctures with awareness and gratitude, all medicine becomes spirit medicine.

There are many excellent books and conferences that can help guide individuals in developing relations with plants and their spirits. I wonder, though, haven't you already begun your own journey? Maybe that is why you are holding this book right now. You may have already met a plant spirit but did not have the experience to trust the veracity of your meeting. Requirements are humility, an open heart, and dedication to showing up. If you learn anything about plants, you will know that they care not for drama or intricate ceremonies, unless you are working with a very sacred medicine. At the end of this chapter, I share a powerful process for developing relationships with plants, but there are many ways to do this.

Elements within Plants

When students taste an herb for the first time, they recognize something familiar. They cannot articulate how they know this flavor or energy but are certain they have experienced it before. Indeed, every culture has learned about the world through the five senses—they are a unifying force in our wonderfully diverse human race. Through the senses, we transcend space and time, retrieving information that has been expressed in our DNA for millennia. Thousands of years ago, the bitter flavor of a plant told foragers to avoid ingesting large quantities of that plant. Today, when we taste the bitterness of goldenseal (*Hydrastis canadensis*) for the first time, we have the same instinctive reaction as our ancestors of long ago and know that a small amount will suffice.

Using the senses is a natural way to understand the language of plants and to discern the elements they contain, such as earth, air, and water. Nibbling on a piece of cayenne (*Capsicum annuum*) clearly reveals the element of fire. Drinking licorice tea (*Glycyrrhiza glabra*), you discover that this root has a fair amount of sweetness or earthiness. These experiences express the medicine and effect each plant has in our bodies. There are ways to know the elements of earth, air, wood, and others that may not be so obvious.

Accessing the realm of herbal energetics through our senses shifts the process from an intellectual journey to an experiential one. Our bodies remember impressions more readily than our minds hold onto facts. During Sacred Plant Traditions classes, we introduce students to plants in a variety of ways; one is called a *proving* or a *tasting*. Without knowing the name of the plant, students sit, take a sip of tea, close their eyes, open their senses, and allow the plant to move within. I suggest that they follow the direction and energy of the plant. Do they feel warmer, or cooler? Do they feel energy in the head or their extremities? They sip again and take time, listening to the internal shift. After a half hour of exploration, rarely do they forget the energy of that plant.

When students taste nettle (*Urtica dioica*) for the first time, one common response is, "This is what the color green tastes like." The first sip reveals the taste of earth, as nettle has the flavor of minerals. There is a sweetness to this mineral-rich brew, enhanced by the amino acids that make this a deeply nutritive herb. Upon further tasting, students notice the presence of salt and a resemblance to the scent of seaweed. (Open a bag of dried nettle and you will discover that it smells remarkably like seaweed.) Upon finishing the cup of tea, they may discover a need to excuse themselves—nettle leaf is a diuretic. I may mention the maxim "water follows salt," and now my students can ground this teaching in their own sensual experience. Herbal diuretics usually are rich with salt and other minerals, and a practice from Chinese medicine is to add salt to herbal formulas to direct the medicine to the kidneys.

One field of study in herbalism is Goethean science, named after the poet, playwright, and scientist, Johann Wolfgang von Goethe (1749–1832). Goethe's science was characterized by taking into account the appearance and structure of plants as a whole entity. This approach is different from the method employed in the taxonomy of Carl Linnaeus, an eighteenth-century natural historian who focused on specific parts of the plant in classifying them. The foundation of Goethe's method is that we enter into the experience of the *phenomenon* (plant) itself through repetitive visits to the plant that is being studied. This method gives credence to the sensory experience as a reliable source of true information. His methods require rigor and consistency, yet we can learn much from his teachings and apply them to how we experience and understand our plant medicines.

Sight

When you first meet a plant, notice every detail. Are the leaves serrated, toothed, smooth, or heart shaped? Do they form a coil or spiral around the plant stem, or are the leaves arranged in pairs? Use a loupe or magnifying glass to look at the parts of the flower—no need to use botanical terminology here, just collect impressions. Look at the ecosystem, where it is growing and who is growing around it. Choctaw herbalist Karyn Sanders says that in her tradition, plant families are based not on genetic mapping, but rather on the choices the plants make to grow together in a particular soil and environment. This is the ultimate expression of kinship.

After noticing the fine details, try drawing or sketching the plant, which is a way to truly sense the plant by moving out of a pattern of linear thinking. The encounter is less about delineating botanical structures and more about sensing who the plant is. The contemplative nature of drawing allows us to access our imaginations, and this practice of seeing allows subtler energetic information to reveal itself. This is part of the technique described later in this chapter for getting to know the spirit of a plant. It is important to draw with the comfort that this sketch is for your eyes only and abandon judgment of what makes a "good" drawing.

Study the plant's hidden parts as well. Dig up the root. This may be quite a project if you are observing a plant like burdock (*Arctium lappa*) that has roots that burrow two feet below the surface, but even this experience gives information about its medicine. Burdock root works steadily and reliably through deep, chronic metabolic issues such as diabetes. Harvesting Joe Pye weed (*Eutrochium purpureum*) in the wild, we usually find ourselves on the edge of a meadow with wet, boggy soil. This is a challenging harvest as it is deeply mired in dense, rich, soggy soil, but this reflects its medicine for working with solids and water, as it is a reliable remedy for kidney stones.

Taking the time to see a plant deeply can reveal clues about its healing nature. In the sixteenth century, German mystic Jakob Böhme wrote *The Signature of All Things*, which gave rise to the practice of the doctrine of signatures. The doctrine states that a plant's shape, color, markings, or essence is a visual clue to the organ or bodily function that the plant has the capacity to heal. While seemingly simplistic, this practice is profound; it arises from working with *archetypes*. An archetype is a prototype, a model, the primal essence of an object that represents its foundational form. This doctrine was discounted centuries ago as pseudoscience, as it was generally thought that the signatures referred to physical similarities alone. However, Paracelsus and other European alchemists of the Renaissance were working with the energetic signature, the impression and essence that the material was providing. Author and herbalist Sajah Popham wrote, "Signatures are the living language through which we read the energetic architecture of life as it is inscribed within matter, and they communicate a being's particular function and character. . . . Signatures in their essence are patterns perceived by the heart."[1] A healthy oak tree (*Quercus* spp.) is an archetype of might and vigor. Based on appearance alone, we are not surprised when we learn that oak medicine imparts immense strength and integrity to our bones as well as souls. This doctrine is still a part of many traditions in herbalism today.

Touch

Touch is our most primitive sense. It is the first sense a fetus develops while in utero. Touch informs us of our environment. Nerve receptors in the skin transmit signals that the brain interprets as sensations such as heat, cold, pleasure, or pain. One of the greatest strengths of herbal medicine lies in the topical medicines we apply to the skin. We can bring heat and move congestion in lung tissues through an application of a mustard plaster. Cooling, soothing chickweed (*Stellaria media*) has mucilaginous properties that draw heat from infections. Plantain (*Plantago* spp.) and slippery elm (*Ulmus rubra*) have potent properties of drawing toxins as well as even small debris (splinters) out of tissues. The sting of nettle is therapeutic as it moves circulation to clear stagnation and pain. Even the thorns on hawthorn (*Crataegus* spp.) and many other members of the Rosaceae family are a signature for the protective qualities of its medicine.

It is a pattern in Nature: Plants that serve as a remedy for toxic effects of other species often grow close at hand. One common example is yellow dock leaves (*Rumex crispus*), which are a good antidote for the sting of nettles. These two plants often will be found growing close to each other in a field or barnyard. I experienced this kind of welcome "partnering" while studying in Belize, where the jungle holds exotic and sometimes dangerous medicines. One day while deep in the jungle, I was distracted by an amazing bromeliad, and unknowingly I leaned up against the famed black poisonwood tree (*Metopium brownei*). The immediate sting and welts that erupted on my arm were painful. Fortunately, I was with a friend, guide and bushman Winston Harris, who is native to Belize. He immediately reached for the gumbo limbo tree (*Bursera simaruba*) that is usually close at hand and quickly made a leaf poultice to relieve the swelling.

Smell

The sense of smell is hard-wired into some of the most sensitive parts of the brain, including the amygdala, which is responsible for governing emotions, and the hippocampus, which relates aromas to memory. This means that scents go straight into our limbic system, bypassing mental processing, thereby accessing primal places that hold information not readily available through everyday cognition. This is the basis of the art of aromatherapy.

Once we know the distinctive smell of an herb, we can determine the elements or pattern the plant may hold. The aromatic oils of thyme (*Thymus vulgaris*) or rosemary (*Salvia rosmarinus*) provide the sensation of lifting or awakening, thus bringing the element of air into our being. The scent of sweet cicely roots (*Osmorhiza longistylis*) informs us that this plant has building, nutritive qualities. The bitter aromatics from *Artemisia* species such as wormwood (*Artemisia absinthium*) signal a stronger medicine.

Oftentimes we can bruise or rub a leaf between our fingers to detect the scent. Other times scents can be perceived only after the plant has been dried. This is the case especially with salty, nutrient-dense plants such as borage (*Borago officinalis*) and nettle. As you start creating your apothecary, take the time to smell the herbs that you gather and get to know what good-quality, freshly dried herbs smell like.

It is fascinating to note recent research by plant ecologists revealing that plants also use scent to communicate with each other. It has been shown for example, when insects damage sagebrush (*A. tridentata*), it broadcasts the invasion by releasing a scent to notify others in its family of the impending danger.

Those plants, in turn, mobilize their defenses. The idea that plants "smell" other plants as a form of communication is awe inspiring and exhilarating.

Sound

The sense of hearing does not directly provide elemental information about plants. Nonetheless, it is a vital aspect of traditional energetics. A Costa Rican medicine person, Jose Ramon Campos, once explained to me that before he could harvest the medicine plants, he had to learn their songs. Beginning at age three, he shadowed his grandfather, devoting himself to learning the simple chants, some of which were only two or three notes. This healer spent eight years listening in effort to discover who the plants were and how to be in right relationship with them. This is how Indigenous people maintain the integrity of the web of life. They sing before they take. They ask before they harvest.

The idea of spending eight years preparing for a simple task such as harvesting leaves or roots may strike you as eccentric. It is not the modern way of thinking about Nature and our place in the world. But medicinal plants are disappearing from the wild at an alarming rate, and as herbalists and plant lovers, when we open ourselves to the language of the sacred, we see this language is one of intimate relationship. Imagine if your partner, friend, or family member spent years learning your essential "song." Imagine the secret places you would yield over time and how you would give deeply from your essence. When we work with plants in this way, we discover that we need less plant material to bring about a therapeutic effect, because the plant has gifted us with more of its essence.

Agricultural scientist George Washington Carver was cognizant of the knowledge that could be accessed by listening to plants. Carver wrote, "Anything will give up its secrets if you love it enough."[2] The historical record tends to celebrate Carver primarily for his work with peanuts, and he was an outcast from the scientific community in his own time because of his honest revelation of his inspiration from Nature and God. Carver attributed his successes to listening to Nature and believing what he heard. Carver would rise at four in the morning to walk in the woods and listen to what the Divine, as well as plants, would tell him.

Taste

Taste is the sense that herbalists and plant lovers revel in. This sense can bring us so much information about the medicines we work with. Plants have developed unique flavors by producing a diverse range of phytochemicals. So much of what we taste arises not only from the plant's direct effect on our taste buds but also from the aroma or sensation the plant imparts. The flavor signals the presence of a constituent of a plant that initiates a change in our bodies. For example, bitter plants increase saliva, salty ones direct energy to our kidneys, and pungent spices move circulation. The acids in sour fruits bring us cooling flavonoids or antioxidants, and sweet herbs are building because the carbohydrates they contain are nutritive. However, it's important to identify any unknown plant and its potential toxicity before you taste it.

While most energetic traditions share five basic tastes of spicy, sweet, bitter, sour, and salty, there are slight variations, such as the addition of astringency in Ayurveda. Let's consider each of these, plus a few others that are useful for understanding energetics of a plant.

Spicy/Pungent
ENERGETICS: WARMING, MOVING, DRYING

Stimulating, spicy plants increase circulation and wake up our senses. This is why most culinary herbs are pungent: They help increase digestive action. Aromatics like rosemary and thyme are warming and drying, reflecting the Mediterranean ecosystem they come from. The energy of fire and air from pungent medicines is also specific for lungs, as these elements disperse energy in an outward direction. Eating spicy foods, such as horseradish or cayenne, can initiate a sweat, which is a common expression of dispersing energy outward. These herbs can be quite stimulating, so usually they are used in low doses. Pungent examples include black pepper (*Piper nigrum*), ginger, garlic (*Allium sativum*), cinnamon (*Cinnamomum verum*), and cayenne.

Sweet
ENERGETICS: BUILDING, NUTRITIVE, BALANCING

Sweet is the subtle flavor of grains and roots. Traditionally, even honey would have been considered excessively sweet and used in moderation. Energetically speaking, the direction of this flavor is upward because these plants tonify, build, and energize. Nourishing roots and adaptogens are sweet-tasting plants due to the presence of complex sugars called polysaccharides. Sweet herbs tend to be anti-inflammatory and demulcent, especially when the content of mucopolysaccharides is high. Most saponin-rich adaptogens are sweet as well. This is the energy of earth and water. Examples of these tonics are American ginseng (*Panax quinquefolius*), licorice, and astragalus (*Astragalus membranaceus*). Blood-building herbs such as red clover (*Trifolium pratense*) and burdock are also sweet.

Bitter
ENERGETICS: CALMING, COOLING, CLEARING

Bitter flavor has a downward, drying, and clearing action. Bitter cools and clears heat from the body and aids in cases of inflammation. The bitter principle stimulates bile and helps with digestion as well as elimination. In Chinese medicine, this flavor is said to go to the heart. In *Out of the Earth*, British phytotherapist and author Simon Mills wrote, "Repeatedly in the records of traditional plant medicine, we find that bitter remedies are the 'true stimulants', a notion surviving in the modern idiom that 'nasty-tasting medicines are the best for you'."[3] The bitter receptors on the tongue stimulate a reflex response that provokes an amazing array of actions: increased appetite, increased bile flow, production of hydrochloric acid and digestive enzymes, protected gut tissues, balanced blood sugar, clearing of dampness from the digestive tract, and a low-level antimicrobial action. Bitter herbs include dandelion (*Taraxacum officinale*), blue vervain (*Verbena hastata*), and motherwort.

Sour
ENERGETICS: COOLING, ASTRINGING

The direction of sour moves energy inward and downward. Think cooling, natural lemonade in expansive summer heat. The sour flavor of herbs, though, is more subtle than the intensity of lemons. This flavor is represented by herbal fruits such as bilberry (*Vaccinium myrtillus*), sumac (*Rhus* spp.), and schisandra (*Schisandra chinensis*). Their energies astringe tissues or bind excesses. Sour antioxidants (flavonoids) cool the tissues and are actually protective against oxidative stress (heat). Sour foods include vinegar and limes, as well as most fermented foods.

Astringent
ENERGETICS: COOLING, DRYING

Astringent is recognized as a taste in Ayurveda, but in other systems it is considered more as a sensation rather than a flavor. Either way, the mouth definitely recognizes the presence of an astringent food or herb. Astringent herbs are drying to the body and tonifying to the skin and mucous membranes. Most herbs are slightly astringing due to the presence of tannins. These compounds are prevalent in plants because they are part of the plant's immune response to disease. As discussed later in this chapter, these compounds precipitate protein and tone inflamed or boggy tissue. Astringent herbs are offered to people who have diarrhea or excessive bleeding and who tend toward dampness, excessive sweating, and secretion. Herbs include witch hazel leaf (*Hamamelis virginiana*), black tea leaves (*Camellia sinensis*), and blackberry root (*Rubus fruticosus*).

Salty
ENERGETICS: COOLS, MOISTENS, SOFTENS

This flavor is described as having a downward direction and is specific for directing energy to the kidney. Because water follows salt, these plants are used to soften hard swellings. In herbalism, salty herbs such as dandelion leaf, chickweed, plantain, and nettle are also mineral-rich plants that are packed with nutrients. Common salty foods are seaweed, kelp, miso, and soy sauce. Herbs with this flavor can also be drying; there are many diuretics in this group. However, other mineral-rich plants, such as chickweed, moisten tissues. Traditionally, salt was a tonic for the heart because it increases fluid and improves blood volume, especially in hotter weather where fluid loss can lead to mineral deficiency.

Acrid
ENERGETICS: WARMING, MOVING, DISPERSING

Acrid plants are the main category of herbs to release patterns of tension. This flavor is actually more of an experience, as it provokes a reaction in our tissues. The felt impression is one of warmth and tingling, a prickly and some may say nauseating reaction. These herbs are generally offered in low doses, yet have a profound physiological effect. Lobelia (*Lobelia inflata*) is the quintessential acrid herb and is that perfect blend of contradiction—it is dispersing as well as relaxing. Many of the antispasmodic herbs are acrid, such as kava kava root (*Piper methysticum*), black cohosh (*Actaea racemosa*), and cramp bark (*Viburnum opulus*).

Bland
ENERGETICS: NEUTRAL, MOISTENING

Bland herbs are as they sound, mostly neutral in energy. It is said they move through the body with relative ease, thus having their effect on the urinary system. Hence, they can act as diuretics. Often, they are demulcent in nature and have a slippery texture associated with mucilage. Bland herbs are oatstraw (*Avena sativa*) and corn silk (*Zea mays*).

Qualities and Actions of Plants

The vocabulary of taste in herbal medicine offers significant clues on how to choose effective and energetically appropriate herbs. For someone who runs colder, for example, we would look to the pungent, warming herbs. If this person tended to run dry, such as dry eyes and constipation, we would want to add a sweet, moistening herb so as not to aggravate dryness, because pungent herbs also tend to be drying. I discuss this vocabulary in great detail in chapter 6.

Most traditions of herbalism recognize four basic qualities of life and natural systems: hot, cold, damp, and dry. These energetic qualities in plants are similar to those in humans, and this is why energetic herbalism is an elegant way to match the right herb with a particular person or situation. Essentially these qualities are based on the elements of fire, water, earth, and air that are explored in detail in upcoming chapters. (In chapter 6, I also discuss two other qualities: relaxed and tense.)

Qualities or energetics of plants can vary depending on where they are grown (sandy soil vs. organically rich), method of preparation, and whether they are used fresh or dried. Fresh ginger has a lovely warming essence while dried ginger is hot. Fresh lemon balm (*Melissa officinalis*) presents an aromatic, uplifting energy. Dried lemon balm has similar properties, but the dried form also brings a depth of minerals not found in fresh. While the nuances may seem limitless, once you begin to develop relations with plants, you will begin to discern patterns for different preparations. Another reason to start with a small apothecary!

Herbal *actions* are different than their qualities, but equally important. These actions are the definitions of how herbs do their work in the body. You may be tempted to gloss over the vocabulary of herbal actions because some of the terms may seem static and a bit incomprehensible at first. Yet these are the terms of herbalism, foundational concepts that reveal vital information for choosing the right remedy. Plus, how cool to master the language of a healing tradition that is hundreds of years old! Before you know it, you'll become a plant geek who knows exactly how to pronounce words like *sialagogue*, *vermifuge*, and *vulnerary* and use them with ease.

Many herbal actions are expressed with the prefix *anti-*, such as anti-inflammatory and antimicrobial. However, for energetic herbalists it is important to remember that our aim is to support the body's inherent system of self-correction. Using an herb, such as blackberry root, that works against the body's natural response may be useful for acute and short-term situations such as acute diarrhea. Our overall goal, however, is not to work against an imbalance, but rather to guide our innate wisdom to return to center. We are tasked then with working with our understanding of a person's tissue states or doshas to remove obstacles to the flow of vital energy. The approach of conventional medicine is all about killing pathogens, and as herbalists we are given the plants to do that as well. In fact, there are very potent examples of antimicrobials in the plant realm, but in natural healing the goal is to promote the health of the terrain so it becomes inhospitable to the offending critters.

More often than not the quality of a plant is implied in its action. For example, most carminatives—herbs that aid digestion and "move" wind (gas)—are warming and relaxing in order to ease digestion. With demulcents (moistening herbs), the plants are rich in sugars, which serve to nourish and cool the tissues.

Energetics of Phytochemistry

At a basic level, chemistry informs energetics because many phytochemicals have a strong flavor or create a physical reaction that informs the senses of the effect they have on the body. Herbs that are rich in flavonoids often have a sour flavor, hence a cooling effect on the body, preventing oxidation due to heat from stress or inflammation. This is the beauty of energetic herbalism. Herbal medicine has flourished for thousands of years without the stories told by scientists, but science is a fascinating storyteller.

Phytochemistry 101

This extremely brief description of plant chemistry is to whet your appetite (no pun intended) to the biochemical worlds that lie beyond and within the cell walls of plants. These chemicals are part and parcel of what is stimulating and affecting our senses.

First things first. The chemistry of a plant serves the needs of the plant, not those of humans. In their love for us though, plants give of themselves so generously. Their deep medicine is nothing short of astonishing. The famed American ginseng and many of the Aralia family are ancient plants that survived the Ice Age. American ginseng is called an adaptogen, an herbal remedy that helps the body adapt to the damaging effects of stress. As I write this book during the fall of 2020, the times seem bathed in nothing but stress, yet imagine surviving an ice age when you are a rooted creature! Perhaps its survival is due to the wonderful steroidal compounds and saponins called ginsenosides, compounds that give great strength to the plants and to us as well. Perhaps it is the thousands of years of gathering medicine stories in old growth forests as they cycled through multitudes of seasons. Whatever blend of forces produced that miraculous evolutionary feat, this plant family gifts humanity with the highly aromatic and earthy sweet taste of ginseng roots.

Presented in the most basic terms, plant biochemicals can be divided into two categories: primary metabolites and secondary metabolites. Primary metabolites are compounds produced by all plant cells for purposes of growth, development, and reproduction. These include proteins, starches, oils, and hormones. Secondary metabolites are primarily concerned with plant defense and serve to help the plant deal with stress. There are three classes of secondary metabolites: terpenoids, phenolics, and alkaloids.

Miraculous Secondary Metabolites

All plants produce terpenoids, the largest grouping of secondary metabolites by far, with over twenty-two thousand known compounds. The simplest terpenoid is a volatile gas emitted during photosynthesis as a way of protecting the cell membranes of a plant from high heat or intense light.[4] More complex forms are the highly volatile compounds called essential oils, named for the fragrance (essence) they emit. These compounds function as attractants for pollinators, deterrents to pest insects, and protection against fungal and bacterial infection. Highly aromatic sage (*Salvia officinalis*), thyme, rosemary, and oregano (*Origanum vulgare*) are revered for their clearing, disinfecting, and antimicrobial applications. The tradition of stuffing meat with these herbs pre-dated refrigeration and was a form of preservation. My favorite throat spray for protection against viral or bacterial agents is a tincture blend of sage, thyme, rosemary, echinacea (*Echinacea* spp.), and propolis (an antimicrobial resin that honey bees produce to protect their hives). Citronella, often added to candles to repel mosquitos, is extracted from *Cymbopogon nardus*, which is related to lemongrass (*C. citratus*).

One of the most antimicrobial plant substances is myrrh resin (*Commiphora myrrha*), which contains up to 10 percent essential oil.[5] So great are its medicinal attributes that Hippocrates, commonly regarded as the father of medicine, mentioned myrrh more times in his writings than any other plant.[6] The resin is harvested by cutting or wounding the tree, which provokes sap to ooze out of the cut in an effort to provide antibiotic protection for the tree and to cover the wound. This liquid then hardens into a waxy resin, which is how myrrh is then gathered and stored. This resin is so effective at preservation that it was a major ingredient in the herbal mixtures used for embalming in ancient Egypt as well as in Medieval Europe until the sixteenth century.

Phenolics are another large class of secondary metabolites vital to plant survival. One of the largest classes of phenolics are flavonoids, which perform a multitude of functions from immune response to chemical messaging. *Flavus* is the Latin word for yellow, and many flavonoids are yellow in color. This compound is found in flowers, where its color helps to attract pollinators. In leaves it provides protection from ultraviolet light. Flavonoids are antioxidants that prevent tissue breakdown in our bodies as well. More often than not the flavor is sour and the effect is often astringing and cooling. In autumn, leaves of the ginkgo tree (*Ginkgo biloba*) dramatically turn a golden yellow and, seemingly overnight, drop from the tree, making harvest quite easy. Because of its high-flavonoid content, this ancient tree provides a multitude of medicinal actions, such as immunomodulating, tonifying for tissues, neuroprotection, and is wonderful at wound healing. The flavonoids are quercetin, rutin, and many other antiaging compounds.

The blues and reds we see in flowers and fruits are from another group of flavonoids called anthocyanins. ("Antho" means flower and "cyano" means blue.) This is the spectrum of polyphenols now so popular in health food products, and for good reason. Blueberries (*Vaccinium* spp.), pomegranates (*Punica granatum*), elderberries (*Sambucus canadensis, S. nigra*), hawthorn berries, and many other plants are being studied for their potentially significant benefits in alleviating the metabolic challenges of inflammation and toxicity. Again, the sour flavor cues us to the energetics of these compounds.

As mentioned above, almost all plants contain phenolic compounds called tannins. These chemicals astringe tissues and precipitate proteins. This is what happens in the tanning process, which is named after these compounds. Fluids high in tannic acid are applied to animal hide, which changes the proteins in the hide in a way that makes the skin less permeable to water and thus more resilient. Unfortunately for insects, but protective for plants, water-soluble tannins bind digestive proteins in an insect's gut, preventing it from extracting nutrients from what it consumes, which accelerates its demise. Oaks have high tannic acid content, and the astringent taste of red wine is due to aging the wine in oak barrels. For medicinal properties, nothing astringes as quickly as a few drops of white oak tincture. The English favor drinking their strong black tea with cream, which contains a protein called casein that prevents the high tannins in the tea from "tanning" their stomachs.

Most alkaloids are bitter-tasting compounds that have a reputation as the troublemakers in herbal medicine, which also means they can be exciting. Many of their tastes are bitter or acrid, alerting us to take care with these plants and work with them in small doses. The names of these compounds often end in "ine," such as caffeine, morphine, mescaline, cocaine, and nicotine. Caffeine is toxic to many types of insects, and high levels produced by coffee seedlings can even inhibit the germination of other plants in their vicinity. This phenomenon, called *allelopathy*, is the production of secondary metabolites to defend against other plants that may compete for space or nutrients. Many of the nightshades or Solanaceae family plants produce alkaloidal compounds. This includes belladonna (*Atropa belladonna*), an herb that is medicinal in very small doses but can be fatal in larger doses. Capsaicin, produced by members of the *Capsicum* genus, is a low-dose alkaloid known for its hot and spicy effects, both internally and topically. Exciting plants indeed.

These days, herbal medicine is celebrated for its use of immunomodulating plants, those medicines that deeply nourish and stimulate our immune functioning. These plants generally share the constituent of mucopolysaccharides, which are many (poly) chains of sugars (saccharides) that have a relationship with fluid (muco). Plants and foods rich in these compounds have a specific effect of building and restoring our deep reserves. Many demulcent herbs (herbs that are slippery when processed) belong in this family, as do sweet tonic herbs such as astragalus and licorice. Medicinal mushrooms from reishi (*Ganoderma* spp.), shitake (*Lentinula edodes*), and maitake (*Grifola frondosa*) to turkey tail (*Trametes versicolor*) and others have complex biochemistry that includes terpenes and alkaloids, but the polysaccharides are some of the major players. Sweet tonic herbs such as burdock, echinacea, and astragalus are immune enhancers because they contain these long-chained sugars. Most of these medicines are roots, the ones who dig deep and gather nutrients.

Distilling Spirits and Developing Relations

While it might seem an odd transition to move from phytochemicals to a guide on meeting the spirit of a plant, the art of alchemy and distillation has always been referred to as accessing the spirit of a plant. There are so many techniques in this magical world of herbalism. For me, the most vital ingredient, the one that makes a tea or tincture good medicine, is the gratitude for the spirit of the plant.

We cherish our close relationships with our human partners, children, and dear friends, but many of us have not experienced our capacity to form extraordinary and vivid relationships with Nature. This is one method I learned a long time ago from author and herbalist Stephen Buhner, whose work has had a profound influence on mine. All of these steps are beautifully explained in his book *The Secret Teachings of Plants*. As stated before, there are many ways to work with developing relations and learning of plant spirit medicine.

Approaching Nature Directly

When first meeting a plant, the hardest task is to unlearn anything you have previously read about the plant or heard from teachers or friends. At this stage you want to approach the plant with a clear palate and observe the plant very closely. This is not the time for translation or extraction of meaning. It is a time for simply sitting with a plant and having the courage to assume you know nothing. Here's a case where being a true beginner—someone new to herbalism—offers an advantage. This is a wonderful opportunity to decolonize your imagination and let go of rules, anatomy, and structures that have been deemed true by authorities. As Henry David Thoreau said, "Nature is a prairie for outlaws."[7]

Sensory Noticing

The second step is coming to your senses and connecting with a plant. Dropping into wide-angle vision will facilitate the shift from your thinking mind into a heightened mode of perception. There are a variety of techniques for learning wide-angle vision, but the simplest is to stand outside in a natural area, raise your arms in front of you and begin to wriggle your fingers. Slowly move your outstretched arms apart and out to your sides, still wiggling your fingers. Continue looking straight ahead, but relax your gaze and allow your peripheral vision to follow your fingers until you cannot see them anymore. Lower your arms, take some breaths, and experience the difference in how you are perceiving your environs. You will likely notice that other senses, such as hearing and smell, become heightened. When you are first learning this technique, you may have to repeat the above experience in order to get used to the new way of perceiving: with softer vision and heightened awareness.

As time unfolds in the company of plants, deeper forms or patterns may begin to reveal themselves to you. You are like a child arriving at a playground of great delight. Everything is interesting and full of wonder as you simply allow it to be. You know how we see a new form and immediately reflect on what it reminds us of? That is partly gut instinct coming through with a neural translation of the object. It is also a natural way to make ourselves more comfortable by bringing in something familiar. Our colonized minds have been taught that order is comfort and anything beyond the edges is dangerous. Why not let something be its wild self, unlike anything we have yet to meet?

At this step, drawing the plant can give you immense pleasure as well as guidance. As stated previously, there is an imaginative space that takes over when you are lost in an artistic activity. This is a time where intimacy is shared as you are allowing images and forms usually not seen to reveal themselves.

In order to understand the nature of plants, it is helpful to meet them where they grow. Study the plant's form and all its aspects. Observe the shape of the leaves and flowers, and the scent, and if you know it is safe, see how the plant tastes and feels on your skin. If the plant is in the wild, observe who is growing alongside the plant, what kind of terrain they have chosen to live in, what the soil is like. If you are limited to a garden or even a container on a balcony, you will still be able to participate in this learning.

Feeling with the Heart

We have come to see new ways in which our heart influences our body–brain systems. Author Joseph Chilton Pearce referred to the "Triune Heart," which encompasses three influences on the heart: electromagnetic forces, neural impulses, and hormones. While all life-forms produce an electrical field, the heart's extraordinary output is said to create an energetic field that extends twelve to fifteen feet away from the body. The medical field of neurocardiology explores the extensive connections between the brain and the heart: Almost 60 percent of the cells in cardiac tissue are neural cells.[8] Research has established that the heart is influenced by a larger range of hormones than previously thought. All of this is to say that science is validating what ancients have said: Our heart perceives the world around us with astonishing accuracy; we need to have the courage to trust our feeling self.

This is when you sit with the plant and *feel* emotions arise within you. Feelings do indeed come from the world to us. I was taught to simplify the vocabulary for describing feelings into sad, mad, glad, and scared. Many times, when I ask clients to describe emotions, they use terms such as disappointment or frustration. When we channel our feeling selves into simple, basic emotional terminology, it gives us clearer information to work with. It also prevents avoiding the reality of the emotion by dressing it in other terms.

The imaginal realm, what French philosopher Henry Corbin describes as the *mundus imaginalis*, is that terrain that exists between the physical, sensory, and spiritual worlds.[9] As a Sufi scholar, Corbin coined this concept to describe this territory of the imagination that is as real as, if not more real than, the physical world we occupy most of our days. Some call the heart the organ of imagination or perception. When we drop into heart space we can imagine shapes, sounds, scenes that may come from what seems like nowhere. Corbin's mundus imaginalis is that place of synchronicities and archetypes. It is the place that many describe with the term *psychic intuition* but it is a realm accessible to all, not just the highly intuitive. When we pay attention, we find ways to access information from the wider soul of the world.

The next stage of the journey will be to ask the plant to reveal itself to you. As you drop into your heart space, begin to notice all sensations in your body. This can take practice, so don't be discouraged if this seems awkward or bewildering when you first try it. With practice, you can develop what is called heart intelligence. For me the simplest way to access this state is wide-angle vision, dropping down into another state of awareness. As you prepare to go into a meditative space to ask the plant more about its medicine or energy, this is the time to make an offering to the plant. This might be an herb, tobacco, a prayer, or a song. The purpose of this offering is reciprocal exchange. Your gift acknowledges your gratitude to the plant as teacher.

When you feel ready, close your eyes, offer gratitude once more, and ask the plant to reveal its self to you. Sit quietly, pay attention to all details of what you experience. This is not the time to interpret what you are being given: simply observe and listen. After fifteen to twenty minutes, acknowledge the plant once more, open your eyes, and notice the energy around you. It is best to journal immediately afterward, because just like a dream, the impressions and memories from this kind of spirit encounter may fade quickly.

Some teachers use drumming, work with rattles, or find other techniques to help participants enter a receptive state. Whatever the method, what is needed is gratitude and an open heart to receive the gifts or messages of the plants. Some folks are visual, others are kinesthetic, and still others are able to hear a plant's story or a song. All in due time and all comes with patience.

Extraction of Meaning

It takes frequent visits to get to know the many facets of a plant's spirit. If some first impression of a plant really strikes you, stay with that as you continue to make visits to the plant and allow the phenomenon, as Goethe says, to make itself known.

As we return again and again to a plant, we come to a deeper place of knowing. This rumination and contemplation may even include returning to draw the plant again during another season of the year. A time will arrive when you feel ready to pause, walk away, and disengage from study. Then, out of the blue, the moment of gestalt, the aha! moment arrives—a recognition of a whole being. The process is nothing short of astounding, and afterward you may never again pass that particular plant and species without experiencing a sense of true kinship. You get the *feeling* that you have *experienced* a truth about this plant. Far from over, you ecstatically realize that you are just beginning a lifelong relationship.

When plant spirit medicine is acknowledged, the potency of the plant as well as the kaleidoscopic nature of what it heals increase dramatically. No longer one constituent, or a bundle of nutrients, the plant's ability to transcend physical form becomes a thing of beauty and reverence.

Sometimes we meet a plant and it will be meant for just one particular person. This has happened to me. As a client was walking into my clinic, I felt the presence of Joe Pye weed, and I sensed the plant's majestic energy. The woman told me her story and related her ailments. All her symptoms related to her recent move from a very different bioregion. My understanding of Joe Pye at that time did not match up with what I perceived her needs to be, but even so, I went to the apothecary and made a formula that included a small amount of Joe Pye. I gave the medicine to my client, and after she left, I looked up Joe Pye in Boericke's *New Manual of Homeopathic Materia Medica with Repertory.* (Homeopathy is a form of herbal medicine that is based on the vital spirit of the plant.) This classic text has provided me with many definitions for the energetic or spirit properties of plants. I was amazed to discover that the first recommendation for Joe Pye was to address homesickness. My client called a few days later. She was deeply impressed by how much more comfortable she felt, but was a bit baffled at how that shift could come about so quickly. I had never heard of that obscure use of Joe Pye in thirty years of herbal practice or lectures, and I have never used that plant in that way since. This is how generous and unconditional plant medicine can be. I was grateful I had taken the time to meet this gorgeous native plant so I could recognize them when they "arrived" at a session.

Another Meeting with Black Cohosh

Three years ago, I was deeply honored to be in a unique apprenticeship led by Choctaw herbalist Karyn Sanders and her partner Sarah Holmes, along with a small group of other experienced teachers. We gathered four times that first year, and the month prior to each session we were told to fast and go without sugar, caffeine, alcohol, and sexual intimacy. Through experiencing these *agreements* (which we lovingly called the disagreements), we came to experience how these substances are medications that distract us from our discomfort. This preparation was like tilling the garden soil so that the seeds, or in this case, Karyn and Sarah's teachings, would take root with greater ease. We were raw and vulnerable, and made ready.

Before studying with Karyn and Sarah, my fellow students and I signed an agreement promising that we would not teach about the use of the plants in the fashion that Karyn and Sarah presented. In asking us to do this, they are protecting the sacred traditions of their people. We are permitted to tell the story of our experiences, but not to guide such sessions ourselves. Through this understanding, Karyn is conveying her traditional ways and showing us the difference between going to a lecture to gain "information" versus being given a teaching. When someone is given a teaching, it means that person has been blessed with the ability to go forward and teach that material to others. But in this apprenticeship, our intention was to receive their healing work, not to learn to teach in this manner ourselves.

After a year of intense, exhilarating personal work, it was time for the final session of the apprenticeship, which was intended to heal ancestral memory. I relate this to the field of study called epigenetics. Epigenetic tags are chemical markers that can turn genes on or off, resulting in disruptions to our normal functioning. Our DNA does not change, but those tags can be inherited. We can inherit traumas experienced by our parents, grandparents, and those that came before them. Nutritional health, toxic environmental exposures, or any lifestyle issues from our ancestors create epigenetic tags on our DNA.

Indigenous people have worked with their ancestors from time immemorial—ancestors that have come before as well as those that are yet unborn. The truth that we can heal wounds from the future as well as the past is mind-blowing, to say the least. That day in northern California, surrounded by the love of my sisters and teachers, my mind was about to be blown.

During the apprenticeship, Karyn and Sarah would give us a few drops of plant medicine and then we would journey silently for an hour or longer, sitting in meditation with the request that the plant spirit takes us on a journey to show what their medicine was about or how their medicine would assist us personally.

At this final session, after receiving a drop of an herbal remedy, I immediately began to experience imagery with such colors and velocity that I had only experienced previously after receiving sacramental entheogenic plants in Peru. Amid the psychedelic visuals, I felt the presence of the plant spirit as a gentle guide. After a while, still deep in this state, I approached a ladder, which I realized was my DNA helix. Upon closer inspection, I saw that one part of the ladder was covered in black smoke and the feeling that came was one of deep grief and shame. Somehow, I instinctively knew that these dark areas stemmed from my father's family, many of whom lived in Germany in the time of Hitler.

My father's father had died when he was very young, so when my father was only four years old, his mother sent him from the United States back to Germany to live with his grandparents. My father had very fond memories of living in Germany. He had a pack of cousins to run with, and he adored the farm life of his grandparents. The year was 1932, and the forces of Nazism were beginning to brew. It wasn't until later in his life that he told me about donning his boy scout uniform and heading to the train station with all of his schoolmates to welcome Hitler. My father returned to the United States when he was twelve, before the United States declared war on Germany. His cousins in Germany fought in the war as U-boat operators and were captured and held as prisoners of war in South Carolina. I had always consciously known of this genealogy, but I felt no connection to it. I had a loving relationship with my father, and he was the most beloved parent in the neighborhood when I was growing up.

This plant journey revealed to me the shame and profound sadness that resided in my father's family. During the journey I was told specifically what plant to use to begin clearing this density from my DNA. In that moment I realized what First Nation peoples mean when they say we work with ancestry for the benefit of the next seven generations. I am still working on this issue and will be for quite some time.

Medicine of Reciprocity

The day after this experience, Karyn told us that the medicine we had been given was black cohosh. Yes, my black cohosh, the plant that initiated me into my sacred walk with these medicines long ago, and of the story I told in the introduction to this book. By the time of this journey with Karyn and Sarah, I had known, planted, harvested, and worked so closely with black cohosh for over twenty-five years and yet never had I experienced this aspect of black cohosh's power. In Karyn's words, "This plant has the ability to be in all time. It rides the patterns of energy that are always spiraling in us and going backward and forward while in present time. This is easier to understand if we don't assume that time is linear! Black Cohosh rides in the space between light and vibration and patterns itself to the interweaving of the two. Black Cohosh is very clear in how it presents your patterns to you. There is usually no question as to what you are being shown! Whether we choose to accept this and work with the understanding of this knowledge to change our patterns is another story."[10]

There I was, an experienced teacher, a director of a clinical school, a well-loved and respected herbalist, and yet this plant I swore I knew so intimately held a pattern in medicine I did not even know was possible. This plant took me to my epigenetic trauma and showed me how to use another plant medicine to begin the long road of generational healing. I tell this story to express the humility that comes from the devotion to this craft. Obviously, the healing was in the hands of skilled medicine women, yet they were merely showing us the spirit and power of these plants. Traditional medicine people have their own ways of building sacred fires, harvesting, and medicine making in alignment with sacred plant traditions, and always with the spirit of gratitude, which is one of the most potent ingredients in medicine—the gratitude with which it is harvested. Author, ethnobotanist, and Potawatomi elder Robin Wall Kimmerer wrote, "For much of human's time on the planet, before the great delusion, we lived in cultures that understood the covenant of reciprocity, that for the Earth to stay in balance, for the gifts to continue to flow, we must give back in equal measure for what we take."[11] Gratitude is not merely saying a polite thank you. Recognition activates a place of responsibility within us, for when we receive, it is only natural to return the gift. The Honorable Harvest is a traditional practice that Kimmerer says is not written down, but if it were, it would read like the following:

> *Know the ways of the ones who take care of you, so that you may take care of them.*
> *Introduce yourself. Be accountable as the one who comes asking for life.*
> *Ask permission before taking. Abide by the answer.*
> *Never take the first. Never take the last.*
> *Take only what you need.*
> *Take only that which is given.*
> *Never take more than half. Leave some for others.*
> *Harvest in a way that minimizes harm.*
> *Use it respectfully. Never waste what you have taken.*
> *Share.*
> *Give thanks for what you have been given.*
> *Give a gift, in reciprocity for what you have taken.*
> *Sustain the ones who sustain you and the earth will last forever.*[12]

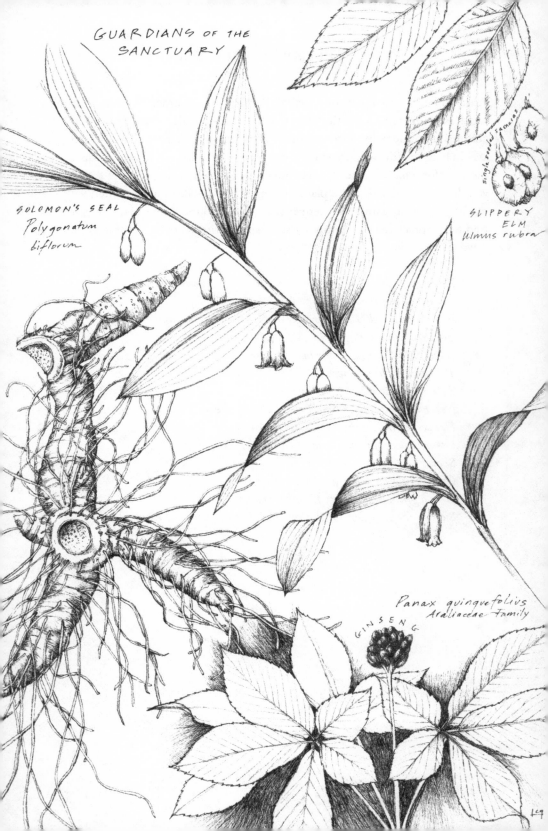

GUARDIANS OF THE
SANCTUARY

SOLOMON'S SEAL
*Polygonatum
biflorum*

single-seeded samaras

SLIPPERY
ELM
Ulmus rubra

Panax quinquefolius
Araliaceae Family

GINSENG

149

CHAPTER 3

Medicine of Place

Plants are the ultimate alchemists, and the land a plant calls home is part of its medicine story. This is where apothecary practices begin. When we harvest and work with a medicine, we are gathering so much more than simply the leaf, flower, or root. Early on in my herbalist journey, as I began observing plant medicines living in their natural habitat, I closed the books and learned to see the patterns emerge. I watched where the trees and plants chose to live. I hiked along streams for days on end where I saw hydrangea (*Hydrangea arborescens*), wood nettle (*Urtica urens*), Joe Pye weed (*Eutrochium purpureum*), and other water-loving plants thrive. Through my observations of where these plants chose to grow, I came to understand that their medicines might affect the kidneys and assist in the flow of the body's water.

Desert medicines have a high content of aromatic oils to protect them from intense heat. Artemisias and plants in the sage family bring astringency and clarity, qualities that many seek from desert venues in times of visioning. These are the physical offerings plants gift us from their unique environment. We can taste and smell the very topography that these plants call home. This is one way in which place becomes medicine. Author and acupuncturist Eliot Cowan wrote, "…Place is more than an incidental backdrop: place has spirit, personality, and sacred purpose. Place is the starring actor in every drama, and without the star the show can't go on."[1]

Every year I take students to visit Robbie Wooding's herb farm in southwest Virginia. Robbie is a fifth-generation farmer who has tended this land using the same tools and drying sheds from generations past. The purpose of the trip is to meet the endangered American ginseng (*Panax quinquefolius*) and goldenseal (*Hydrastis canadensis*) who preceded his family's arrival on the land and also to witness and experience what a generational farm *feels* like. It doesn't take long for the palpable energy created by continuous habitation of place by generations of loving stewards to touch the students' hearts. Boundaries begin to soften. They drop out of the routine of modern life and sink into a world held by stories from traditions born of the land. Robbie's ginseng is some of the finest I have ever tasted. It is medicine from multitudes of seasons creating rich woodland humus as well as the personal relationship of tending the wild beds. We acknowledge the work done by this generation and the stories of the Black, Indigenous, and other people of color who tended this land. We engage in conversations of how to make reparations for this unceded territory of Occaneechi band of the Saponi Nation and then how to turn these thoughts into actions.

Sadly, it is no longer the norm for families to live on the land where their grandparents, or even their parents, lived. The reasons for dislocation from one's family/ancestral home are many. There is no requirement to "own" land to begin to relate to place, and *where* you begin to relate to place does not matter. Whether you live in an apartment complex, subdivision, or a home in the country, home ownership is far from a prerequisite. The destructive concept of owning land has been part of Earth's history but for a blink of an eye. We honor, nourish, and sing to plants anywhere.

First Nations, First Teachers

While there is vast cultural and linguistic diversity among Indigenous peoples, they share the common denominator of developing an intimate relationship with the land for generations on end. Customs, art, music, and ways of life became inextricably bound to the land. The land, Mother Earth, reciprocates with medicine, food, and most of all the story of that peoples' creation. These origin stories are not tales for the imagination. They are sacred stories of how the world came into being for that nation. Creation stories define relations among all species: Rocks, rivers, and trees take part in the web of life as kin, teachers, and ancestors. *Animism*, the belief that everything has consciousness or a soul, enlivens the landscape to unimaginable realms. When this belief becomes a way of life, we realize we are never alone. Just as we begin to become aware of a tree in our yard or in a city park, so, too, is that tree aware of our actions and presence. Creation stories are roadmaps to remember the way home and ensure one never feels alone.

The Dreaming describes the cosmology of the first people of Australia.[2] In many Aboriginal creation stories, the spirits come in human form, and it is believed that when a woman conceives a child, spirits inhabiting the area of the land pass into the infant in utero. This child carries the spirit quality of that place, and when that child dies, Aboriginal people feel the spirit return to the land. This profound relationship indicates the land is generative of humans and humans in turn reciprocate through ceremony, dance, and life itself. The Dreaming is the environment Aboriginal people live in and always comprises the significance of place.

Indigenous creation stories often feature humans playing a vital role in the web of life. Richard Bugbee from the Kumeyaay tribe of Southern California said, "The biggest misconception is you take humans out of nature and nature comes back. That is not true. You take humans out of nature and there is something missing."[3] The Earth delights in all of our sounds. How long has it been since land heard the sound of a birthing woman? A grieving father? *Solastalgia* describes the experience of emotional distress brought on by environmental losses and the subsequent dis-*place*-ment that often follows. This phenomenon has been studied clinically for over fifteen years.[4] Coined by environmental philosopher Glenn Albrecht, the term *solastalgia* refers to the homesickness that can be experienced while still at home but in surroundings that have been radically altered by environmental degradation and loss. The Earth experiences the same loss of our presence in her own way.

Our notion of wilderness calls for reexamination because it is perpetuating the misconception that for land to stay pure and pristine, humans are not permitted. With the world's population continuing to rise, conserving some lands as wilderness is vital. The word *wilderness*, however, does not appear in many Indigenous languages. Indigenous beliefs are that when land is left in wilderness status, that is kin to abandoning that land.[5] Intricate systems of land management where Indigenous practices flourish are at long last being recognized for the brilliant designs that they are. For thousands of years First Nation people have watched and read the landscape to note changes and developed technology for adaptation. Lyla June Johnston, Diné (Navajo) and Cheyenne Indigenous water protector and environmental scientist, said, "The reality is, indigenous nations on Turtle Island were highly organized. They densely populated the land and they managed the land extensively. And this has a lot to do with food, because a larger motivation to prune the land, to burn the land, to reseed the land and to sculpt the land was about feeding our nations."[6] Government agencies are beginning to consider the role of these practices as a viable way to offset climate change. In Africa, a field of science called Indigenous knowledge systems (IKS) is slowly being recognized by those responsible for defining environmental policy.[7] In North America, the Indigenous-led field of traditional ecological knowledge (TEK) is being taught at colleges and universities as a type of land management practice.[8] Ironically (and tragically that it took this long), the federal government is asking First Nation consultants of traditional knowledge for guidance on best practices for restoration of federal lands following devastating fires and in the face of rapid loss of species. Could this be the seed that begins the realization that rematriation of land is the ultimate act of decolonization?[9] The native land return or the land back movement are powerful living actions that are working to reclaim Indigenous sovereignty.

In the decade of 2010 to 2020, there was unprecedented growth in the numbers of people drawn to plant medicines to help ensure good health for their families. While this outpouring of interest has had negative consequences on wild plant populations, could this call of the plants be one of Earth's self-correcting mechanisms, a part of the Gaia hypothesis? Is this a way Earth is mobilizing humanity to begin to seriously defend the ecosystems that are our life's blood? If there is such widespread interest in these medicines, a primary task is to educate consumers to the fact that these plants are integral species for the functioning of the whole ecosystem, maintaining many life-forms beyond humans. We know of many strategies that combat climate change, including carbon sequestration, alternative energy generation, and a host of community-centered innovations. The technology needed to complete the effort is to restore sacred relationships with the Earth and with the plants.

Tending Land Close to Home

Tending land is much more than planting a garden or mowing a lawn. It also includes protecting resources so regeneration happens naturally. For example, when you walk through the woods or along a beach, you may spot a beautiful natural object that seems meant just for you, as a special sign or a bit of magic. You may want to take that turtle shell or bone or rock home with you. It's possible that the object truly is a gift that the Earth is bestowing to you. But just as it's important to listen for a plant's permission to harvest it, the same goes for all of creation. Shells and bones provide necessary nutrients and minerals that nourish our beleaguered soils. The more life-forms we allow to remain in the matrix of nature, the healthier our ecosystems, and thus our plant medicines, will be.

Preservation of Resources

Whether harvesting in our gardens or the wild, we are tasked with noting the condition of the environment. For example, water-loving nettles heal our kidneys, so we need to ensure the water they are growing near is clean and pure. Plants belong to the land where they burrow. Just as we go out with our gathering baskets and tools, so, too, do plants summon nutrients from the soil to nourish the leaves above, who in turn harvest sunlight and give us breath. Plants ingest nutrients of their kin as the mycelial and fungal worlds create life from death. The health and nutrition of the soil are part of our tasks in preserving resources and enhancing the terrain for future gardens.

Practicing Bioregionalism

Bioregional farmers and herbalists are just beginning to reap benefits from society's increasing awareness of the importance of sourcing food and herbal medicine close to home. There are other significant reasons to look to our local environments for our medicines.

There is an interesting phenomenon I have witnessed for over thirty years: an uncanny relationship with where people live (rent or own) and the plants that are growing there. I cannot tell you how many times I have heard a client's story and when they tell me what is growing in their yard it happens to be exactly what they need. In part, this is because many of our favorite medicines are prolific common weed species, but there is a relationship that transcends reason. I have heard so many client stories like this one. A mother of three boys tells me she is worried about allergies for two of them and recurring muscle aches for the third. When I describe the uses of gold-enrod (*Solidago* spp.) for clearing sinus congestion and for treating strained muscles, her face lights up. She tells me that goldenrod grows all along the fence line by her home. This is a pattern witnessed by many herbalists, not just me. And a related phenomenon: Plants have appeared in my garden that I am certain I did not plant, and not long after they showed up, a need arose for that very medicine. This is the ultimate act of reciprocity, where the gift being given (our medicine plant) arrives before we realize we are in need!

Another reason for harvesting close to home has to do with potency. Author and acupuncturist J. R. Worsley famously taught that plants growing within a fifty-mile radius of a person's home will have significantly greater healing power for that individual. Herbalist Phyllis Light taught that it is an herbalist's task to observe which plants are in greater profusion than usual each season and to gather those medicines, because they will be especially needed for that year. In the summer of 2001, I was amazed by all the mullein (*Verbascum thapsus*)—it seemed to be growing everywhere. I dutifully increased the amount I harvested because I had seen Phyllis's teaching prove true in the past. After the shocking and tragic losses of September 11, 2001, an outbreak of prolonged cases of bronchitis such as I had never seen occurred in my area. I was living in rural Virginia, far from the dust resulting from any of the explosions, so physical irritants were not the cause. In energetic terms, though, the lungs are a place where the body processes grief, so the intense cases of bronchitis weren't such a mystery. Mullein is a gentle yet profound healer for the respiratory system. I was glad to have a plentiful supply to address the healing needs of that deeply sad time.

Clearing History

If you have a place where you can plant a medicine garden, whether a backyard or urban community garden, this can be a wonderful experience in building a relationship with the land as well as the plants. When we start a garden, some of the obvious things to evaluate are the condition of the soil, the sun and wind exposure of the site, and the availability of water. The most important aspect of learning about a site is one that is rarely acknowledged by non-Indigenous people. When starting a relationship with a new piece of land, what is often overlooked is the history of that land. What are the stories of the people who have lived there in the past, and how has that land been treated? The laws of thermodynamics tell us that energy cannot be created or destroyed: It simply changes states. Thus the his-story or her-story of the previous occupants remains a force on the land, even after the residents are long gone. We all have experienced this reality. More often than not when we enter a home, a garden, or a forest, we get a vibe from that place. Consciously or unconsciously, our bodies scan our environs for its potential for pleasure, healing, refuge—or danger. This sensing of the quality of a place or a landscape is much like the experience of sensing a plant's vital energy. When we drop into our perceiving hearts, we allow our ancestral navigational skills to come forward. We realize how skilled we actually are at determining whether an environment is healthful or detrimental to our well-being. We listen to the story of the place, the story of the land.

As mentioned in chapter 2, epigenetics can provide a wealth of understanding about how our bodies are affected by trauma that was experienced by our ancestors. Intergenerational trauma is also felt by the land. Gaia is a living, intelligent being, and she, too, experiences effects in the present arising from neglect and violence that occurred in the past.

Recall one of the tenets of the honorable harvest: *Ask permission before taking. Abide by the answer.* The purpose of asking permission is not simply to assure the proliferation of the species being harvested. It is an acknowledgment that these plants serve a myriad of purposes, including many we may not be able to perceive. Maybe these plant medicines are not growing there for our consumption but for the reclamation of the land and the healing of stories past. Keep this in mind if you hear a plant or a stand of plants replying "no," and respect their knowledge. My experience gathering plants from the wild here in Virginia has taught me how to sense the landscape and notice the stories rising from the land. More often than not I have come upon a field of the wound-healing yarrow (*Achillea millefolium*) or the protector plant St. John's wort (*Hypericum perforatum*) close to sites of battles during the Civil War or even farther back in history. Virginia has such a history of trauma and violence—could this be why an abundance of medicinal plants grow in our commonwealth?

Many have written about the complex role that invasive plants can play in the healing of an area. In *Gaia's Garden*, permaculturist Toby Hemenway wrote, "Evidence is mounting that the vigorously growing blends of native and non-native plants that 'invade' damaged land are yet another example of nature's wisdom and resourcefulness. Nature creatively mingles native and exotic without prejudice, using all resources available."[10] Sometimes plants show up in ways that are remedial to that land. But at other times, we are asked to directly engage with helping to clear the land of trauma.

Reclaiming Sacred Space

When I became a steward of a home and property in Charlottesville, one of the main attractions was the woods behind the house. In this downtown spot, the large wooded area was a rare find. In short order I got to know the hawk, cedar waxwings, fox, and many other creatures who resided there. I had heard that a building project would be taking place, but mistakenly, I thought it would provide a fair amount of green space. Part of this land belonged to the city, and the only way the developer acquired this prime real estate was through a promise to build a city park—but then he did the opposite.

I will spare you the gory details, but the trauma, deceit, and stress during construction was relentless. My neighbors and I tried desperately to work with the developer to mitigate the extensive degradation of the woodlands but to no avail. As a final gesture of helping the land, I posted a United Plant Savers Botanical Sanctuary sign in the woodlands. I did this on Winter Solstice, the time of year we seed our dreams, rest for the winter, then watch the new visions come forth in the spring. Working with the energy of the land was the only recourse I had at that time.

That following spring, after residents moved into the new development, they asked me to help them with their own landscaping because they thought I was a landscape designer. They felt awful about the destruction carried out by the developer. I explained I wasn't a professional gardener, but that my gardens were vibrant and plentiful because of my use of local weeds, my love of plants, and my knowledge of permaculture design (aka Indigenous farming). I told them I would help them only if I could turn the landscaping installation into an educational project. Accepting their mission, I partnered with a skilled permaculture teacher, Christine Gyovai, to create a course called Healing the Land, Healing Ourselves. Over the course of seven months, we worked with the students to restore the site. Our first engagement with the land was to practice listening. This arises from my belief that before the usual soil analysis, mapping, and design processes, every landscape design needs to begin with listening to the story that resides in the land and to what the needs of the land are. I had learned about listening from the work of Australian elder Miriam-Rose Ungunmerr-Baumann, of the Ngangikurungkurr language group, who has said that in her culture, from a very early age, learning is about waiting and listening, not asking questions.[11] We spent time letting the land find us and sit with us as much as we with it. One of the concepts I shared with the group is from mythologist and author Sharon Blackie, who describes her personal practice as "sinking so deeply into the bones of the land that you dream what it dreams."[12]

Next we followed the steps I described in chapter 2 for developing relations with a plant, but our focus was on the whole site, not a single plant. We also worked with a process taught by Stephen Buhner on how to read landscapes, which is presented in his book *The Secret Teachings of Plants*. What was fascinating was that our whole group came up with the same pattern of stories, or clues to what happened in the location. The common thread through all the observations was a deep history of conflict and anger. Researching the land through county records and interviews of long-term residents revealed that this spot was where cockfights had been held for many years. It was notorious for fights breaking out among gamblers and other groups that would use the woodland lot. This kind of energy (history) does not simply dissipate; it rests in a landscape, waiting to be transformed. There was a parallel of fraught energy among my neighbors, too. They were wonderful people, yet they had major issues with boundary lines and whose trees were on whose property. This all seemed out of character for their genial personalities. Who knew all the dimensions of the land we would be transforming?

I offer this story as a message of support if you find out that the parcel of land you are stewarding has a challenging past. That could be why you are there. When folks are struggling in a search for the perfect piece of land, I like to remind them that land is also searching for the perfect steward.

There are many techniques for clearing energy from a site, but truth be told, simply our presence, love, and respect for Nature can be very effective. We also chose plants we felt were being requested by the land and were appropriate for the woodland where we were working. Consider the life of Jadav "Molai" Payeng, also called the forest man of India. For thirty-five years, single-handedly, this farmer started his day at 3:30 in the morning by walking an hour to a boat, then paddling for half an hour, then riding a bicycle for over another hour to plant cuttings from trees. Over the decades, he planted 1,360 acres of dense green forest in a remote district of Northern India. The barren land has grown into a forest teeming with life: Tigers, rhinos, and elephants now have sanctuary. On a very different scale, the woodlands behind my home have been repopulated with once familiar families of fox, hawks, and a greater sense of stewardship from surrounding neighbors.

When you undertake an energetic land clearing, what is most important is to approach the land with a spirit of respect. Committing to caring for the soil and planting and tending plants is an age-old form of reverence. Humans are dependent on the land and the land in turn needs human ritual to maintain vitality. Ritual takes many forms and one of the most magnificent ceremonies is planting the plants.

The Rise of Botanical Sanctuaries

Another compelling reason to seek out land where you can grow medicinal plants is that many of these plants are rapidly disappearing from the wild due to overharvesting or destruction of their habitat. To understand what is at stake for the world of botanicals, we need to appreciate the scale of the global marketplace and how it impacts wild populations of herbs, farmers, herbalists, and fragile ecosystems all around the world. This was the topic at a significant gathering of world-renowned conservation scientists and organizations in 2016 sponsored by the Royal Botanic Gardens in Kew, England. The wildlife trade-monitoring network called TRAFFIC was one of many participants, along with the World Wildlife Fund and the International Union for Conservation of Nature (IUCN), the creator of the respected Red List of Endangered species. TRAFFIC is the world's leading nongovernmental organization monitoring wild populations of plants and animals. This symposium launched Kew's ground-breaking study *State of the World's Plants and Fungi*, and as of 2020, Kew has published four reports as part of this study. According to the 2018 report, *Wild at Home*, it is estimated that there are four hundred thousand plant species worldwide and thirty thousand to sixty thousand of these have well-documented commercial use in medicine and cosmetics. A staggering 60 to 90 percent of these documented plants are harvested from the wild. Since 1999, the trade in aromatic and medicinal plants has tripled. Production of essential oils in particular requires vast amounts of plant material, and this is having a drastic impact on plants in the wild. It is estimated that by 2025 the United States will see $14–15 billion in trade for essential oils.

Worldwide, only 7 percent of known medicinal plant species have been assessed for extinction status. That leaves the status of 93 percent of wild species unaccounted for. Of the 7 percent that have been studied, one out of five is facing extinction. For all we know, many of the species not yet assessed may be threatened or endangered as well. Within the next decade, we may see the last harvests of some of these medicines. This might seem like cause for despair, but I believe it is a clarion call to action.

Conservation through Education

Over twenty-five years ago, beloved author and teacher Rosemary Gladstar had the vision to start United Plant Savers (UpS), an organization whose mission is "to protect native medicinal plants of the United States and Canada and their native habitat while ensuring an abundant renewable supply of medicinal plants for generations to come."[13] As the founder of the California School of Herbal Studies, the oldest continuously run herb school in the United States, Rosemary has educated thousands of herbalists who have gone on to educate other communities all across North America. Rosemary came to realize there was a growing need to begin replanting and preserving herbs that were being harvested on a commercial scale. For the past forty years, herbalists have worked to educate their communities on the safety and value of plant medicines. Now the teachings are very different. I don't think many of us would have foreseen today's multi-*billion*-dollar industry based on natural supplements from plants. Two of the most threatened plants are American ginseng and black cohosh.

The criminal activity of illegal harvesting, known as poaching, is occurring at unprecedented levels. International markets are insatiable for American ginseng. The extraction of native medicinals is the tale of rape and pillage—plain and simple. Often there is little to no oversight of timing the harvests, no sustainable practices employed, and no other measures of accountability. Economic hardships exacerbated by the tragic opioid crisis in Appalachian communities are forcing many local harvesters to abandon sustainable harvesting practices in order to collect greater amounts so they can earn more money.

According to the US Fish and Wildlife Service, more than 360,000 tons of black cohosh were sold in 2015. That does not include the tonnage that was ripped out of the earth and sold on the black market. A digger friend of mine, Laurie Quesinenberry, tells me that it takes six to ten fresh plants to make up a pound of cohosh roots. Doing the math, one ton of cohosh is fifteen thousand roots, at the minimum. Each root represents the life of a plant. The annual tonnage sold represents *many millions* of black cohosh plants. Picture a vast forest with millions of black cohosh plants growing. Then, imagine that woodland with all of these treasures gone, within the span of a single year. How in the world is that possible?

UpS has compiled a plant list that has become the gold standard for conservation efforts in the United States and Canada. On the UpS At-Risk List are those medicinal plants that are deemed the most vulnerable to overharvesting. The list is based on an assessment tool that encompasses a variety of factors, including life history, effect of harvest on the plants, abundance and range, habitat, and how much is needed. As plant stewards, it is important to understand these criteria as well as variables that affect the safety of a plant species. (See appendix 1, "At-Risk Assessment Tool Scoring Sheet," on page 317 for more information about the assessment tool.) Although there may be abundant stands of a certain plant in your locale, the nature of that plant's life cycle or the degree of demand for it

The United Plant Savers At-Risk List

American ginseng	*Panax quinquefolius*
Arnica	*Arnica* spp.
Black cohosh	*Actaea racemosa*
Bloodroot	*Sanguinaria canadensis*
Blue cohosh	*Caulophyllum thalictroides*
Butterfly weed	*Asclepias tuberosa*
Cascara sagrada	*Frangula purshiana*
Chaparro	*Castela emoryi*
Echinacea	*Echinacea* spp.
Elephant tree	*Bursera microphylla*
Eyebright	*Euphrasia* spp.
False unicorn root	*Chamaelirium luteum*
Gentian	*Gentiana* spp.
Goldenseal	*Hydrastis canadensis*
Goldthread	*Coptis* spp.
Kava kava	*Piper methysticum* (Hawaii only)
Lady's slipper orchid	*Cypripedium* spp.
Lobelia	*Lobelia inflata*

in the marketplace might cause the medicine to be more vulnerable in the big picture. Therefore it may be ranked higher (more at risk) than you might imagine.

Conservation through Relationship

As with most conservation issues, determining the optimal way to protect wild medicines is a labyrinthine path. It might seem prudent to fervently say no to the harvest of any species of threatened plants. But what effect might that have on those who make their living by collecting wild plants, or on even the plants themselves? Keep in mind that humans are a keystone species that serves multiple roles in relation to other life-forms—and we do not have a complete understanding of what all those roles are.

From a cultural standpoint, it's important to recognize that there are generational harvesters in the mountains of Nepal, the hollows of Appalachia,

Lomatium	*Lomatium dissectum*
Osha	*Ligusticum porteri*
Peyote	*Lophophora williamsii*
Pink root	*Spigelia marilandica*
Pipsissewa	*Chimaphila umbellata*
Ramps	*Allium tricoccum*
Sandalwood	*Santalum* spp. (Hawaii only)
Slippery elm	*Ulmus rubra*
Squirrel corn	*Dicentra canadensis*
Stone root	*Collinsonia canadensis*
Stream orchid	*Epipactis gigantea*
Sundew	*Drosera* spp.
Trillium, Beth root	*Trillium* spp.
True unicorn root	*Aletris farinosa*
Venus fly trap	*Dionaea muscipula*
Virginia dutchman's pipe	*Aristolochia* spp.
White sage	*Salvia apiana*
White indigo	*Baptisia tinctoria*
Wild yam	*Dioscorea villosa*
Yerba mansa	*Anemopsis californica*

and other regions who are the sole income providers for their families. Many of these collectors are women who may have few opportunities for other sources of income. Collecting wild plants can be grueling work that involves climbing steep gorges and carrying heavy bags of plants over long distances. This intense labor can be a source of pride and a trade to pass on to younger generations.

One way to engage in forward progress on plant conservation work is to support advocacy and regulatory agencies that are trying to understand and reconcile the complexities of these issues. As an individual, your mission is clear: Plant the plants if you have access to land, and protect the plants that are growing wild in your area. Consider that it was humans who decided to define wild as something separate from us. You can change that definition. Allow the wild plants back into your gardens. They may be weedy, but remember that it is about relationship and you can craft your garden with skill as well as heart. Before you cull plants from your garden, observe the patterns or stories they are presenting. It is now time to welcome species that we once relegated to outside the borders of our gardens.

Botanical Sanctuaries

One of UpS's most successful programs has been the establishment of the Botanical Sanctuary Network. All gardeners are encouraged to join in this ever-growing network and the requirements to start a sanctuary are quite simple (go to www.unitedplantsavers.org to learn what it takes). These sanctuaries serve three essential functions in the preservation of native medicines. First, they are rich depositories of native medicinal plants. Second, they are an educational resource, because sanctuary stewards commit to educating their local community about medicinal plants through informal classes. Third, botanical sanctuaries serve as important seed and germplasm repositories. This last function is the most important, especially if we have acquired plants endemic to our bioregion. Our sanctuaries then become a place of exchanging genetic material appropriate for our own areas, strengthening local populations.

The early vision of a network of botanical sanctuaries weaving North American bioregions together has become a reality through the efforts of farmers, herbalists, and plant enthusiasts from all walks of life. From Ontario to Arizona, from tribal lands to urban lots, members of UpS have shared their stories generously for others wondering how to take on the task of converting their woodlands or lawns into a plant sanctuary. A sanctuary supports multilayered natural systems of pollinators, wildlife, and companion plants that find their way to healthy ecosystems.

Medicinal plants are so resilient. If you are new to gardening, start slow and plant just a few plants. Before you know it you revel in the success and joy of growing amazing medicines. Our lot is less than a quarter acre of land, and the profusion of species and pollinators that live there has more to do with the resilience of these plants rather than my gardening skills. Perhaps it is my intention and presence with them daily that makes up for lack of horticultural knowledge, but isn't that the first ingredient in a good soil mix? Our approach is very low tech. The wild gardens are never watered save possibly the first few days after transplanting.

Over the years my community of staff and students have planted native species such as witch hazel (*Hamamelis virginiana*), fringe tree (*Chionanthus virginicus*), winterberry (*Flex verticillate*), hornbeam (*Carpinus* spp.), flame azaleas, and more. Goldenseal is taking over the walkway, and black cohosh, when in flower, waves to neighbors walking by. At the first sign of spring, bloodroot unfurls along the path that is also home to the Joe Pye, blue vervain (*Verbena hastata*), teasel (*Dipsacus* spp.), and Solomon's seal (*Polygonatum biflorum*). We estimate that our garden includes over two hundred species of North American plants, European natives (weeds), and a few ragamuffins, all welcome from unknown parts. Goldenseal is on the United Plant Savers At-Risk List, and that made me reluctant to include it in my materia medica for a while. Now that I see how easy it is to grow, I have returned this wonderful medicine to my materia medica. Most home gardeners can grow goldenseal, no matter their locale, and the same is true for the majority of the plants in my materia medica (see chapter 9).

How beautiful that one of the first responses to modern-day pandemic was a dramatic increase in family gardens. Burpee Seeds and Plants sold more seed in 2020 than in any other single year in its 144-year history. Imagine if we planted medicinal sanctuaries with the same fervor Americans planted gardens in 2020. Or perhaps not unlike Victory Gardens during World War II. One-third of all vegetables produced in the United States at that time came from Victory Gardens.[14] Started in Canada in 1917, this garden movement was a collective response in support of the efforts at home and abroad during the two world wars. It was estimated that in 1942 the harvest of fruits and vegetables from these community plots approximated a staggering eight million tons, which was thought to be almost half of the fresh vegetables and fruits eaten in the United States that year![15] If war can galvanize a nation to respond with such vigor and success, we can surely mobilize in a similar fashion against global climate crisis.

The goal in supporting the establishment of the UpS botanical sanctuaries is not simply to serve as an isolated retreat for at-risk plants. Plants are responding to climate change in ways we cannot begin to imagine. This is what artist, scientist, and anthropologist Natasha Myers refers to in her discussion of renaming the Anthropocene epoch to the Planthropocene.[16] By this she means redefining this geological time placing plants at center stage, allowing them to define technological directions. We need to follow their lead and engage in research and models of investigation that give space to observe adaptations by the plants. We need to give plants agency as intelligent evolutionary beings that have infinitely more experience at adaptation than we do.

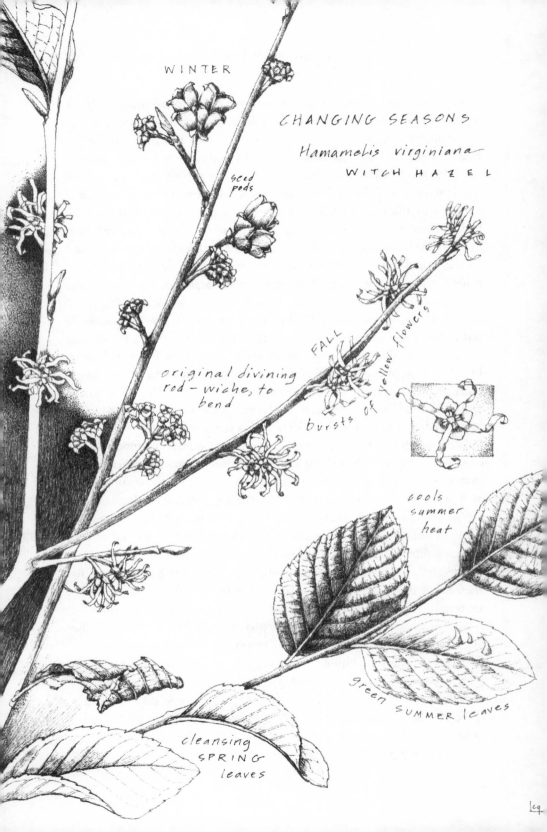

WINTER

CHANGING SEASONS
Hamamelis virginiana
WITCH HAZEL

seed pods

FALL

original divining rod – wiche, to bend

bursts of yellow flowers

cools summer heat

green SUMMER leaves

cleansing SPRING leaves

Lcq

CHAPTER 4

Medicine of the Seasons

E very season has its medicine—joyful moments that stir our emotions and spirit. There is nothing more exhilarating than watching the first bloodroot (*Sanguinaria canadensis*) offer its leaves furled like praying hands rising through newly thawed soil. Perhaps you relish those long sultry days of summer when even after the workday ends, you have many daylight hours left to garden, play, or relax outdoors. As day length shortens in the fall, deciduous leaves lose their chlorophyll, and the brilliant colors of yellow flavonoids and orange carotenoids become the alchemical magic that makes autumn so sensual and comforting. Leaves and daylight hours fall further still, as we enter the winter season with its cold, clear, crisp nights. Time to stargaze and incubate our winter dreams while closing in for the season's hibernation. By living with these forces, we begin to find our way again to a place so familiar it can startle us with its beauty. The expression of the seasons is another way in which we understand patterns.

It was out of necessity that our ancestors learned to read the skies, note changes in the winds, and smell the coming rains. Their lives were inextricably bound to the seasons. Shelter, food, and being in concert with the rhythm of the world around them were a matter of survival. Today, many of us spend most of our lives in a one-size-fits-all indoor environment. And yet, we suffer more from allergies and asthma than ever before. One exciting and effective way to restore our relationship to the natural environment is through the medicine of the seasons with the lens of Five Phase (Five Element) Theory. If we are the microcosm of the macrocosm, then we are the reflection of the seasons. The elements within us transform as they do in Nature.

The Basics of Five Phase Theory

While many practitioners refer to this energetic system as Five Element Theory, the translation that corresponds most closely to the original teaching is Five Phase Theory. This name reflects processes that are occurring in Nature and therefore in ourselves. The movement from one element or season into another is a dynamic relational process. This dynamism applies not only to the phases of the year, but to those of our lives as well. This is reflected in these words from the *Nei Ching*: "When speaking of one day, the morning is governed by Spring, afternoon by Summer, evening by Fall and night by Winter. The Spring energy gives birth; the Summer produces maturity; the Fall is the time for gathering in; and the Winter is the time for Storage."[1] This text, also called the *Inner Canon of the Yellow Emperor*, is said to be the oldest medical text written. These ancient writings provide wonderful phrases that are extremely helpful for Westerners to grasp the concepts presented in this model. I make use of these phrases myself in my teaching and in this chapter. Also note that in this chapter, and throughout this book, I capitalize the names of elements and Organs of Chinese medicine that are distinct from Western concepts.

The art of Chinese medicine includes complex and very intricate practices that require in-depth training and years of study. I am still very much a student of this art, not an expert. What I offer in this chapter are teachings that I have found invaluable in helping Western herbalists engage their health through their senses and the elements of Nature. This chapter is an invitation to begin to experience the seasons as well as our emotions in a new light. This chapter is not intended as a guide for diagnostic purposes, but instead serves as an introduction to observe the patterns of the seasons and their medicines, which are available to everyone. As stated in chapter 1, most acupuncturists follow Classical Chinese Medicine Theory or the more contemporary Traditional Chinese Medicine (TCM), and many of them blend Five Phase with those systems. Many practitioners who work only with Five Phase Theory call themselves Five Element acupuncturists.

Chinese philosophy conceptualizes human beings as microcosms of the world around us. We require the same elements as seeds do to germinate and flourish: moisture, warmth, light, and air. When these forces are present and in right relationship with each other, health ensues. If the elements are imbalanced, disease occurs. Too much fire in the body depletes and debilitates, just as extended summer heat depletes the landscape. Too little

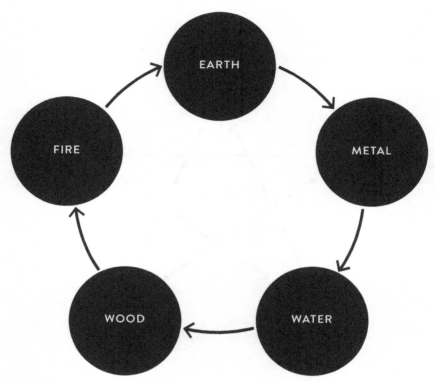

Figure 4.1. The generating cycle.

water in the body dries out membranes, as do the dry days of autumn. The process of the Five Phases follows all life through birth (Wood/spring), growth (Fire/summer), maturation (Earth/late summer), harvest (Metal/autumn), and storage (Water/winter).

In our daily lives we constantly access elemental energy as we birth an idea (Wood), activate it (Fire), make it manifest (Earth), communicate our idea (Metal), then pause for reflection (Water). This is referred to as the Generating or Mother–Child cycle (figure 4.1). In the same way a mother nourishes her child, each element supports another. Wood easily burns to make Fire. Fire produces ash, which becomes Earth. Earth generates Metal. When Metal is heated and cooled, condensation results, producing Water. This is another way of expressing the interrelatedness of our systems. There is a saying in Chinese medicine that to treat a child, first treat the mother. If we see an element out of balance, it is helpful to see if the "mother" needs support.

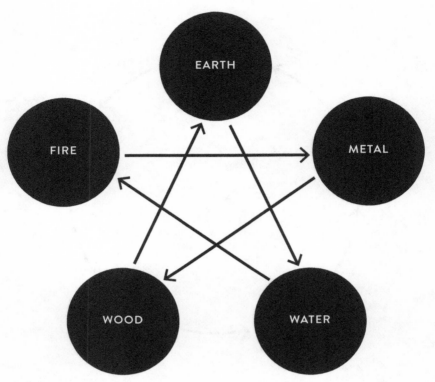

Figure 4.2. The controlling cycle.

Another cycle, called the Controlling cycle, delineates interrelationships among the elements that keep the system in check (figure 4.2). Wood depletes the Earth's nutrients, thus controlling Earth. Earth controls Water by damming the flow. Water extinguishes and therefore controls Fire. Fire controls Metal through its power to melt it. When turned into an axe, Metal can cut Wood, thereby controlling that element. While a deep exploration of these relationships is beyond the scope of this text, it is interesting to understand what these common diagrams are referring to, as they are used frequently in Chinese texts.

It is impossible to grasp all the information and underlying meaning presented in this chapter in just one sitting. So after you read this chapter for the first time, give yourself time to reflect. Then, with each approaching change of season—winter to spring, spring to summer, and so on—revisit the appropriate section of the chapter. Observe or journal what you notice, both inside your body and externally. Once you begin to experience the truth that these forces and elements make us who we are as well as our outer landscape, there is an excitement, kismet, a relating to the world with such meaning that you cannot help but feel part of the sacred dance of life.

Yin and Yang

The first time I learned wide-angle vision, it was taught to me by my teacher of Chinese medicine, Robert Clickner, as a way to explain yin and yang. My teacher explained that the yin/yang theory is not a mental concept but rather an expression of how the universe is in constant motion, transition, and transformation based on the relationships of yin and yang. Through millennia of observing Nature, this theory describes the way phenomena naturally group in pairs of opposites—night and day, inside and outside, Heaven and Earth, yet also represents the ever-changing nature of all life.

Yin and yang were initially defined as two sides of a mountain.[2] Yin is the dark side of the mountain, which is shaded and moist. Other qualities of yin are nighttime, inward, cool, resting, downward, and feminine. Yang, the sunny side of the slope, relates to daytime, outward, warm, active, upward, and masculine. Yang represents the active processes such as digestion, libido, and circulation, all activities that need warmth. As in the other energetic models discussed in this book, these concepts reflect that life is not static and that opposites give rise to one another. Day transitions into night, hot moves to cool, feminine dwells within the masculine.

The famous yin/yang symbol (figure 4.3) depicts a white swirl and a black swirl that mirror one another. The black swirl represents yin, yet has a white dot within it, which conveys that yang is held within yin; the white swirl represents yang, with a black dot (yin) within. At first glance it appears to be a concept of dualism, however it is seen as a profound expression of the dynamic inter-relationships found in the natural world. The small black dot residing in the larger white space expresses the necessity of darkness to define the light, and vice versa.

This symbol is also a beautiful expression of transitions and transformation. When yin expands

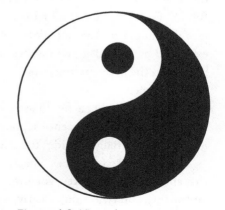

Figure 4.3. Yin and yang.

(moisture increases), yang contracts (heat decreases), and vice versa. These transformations also occur at the transition from one season to the next, one moon cycle to the following, and every minute of every day.

Five Fundamental Substances

The language and lens of Chinese medicine is very different from that of the Western medical model. Here, I offer some brief definitions of terms to help increase understanding of basic principles. These definitions are just a starting point. If you'd like to read more about Chinese medicine, see "Recommended Reading" on page 331, where I've included some of my favorite texts for deeper study of Chinese medicine.

Qi (pronounced chee) is often used as another word for the vital force, yet Qi includes even more qualities to the Chinese practitioner. As professor and scholar Ted J. Kaptchuk states in *The Web That Has No Weaver: Understanding Chinese Medicine*, "Neither the classical nor modern texts speculate on the nature of Qi, nor do they attempt to conceptualize it. Rather, Qi is perceived functionally—by what it does."[3] The main functions are: warms, transports nutrients, protects from environmental influences, transforms food into usable nutrients, contains Blood in the vessels, holds Organs in their place. You can see this is more than simply providing energy. The *meridians* are a network of pathways throughout the body that Qi follows; it is the points along these meridians that an acupuncturist works with in managing the flow of Qi, Blood, and Fluids.

Blood in Chinese medicine has some similarities to the blood in Western modalities, but it is inseparable from Qi. Qi is indispensable for the production and movement of Blood; the *Nei Ching* says, "Qi is the commander of Blood." For Qi to enable all parts of the body to carry out their functions, it is dependent on the nutrition and moistening nature of Blood. This is expressed as "Blood is the mother of Qi." Blood warms the body and is born from the bone marrow, which is why nutrition is so important for this vital substance.

Essence, or *Jing*, is a fluidlike substance that is the foundation of life. Stored in the Kidney, Essence supports reproduction, growth, and development and essentially provides the strength of our constitutions.

Shen is best translated as "spirit." It is said that "Shen is the awareness that shines out of our eyes when we are truly awake." Shen also reflects our personality, ability to think clearly, act appropriately, and provide the joy to live a full and satisfying life. Shen is directly connected to the Heart.

Fluids are essentially as they sound: saliva, tears, urine, lymph, and bodily secretions such as mucus and phlegm. They are responsible for moistening tendons and joints and make up spinal fluid.

Spirits of the Organs

For thousands of years, Chinese practitioners observed health and illness through astute observations in relation to natural elements. The practice of autopsy was forbidden, so the articulation of functions and roles of Organs by Chinese practitioners of long ago was remarkable. In Chinese medicine, the Organs are viewed in energetic terms, rather than by their anatomical structure and physiological functions, as they are in Western science and medicine. These energetics are seen as dynamic, interrelated processes that occur throughout the whole body versus in a localized area.

The Organs are paired into solid and hollow, or yin and yang. The Chinese classics view the yin Organs to be more precious (vital) because yin provides life or nourishment. Yin Organs are Heart, Spleen, Lungs, Kidney, and Liver. Yang Organs are the motive force for transformation and change (function). These are Small Intestine, Stomach, Large Intestine, Urinary Bladder, and Gallbladder. I give examples of these pairings below in the description of each of the five seasons.

Correspondences

Each of the five elements in Five Phase Theory has traits and characteristics that offer significant information about how to support each phase. These traits include season, taste, yin Organ, yang Organ, tissues, emotions, color, climate, voice, sense organ, and time of day. For example, as shown in table 4.1, the climate that affects the Earth element of Stomach/Spleen is dampness. To optimize digestion and assimilation, it is best to avoid damp foods such as dairy and sugar. I provide many examples of these relationships of the traits and characteristics as I discuss each of the five elements in turn below.

The times that are listed in the "Time of Day" sections for each element refer to what is called the Chinese body clock or Chinese meridian clock. As mentioned above, the meridians are the energy pathways that allow Qi to flow. This clock describes the flow of Qi over a twenty-four-hour period. The two-hour intervals are those periods during which the energy is most active in that Organ. For example, Liver time is 1 a.m. to 3 a.m. This is when the Liver needs deep rest to tend all the important functions that are taking place at this time. When one Organ is at its peak, the Organ

Table 4.1. The Elements and Their Qualities

Quality	Wood	Fire	Earth	Metal	Water
Season	Spring	Summer	Late Summer	Autumn	Winter
Yin Organ	Liver	Heart and Pericardium	Spleen	Lung	Kidney
Yang Organ	Gall Bladder	Small Intestine and Triple Heater	Stomach	Large Intestine	Bladder
Emotions	Anger	Joy/Over-excitement	Sympathy/Worry	Grief	Fear
Tissues	Muscle, Tendons, and Ligaments	Blood Vessels	Flesh and Muscles	Skin and Body Hair	Bones and Bone Marrow
Taste	Sour	Bitter	Sweet	Pungent, Spicy	Salty
Time of Day	11 p.m. –3 a.m.	11 a.m.–3 p.m.; 7 p.m.–11 p.m.	7 a.m. –11 a.m.	3 a.m. –7 a.m.	3 p.m. –7 p.m.
Color	Green	Red	Yellow	White	Blue/Black
Climate	Wind	Heat	Dampness	Dryness	Cold
Sound	Shouting	Laughing	Singing	Weeping	Groaning
Sense Organ	Eyes	Tongue	Mouth and Lips	Nose	Ears

opposite (twelve hours later or earlier) is at its weakest. For example, twelve hours from Liver time is Small Intestine time. Thus, we can understand the detriment of late-night meals or snacking, because the function of the small intestine is at its weakest in the hours just after midnight. This clock is simply a tool to observe patterns and understand our nature in relation to our natural cycles through day and night. The other correspondences will be described with each element.

Spring

At the spring equinox, there is an awakening from the depth of winter's sleep. Usually this season is described as the gentle unfurling of leaves. At

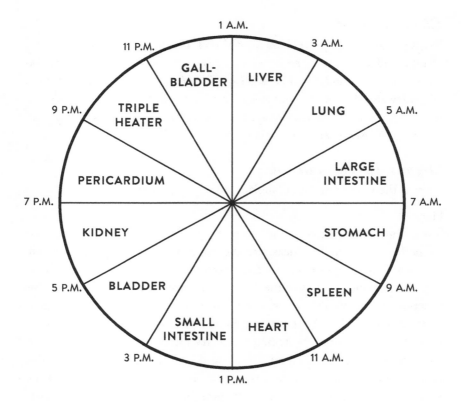

Figure 4.4. The Chinese body clock.

the same time, this season has a power that is commanded by life as it surges to the surface, breaking through the dormancy and cold of winter. The uprising energy of spring is the indomitable spirit of regeneration that renews life. Emerging from the dreamtime of winter's hibernation, the quickening of blood and the flowing of juices ignites our vision. Spring is the season to move forward, have plans, create new designs, and make clear decisions. The seeds we plant now are not only in our gardens but in the life we wish to cultivate.

The *Nei Ching* states: "The three months of spring are the period of commencement; Heaven and Earth are born, and all living things are flourishing. Get up early in the morning, walk around in the courtyard, loosen your hair and relax your body. By doing so you will generate mental strength and act in harmony with the qi of spring, thus following the way of nourishing life."[4]

Element: Wood

Spring is governed by the element of Wood. This is the element of growth, change, and a force to be reckoned with, like a mighty oak tree. This is also the energy of a dandelion (*Taraxacum officinale*) as it pushes up through a city sidewalk. We speak about spring as a time when the sap is rising—we feel rambunctious. Shoots are sprouting everywhere. There is an upward, reaching, focused energy; a quickening in our bodies and thoughts.

Organs: Liver/Gallbladder

Liver is the yin Organ and Gallbladder is the yang Organ.

Liver

The Liver maintains the smooth flow of Qi in our bodies. This flow can be in the form of thoughts, ideas, and digestion, as well as fluids to lubricate tendons. Liver health supports the flow of emotions. Extreme emotions and fluctuations can injure the Liver or indicate a need to support this function. The Liver also stores blood and regulates the amount required at various times during the day. For example, when you exercise, blood flows to muscles and tissues, providing necessary nutrients and oxygen. When you rest, blood returns to the Liver to be stored again. This balance is also reflected in a woman's reproductive cycle. Excessive or scanty menstrual flow may not be due to hormonal influences but rather due to Liver imbalance. More often than not, supporting Liver function will alleviate many reproductive challenges in order to reinstate healthy flow.

The spring cleanse is a longstanding tradition, serving an important function as people emerged from the dark and dank of winter when fresh foods were not available and they were more prone to stagnation and winter illnesses. A spring cleanse is a great practice to help minimize spring allergies as well.

The Liver is in charge of planning. This function involves the whole body and plays a significant role in regulating processes from the emotional down to the cellular. The flow of all physiologic processes needs to happen according to plan. Since this is all encompassing, we can see why Liver health is so important, especially today when there is so much exposure to environmental toxins.

Gallbladder

As the yang Organ in this pair, the Gallbladder is in charge of executing the decisions needed to carry out the Liver's plan. The Gallbladder makes determinations on the best way forward. Someone who is able to execute clear plans has sufficient gall to speak their mind to carry through with their vision. Stimulating the Wood element through the use of bitters or digestive enzymes can be incredibly helpful for those struggling with decision making. I find it significant that the majority of people who have had their gallbladders removed are women.[5] Gallstones are two to three times more prevalent in women than men. Consider that, traditionally, men are more encouraged and allowed to express their gall. There is a hormonal component to the prevalence of gallstones in women, but it's also true that, historically, women have been denied the role of decision-maker in so many aspects of life. This lack of participation and acknowledgment creates stagnation and frustration. Fortunately, change is happening on this front, and more women are creating opportunities to honor their vision and move forward with their plans.

Emotion: Anger

Many people in Western cultures struggle to understand the purpose, need, and utility of anger. This emotion is an energy that we need to recognize, honor, and allow to be expressed in an appropriate fashion. Anger serves as a defense mechanism, an energy that protects us when we feel threatened.

Bitters for Better Decisions

This tincture can be extremely helpful in gaining clarity as well as enhancing assimilation of food. Digestive enzymes are also available as commercial supplements and can offer similar benefits. Choose a product that includes amylase, lipase, protease, bromelain, and papain.

Blue vervain *Verbena hastata*
Dandelion root *Taraxacum officinale*
Motherwort *Leonurus cardiaca*
Wood betony *Stachys officinalis*

Combine the tinctures in equal parts. Take as needed, 10–15 drops at a time.

Anger is meant to be short-lived, to last only long enough to remove us or our loved ones from danger. Anger is also an instinctive response when we feel frustrated and life is not flowing according to plans. Unfortunately, our Western culture does not provide many examples of healthy expression and for the most part anger goes unexpressed. This builds heat in the Liver, and Liver heat rises in the body—hence if a person has "hotheaded" tendencies this may indicate a need to address Liver health.

The energy of Wood/anger needs to be expressed and then released through physical movement. Anger can also be released through deep breathing as well. When this energy gets stuck it can lead to stagnation in the Gallbladder. If anger is repressed for a long period of time, the energy required can extinguish our fire; eventually our ability to make and carry out plans will be dissipated. Repression of anger is one of the main causes of depression, especially in women.

Tissues: Muscles, Tendons, and Ligaments

The phrase from the *Nei Ching*, "The Liver governs sinews," means that when there is sufficient blood moistening tendons and muscles, smooth flow of movement is ensured. If there is blockage or congestion, it will manifest as stiffness and difficulty in moving. The saying "the nails are the Liver's bloom" indicates that when blood is flowing, nails will be healthy and pink. If the nails are brittle and pale it may indicate blood deficiency from Liver stagnation.

Taste: Sour

Sour is the flavor of spring and nourishes the Wood element. Drinking lemon water during this season is beneficial. If a person is attracted to an excess of sour, such as adding large doses of vinegar to all foods, an imbalance in the Wood element might be the cause.

Time of Day: Gallbladder and Liver
Gallbladder, 11 p.m.–1 a.m.

It's been said that the Gallbladder is the "night train" that takes us to a place of deep rest for the night. Many people find that if they stay up past 11 p.m., they find it hard to fall asleep. Some endocrinologists explain the value of getting to sleep at the right time of day by noting that our bodies experience as much benefit from *one* hour of sleep *before* midnight as they would from *two* hours of sleep *after* midnight.

Liver, 1 a.m.–3 a.m.

When someone says, "Let me sleep on it," they may not be aware of how important sleep is for the processing of decisions. A good night's sleep will support a deeper dream state, where our unconscious can unravel the day and plan for the next. This rest nourishes the Liver, enhancing its visioning function.

Color: Green

Springtime is the greening of our landscapes when the branches leaf out once again. An acupuncturist who is experienced in Five Phase Theory can see a green tint to a person's face when the element of Wood is out of balance.

Climate: Wind

Wood element is characterized by wind. Wind is the energy to blow away the old and leave a feeling of freshness and clarity. Yet too much wind is considered a pernicious influence in Chinese medicine. Spending too much time outside on a windy day leaves us exhausted, feeling unsettled and unfocused. Wind can disrupt the smooth and easy flow that is governed by the Liver. Meanwhile, we also know that Liver function affects our muscles and tendons, and if there is too much Liver wind then this can manifest as tremors, convulsions, and twitches.

Sound: Shouting

Shouting is the quality that indicates Wood element is out of balance. Perhaps you know someone who talks too loud or seems to shout even during normal conversation. This behavior can indicate a need for Liver/ Gallbladder releasing and relaxing. Conversely, someone who habitually speaks in a near whisper may need more Liver/Gallbladder support—a bit more gall, so to speak. But loud speech is not always a sign of an imbalance. It is simply one aspect of a person's presentation that gives us clues as to what they may need.

Sense Organ: Eyes

In Five Phase Theory, the Liver governs vision—both physical and spiritual —and is also considered the seat of the soul. As we saw above, in order to have a good plan, our vision needs to be clear and strong. The practice of liver cleansing and fasting is associated with a vision quest. However, many drugs (prescription as well as recreational) can affect the Wood element and take away our ability to vision for ourselves.

If the Liver cannot provide enough blood to the eyes, then eyesight will fail or a person may experience floaters or other vision problems. Feeling bleary-eyed at the end of the day is a sign that the Liver has not been nourished enough or its energy was consumed by stress and overwork.

Seasonal Medicine for Spring

Eat spring greens. Chlorophyll itself is medicine. This pigment is built around a structure called a porphyrin ring, which is almost identical to our hemoglobin. The ring in chlorophyll is built around magnesium, whereas iron is at the center of the heme ring in our red blood cells. Spring brings an abundance of chlorophyll in the form of chickweed (*Stellaria media*), dandelion leaves, and violet leaves (*Viola* spp.), and all of these can be eaten raw or cooked. I love to sprinkle redbud (*Cercus canadensis*) and violet flowers onto all of our spring dishes.

Collect and consume nettle. Depending on where you live, the leaves of nettle (*Urtica dioica*) are some of the first to appear in the spring. Drinking nettle leaf tea before the full onset of spring pollen can allay seasonal allergy symptoms. Nettle pesto is also a delicious, mineral-rich addition to this season's diet. Just follow your favorite pesto recipe but substitute fresh nettles for the basil (*Ocimum basilicum*) (although if you have basil available, you can add some for flavor, too). Blending nettle leaves at high speed in a blender generates enough heat to take the sting out. I also make a lot of nettles soup. Use your favorite cream of spinach soup recipe and substitute nettles. If you want to avoid dairy then add a potato and some other vegetables in place of milk or cream to make a delicious spring soup to serve either warm or cold.

Focus on bitter and sour foods. Fermented foods, sourdough bread, and other bitter and sour foods reduce Liver heat. One of the best remedies is apple cider vinegar.

Include detoxifying foods. Other foods that detoxify and cool the Liver are daikon radishes, mung bean sprouts, seaweeds, watercress, millet, mushrooms, celery, and all bright green vegetables.

Try a liver cleanse. Begin the spring by introducing a gentle liver cleanse such as the Master Cleanse Formula.

Move your body! Getting outside can be a welcome change of pace, and for most people, walking is one of the best forms of exercise. My teacher of Chinese medicine told us in class that it was always a good idea to take our livers for a walk after each meal. This stimulation of circulation

Master Cleanse Formula

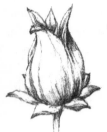

This formula was highly popular in the 1970s and '80s, and I still find it one of the simplest and healthiest ways to do a cleanse. It was developed by Stanley Burroughs, but there are many variations on the theme. I have adjusted it slightly to make it easier to multiply parts if you want to make more than one serving at a time. Just know that this is safest to do for only a couple of days. Lemons nourish the liver and are a great cleanser. They are also high in potassium and vitamin C. The maple syrup supplies calories and energy and helps take the edge off the hunger pangs. The cayenne is warming and helps clear mucus. This can be done for one day or up to a week. If you are on medications it is always best to seek supervision of a health care practitioner because undertaking a cleanse may affect the metabolism of pharmaceuticals.

2 tablespoons fresh-squeezed lemon or lime juice
  (organic is preferable)
1 tablespoon 100% pure maple syrup (less if preferred)
1⁄10 teaspoon cayenne

Mix all ingredients in a cup of pure spring water. Drink six to eight glasses a day.

helps the liver release digestive juices. Spring is a great time to launch an exercise habit, as appropriate for your body. While there are a plethora of gyms, studios, and new movement techniques, nothing beats walking. A brisk, vigorous walk is an affordable form of exercise. If you wish, you can challenge yourself to add arm weights or walk up an incline.

Summer

The seeds sown in the spring welcome the warmth and light of summer as they become the fruit that is to be harvested. The *Nei Ching* states: "The three months of summer are called the period of luxurious growth. The breaths of Heaven and Earth intermingle and are beneficial. Everything is in bloom and begins to bear fruit." Sunshine and warmth bring about the growth and maturation of what was seeded in the spring, whether in our gardens, bodies, thoughts, or emotions. This season of ripening is the time to bring visions and plans to fruition and is the time to gather with friends and families, nourishing the Heart's joy.

Element: Fire

The Fire of summer is dynamic, vital, and provides a spark to ignite and direct creativity. To be fired up, on fire about something, means there is movement and aliveness surrounding an idea. *Enthusiasm* is a perfect word for Fire element in balance: an upward excitement tempered with joy and pleasure. The expansion we feel during the longer, warmer days of summer deeply replenishes our ability to share our gifts and talents with others, manifesting as lasting confidence that sustains our inner light the whole year through.

Fire is the most yang of the elements, representing the sun. Fire is about providing and receiving warmth from relationships. When Fire is low, it is difficult to bring ideas and projects to fruition, and this cold can manifest in many ways, from cold extremities to lack of intimacy.

Organs: Heart/Small Intestine/Pericardium/Triple Heater

The element of Fire has four Organs: Heart, Small Intestine, Pericardium, and Triple Heater. One reason for this is the Heart is seen as the supreme ruler and in order to avoid chaos and confusion, there are safeguards in place to protect this treasure. As herbalists we may not use the Pericardium or Triple Heater in practice, but it is astounding to me that our energetic anatomy has Organs protecting our sacred and tender heart. The Heart and Pericardium are yin Organs and the Small Intestine and Triple Heater are yang. The Pericardium and Triple Heater do not have exact analogous structures, yet there are acupuncture channels associated with them because these are very important functions acupuncturists need to work with.

Heart

In Five Phase Theory, the Heart is the supreme ruler, the emperor, the Organ responsible for seeing clearly and compassionately. The Heart, like the emperor, links Heaven (spirit) with Earth (body) and is said to house the Shen. Shen is the form of spirit that resides in the Heart that sources joy and enthusiasm. It also governs the mind's capacity for comprehension, thinking clearly, and remembering. Often when Shen is disturbed it can affect our memories, as well as our sleep and dream state. Disturbed Shen is seen as agitation, fright, and mania, so you can see why this Organ deserves protection.

Small Intestine

The Small Intestine's main function is to sort pure from impure. Through its transformative capabilities, this yang Organ receives food from the Stomach, sorts the pure and nutritive fluids, and transports them throughout the body. The impure fluids are sent on to the Large Intestine to be cleared from the body. Energetically, the Small Intestine sorts indigestible events, thoughts, and emotions that we absorb daily and transforms what is useful through digestive fire. Tending this Organ also supports the Gallbladder in its decision-making role. Without discernment, it is hard to make a clear choice. I had a dear friend who was generous, warm, beautiful inside and out, yet her choices for partners were always disastrous. A Five Element practitioner treated her Heart/Small Intestine and within three to four months it was as if the veil of discernment lifted.

Pericardium

Also called the *Heart Protector*, Pericardium is the internal defense that protects the Heart. The Heart Protector defends against the fluctuations of emotions and energies that can be damaging to the Heart. It is also the "heart opener" that governs circulation as well as sexual intimacy. If this Organ is in excess, we find ourselves overly protective and isolating ourselves from appropriate relations. If there is deficiency here, we may feel exceedingly vulnerable to other's thoughts, ideas, and actions.

Triple Heater

The Triple Heater is composed of three areas or "burners" in the body. The top burner is the area around the head, chest, heart, and lungs. The middle burner is the solar plexus area or upper abdomen. The lower burner comprises the area below the umbilicus or lower abdomen. The Triple Heater governs even and steady circulation of respiration, digestion, and elimination. It regulates metabolism and circulation of fluids other than Blood. It is remarkable how you can feel these three areas through palpation. Easier to do with someone else but if you place your palm on the three areas of the body you can see if the temperature is the same. Tight-fitting clothes are a surprisingly major culprit of an imbalance in this Organ.

Emotion: Joy/Overexcitement

So many poetic terms that express the breadth of joy or sadness make reference to the heart: halfhearted, wholehearted, brokenhearted, heartfelt, lionhearted, faint of heart. No other organ is used with such frequency in describing meaningful and intimate feelings.

Joy rises from a deep sense of contentment, like watching fireflies on a cool summer's eve. Joy is a fire rising upward with warmth, not a blazing inferno. Many people seem to overcompensate, seeking as many positive experiences as possible. Happiness is more of a fleeting emotion, like the passing thrill of a social media post getting attention. Experiencing too much fire and excitement in an excessive drive for constant bliss is detrimental to the Heart. Excitement can move into mania, which is indicative of this element being out of balance. In TCM, psychological challenges may be treated through this element and are termed *Shen disturbances*.

Tissues: Blood Vessels

The flow and movement of the Blood is under the direction of Fire. This is invaluable, as this fluid nourishes the entire body. The description of the Triple Heater and its functions makes clear that the health and vibrancy of the blood vessels are highly important. Arteriosclerosis, varicose veins, and cold extremities are all under the influence of this element. For more suggestions for keeping the blood vessels healthy, see "Cholesterol Maze" on page 143.

Taste: Bitter

It may surprise you to learn that bitter flavor nourishes the Heart rather than the Liver. However, when we consider the increase in activity and heat typical of summer, we understand why the cooling, relaxing nature of bitter is most appropriate at this time.

Time of Day
Heart, 11 a.m.–1 p.m.

The Heart functions optimally at the peak of the day. It is a time to break from the busyness of the morning and relax and socialize a little more. Making a habit of working through lunch can strain the Heart more than we may realize. It's important to take time to digest what should be the largest meal of the day.

Small Intestine, 1 p.m.–3 p.m.

The Small Intestine begins to process and organize in the early afternoon. It digests the food consumed during the noon meal and begins sorting and clearing the day's activities as well as deciding what to keep and what to discard so the afternoon can be productive.

Pericardium, 7 p.m.–9 p.m.

This Organ is also called the Circulation/Sex function and evening is when this energy is at its peak. This is a good time to socialize and to enjoy love making and relaxation. This is the resting time of the Stomach, and so eating a large meal in the evening can lead not only to suffering in our digestive systems but also in our sex lives. I am certainly not one to limit the time when we come together and enjoy intimacy, but reflecting on the body's natural daily rhythms can support functioning when we are having difficulties with libido and performance.

Triple Heater, 9 p.m.–11 p.m.

In the evening, energy circulates around the body and supports metabolic and endocrine functions at this time. The goal is to lessen the heat and activity from the day and to begin the descent into a restorative sleep.

Color: Red

The color of the Fire element is red, and we see this when a person is flushed in the face, whether from overworking in the outdoors, experiencing anxiety, or even blushing from embarrassment. All of these are examples of heat rising. If someone's face has an ashen hue, by contrast, it's a sign that the Fire has gone out and there is a lack of vitality and warmth.

Climate: Heat

The climate correspondence is indicating an environment that has detrimental effects. Although many revel in the heat of the summer, keep in mind that excess heat is injurious to the Heart.

Sound: Laughing

Conjure up your favorite summer memories and they will probably include laughter. Whether it's a day at the beach, on vacation, or just fun in the park, laughter is part of the sounds of summer. Like Fire, laughter is meant to rise naturally from within and then to descend when the energy of a humorous or joyful event dissipates. After I learned about the concept of vocal sounds representing the elements, I began to notice how many people laugh at inappropriate times. This can show the Heart out of balance, as laughter is used to cover up discomfort and anxiety. Sometimes we make light of a serious issue as a form of self-defense. Or we may act the prankster when we really are masking a wounding of our Heart. Lack of mirth in the voice can indicate imbalance as well.

Sense Organ: Tongue

The *Nei Ching* states: "The Heart rules over the tongue." This expresses the concept that stuttering and many speech impediments can be seen as imbalances in the Fire element and hence in the Heart. This is also the element that governs relationships and matters of the Heart. How we express ourselves is important for tending this vital Organ. To not be tongue-tied and to speak with clarity is a sign of Fire in balance. The color of the tongue can indicate healthy circulation. A pale tongue may indicate deficiency; a purplish tone indicates cold and stagnation.

Seasonal Medicine for the Summer

Enjoy cooling foods. Cooling foods tend to increase yin or fluids in our bodies and this is effective to counteract the drying nature of summer heat. Watermelons are one of the best foods for cleansing as well as clearing heat from the system. One time when I had a case of food poisoning following a meal at a barbeque, a friend gave me watermelon to clear toxic heat. I was amazed at how quickly I returned to the land of the living. Cucumbers are cooling in salads or soups (the Chilled Cucumber-Yogurt soup recipe from Mollie Katzen's *The Moosewood Cookbook* is one of my favorites). Coconut water and the meat of coconuts are very cooling. Harvest as many organic berries as possible and freeze them for the coming months. Avocados are a cooling addition to recipes because they have the highest monounsaturated fat content of all fruits, and this helps to increase moisture. Spicy peppers can actually cool our bodies by stimulating perspiration and releasing surface heat.

Savor cooling herbs. Plants that clear heat and relieve thirst are called refrigerants. Hibiscus flower and leaf (*Hibiscus* spp.) is one of the best. Lemongrass (*Cymbopogon citratus*) is so refreshing and a great pairing with some of the more bitter or astringing cooling herbs such as chamomile (*Matricaria chamomilla*). Most members of the rose family, including apples, lady's mantle (*Alchemilla vulgaris*), agrimony (*Agrimonia eupatoria*), and hawthorn (leaf, flower, and berry) (*Crataegus* spp.), are cooling and astringing, and rose petals (*Rosa* spp.) are so beautiful in a summer brew. Mints (*Mentha* spp.) are cooling: think spearmint (*M. spicata*), peppermint (*M. × piperita*), apple mint (*M. suaveolens*), and lemon balm (*Melissa officinalis*).

Include digestive herbs or enzymes. To support Small Intestine function, look to carminative herbs or digestive tonics such as ginger (*Zingiber officinale*), rosemary (*Salvia rosmarinus*), and chamomile. Digestive enzymes stimulate the breakdown of foods in the small intestine.

Engage in social gatherings. Get together with friends and family in order to nourish and deepen the joy that keeps all functions of Heart in balance.

Enjoy time near the water. Fire is the summer element, but the Water element experienced from a lake or the beach can be meditative and calming, a good antidote for the tendency to be too busy during the summer.

Late Summer

Come late summer, there is a subtle yet palpable shift that occurs at this time of year. In the beginning of August, we sense that the peak of summer is nearing its end. Even though the temperatures haven't yet begun to cool off, folks make comments about how quickly summer flew by or about back-to-school blues. Late summer is the pause following the rising, active seasons of Wood and Fire and the prelude to the descending, resting seasons of Metal and Water.

Element: Earth

Earth is the element of late summer. It is the most grounding element and one that provides nourishment and security. The bounty of the gardens and fields is in full force. We revel in the sensuality, sweetness, and abundance of this time of year. To experience the Earth in all her voluptuous ripening is such a gift. If we are gardeners, we treasure our overflowing harvest baskets as a blessing and gain security from knowing we are tended so lovingly by Mother Earth. Earth literally takes care of us. This element is about groundedness, nourishment, and sense of identity. Our sense of security comes from our first relationship, that with our mother. The mother–child relationship is a manifestation of Earth element. Even if that relationship was strained or nonexistent, through our relationship with the Earth we can begin to heal this loss. This element also asks us to observe our relationship to food and how well we digest or transform that food into usable nutrients.

Organs: Spleen/Stomach

Spleen is the yin Organ and Stomach is the yang Organ.

Spleen

In Western medicine, the spleen is defined as the organ responsible for the removal of old red blood cells and it aids in the production of white blood cells. It is like a large lymph node in that it focuses on cleansing the blood and building immunity. In Chinese medicine, the Spleen plays a central role, as it is in charge of transportation and transformation of nutrients throughout the whole body. This Organ is a key player in metabolism as it moves vitality, fluids, nutrients, and wastes to where they need to be. It is more kin to the functions of the pancreas in Western medicine, as the pancreas produces and releases digestive enzymes so food can be broken down and assimilated properly. The pancreas also has a major role in the balancing of blood sugar, which balances the sweetness of the Earth element.

Healthy Spleen manifests as good appetite, strong digestion, and strong vitality. When the Spleen is not functioning well, there will be bloating, reflux, lack of appetite, poor digestion, obsession, worry, and fatigue. Warming bitters, such as the Warming Bitters Tincture on page 93, can help.

Stomach

Aside from the digestion of food, the Stomach helps us digest emotions, experiences, and all facets of life. This puts new light on the expression, "I can't stomach that." This is important body wisdom that we need to listen to when we are watching a movie or experiencing an event and we get the gut reaction that the event is too much to digest. Repeating this offense over time will definitely have repercussions for the Stomach. This is especially true when media outlets are supplying global news twenty-four hours a day. This Organ is concerned with our ability to take things in, to nurture ourselves, to feel full and satisfied with the fruits of our harvest. When we hear of global catastrophes and areas of great need, we feel conflicted about how to reach out and offer support and nourishment, which this element is all about. What a challenge today as we strive to alleviate so much suffering while tending ourselves. The balance point is different for each person, but retreating from the world and centering in the Mother of Earth (Fire) and tending our Hearts can often serve more than we realize.

Issues with weight control can manifest if the Stomach is out of balance. Perhaps we do not feel satiated because of insecurities. We may continue to feed ourselves unnecessarily, looking for some sweetness in life.

Emotion: Sympathy/Worry

When Earth element is out of balance, sympathy turns to worry. This signifies a lack of trust in the security that Earth will provide. Oftentimes, people will excessively mother others, and present themselves as sympathetic when in reality they are insecure about allowing others to grow on their own. Digestive bitters can help a person with Earth imbalance better process how to best support others.

Tissues: Flesh and Muscles

The tone, texture, temperature, and quality of someone's flesh give clues to the functioning of their Stomach and Spleen. If someone seems overly thin, this may indicate an under functioning of this element. The same can be true if we see flesh that is doughy, lifeless, pale, and without vitality or tone. The Spleen nourishes muscles as well, especially those of the limbs, so wasting diseases may indicate long-term imbalance of the Earth element. Remember, the Mother of Earth is Fire so if there is low vitality here, supporting the Heart can nourish this element.

Taste: Sweet

The taste that nourishes Earth element is sweet. This is the sweetness of root vegetables—the starchy, nutritive foods like carrots, beets, and squashes. The mineral-rich herbal teas such as alfalfa (*Medicago sativa*), nettle, and oats (*Avena sativa*) are sweet and building. The long-chain mucopolysaccharides (many sugars) are found in our adaptogenic tonic herbs such as astragalus (*Astragalus membranaceus*) and reishi mushroom (*Ganoderma lucidum*).

Time of Day

Stomach, 7 a.m.–9 a.m.

In the morning as we rise, Qi has just moved out of the Large Intestine, where it assisted in emptying the previous day's waste, and now moves into the Stomach to ensure optimal refueling for another day. According to Chinese medicine, breakfast should be warm and nourishing in order to supply sufficient Qi for the day. The trend of starting the day with a cold smoothie can contribute to creating dampness in the Earth element.

Spleen, 9 a.m.–11 a.m.
Mental clarity is very high at this time, as the Spleen has converted nutrients from the morning meal into Qi for the whole body to use. We see the importance of this Organ and why this time is for peak performance from this description of the Spleen in the *Nei Ching*: "Five viscera all desire their breath of life from the Spleen; it is the Spleen that is the foundation of existence for the five viscera."[6] (*Viscera* here refers to Organs.)

Color: Yellow
Again, this correspondence is generally used for trained practitioners who can see these hues in a patient's face. This is not the orange/yellow seen with jaundice, but in good daylight when Earth is out of balance, you might see a yellow tint around someone's mouth.

Climate: Dampness
An excess of humidity or dampness injures the Earth element. The Spleen in particular struggles greatly with damp conditions, which is why it is important to keep digestion warm with nourishing broths and warm digestive herbs and by avoiding foods that create damp, like sugar and dairy. Diabetes is a classic Earth imbalance, and so many of the challenges of that disease are due to excess fluids or dampness.

Sounds: Singing
The sound of the Earth element is singing. Someone whose Earth element is in balance will speak with a voice that is gentle, sure, and melodious.

Sense Organ: Mouth and Lips
The mouth and lips are governed by Earth element. Infants derive a sense of comfort from suckling. Dry and cracked lips indicate problems with fluid metabolism in the stomach, and pale lips can represent low metabolic functioning.

Seasonal Medicine for Late Summer
Support your local farmer. Shop at a farmer's market if one is available
   nearby. The nutrients that are available through organic produce are well

Warming Bitters Tincture

This differs from the Bitters for Better Decisions formula on page 79 because that formula is more cooling. This formula is specific for warming a damp Spleen condition.

Dandelion root	*Taraxacum officinale*	40%
Angelica root	*Angelica archangelica*	30%
Yellow dock root	*Rumex crispus*	25%
Ginger root	*Zingiber officinale*	5%

Take 20 to 30 drops of the combined tincture before eating.

worth the extra money you might spend. Not only is organic produce free from pesticides and fungicides that are detrimental to our health, but many organic farmers focus on restoring vital nutrients to depleted soils, which in turn results in food that is more nutrient dense. This added nutrition boosts the quality of the produce.

Begin eating lightly cooked foods. The summer diet emphasizes cooling, raw foods, but late summer is the time to shift. Cooked foods are much easier for these Organs, as they avoid adding cold damp to digestion. Adding warming spices such as a bit of ginger can really help remove dampness. Try some warming bitters.

Connect with nature. Spend more time in a natural area. Nature nourishes us at all times of the year but the Stomach and Spleen especially benefit from contact with the sweetness of the Earth. Worry is the emotion that impacts this element and spending time in Nature is one of the best ways to relax and leave work and stress behind. There is a new term for the age-old practice of simply laying on the earth to relax and rejuvenate. The technique is called *grounding* or *earthing* and is based on the fact that the Earth has a very specific electrical charge. When we ground electrical appliances, we are making sure the system is safe and stable by connecting it with the energy of the Earth. The body's electrical system needs the same kind of connection, and contact with the Earth provides centering, stability, and a greater sense of peace. Multiple studies show the beneficial effects of this technique on stress hormones and our endocrine system.

Add protein to your diet. Eat protein in small amounts throughout the day if there is Spleen deficiency; protein strengthens and regenerates this organ. If you are a vegetarian, you can add more legumes, sea vegetables, or nettles to your diet.

Autumn

Early fall whispers of the coming descent into the cooler months, and even in this era of changing global climate, the shift into autumn is palpable. I love the scent of damp, rich earth ripening with fallen leaves. The spectacle of colors on hillsides where maples, oaks, and beeches hold court is awe inspiring. Even in the desert southwest I have felt a quickening at this time of year. Autumn reconnects us to our essence. Late summer gives us the energy of the sweetness of the Mother, and autumn represents the Father (elements of Heaven) and nourishing the value, integrity, and authority within ourselves. This is the season of letting go, a lesson that trees teach us so beautifully as they release their leaves with ease and grace. In contrast, how resistant we become when it is time to let go of emotions, belongings, and the stuff of life that clutters our homes and thoughts. Trees don't stubbornly hold onto their leaves because they might need them next year. Their bare limbs and branches then take on even more beauty, silhouetted against the autumn sky.

Element: Metal

Metal represents purity, integrity, and connection with an inner authority that brings clarity to thoughts, speech, and writing. This is a highly refined quality of who we are. It is said that by giving us connection to the heavenly realms, Metal gives us meaning beyond day-to-day existence. Metal represents the essence in minerals and the soil that brings about the richness that creates structure and supports life.

Metal is related to the air and ether elements in other traditional systems. In classical Chinese texts, this Organ is referred to as "the working of change," which represents this element's ability to shape other elements and give them new form. A metal knife can transform garden vegetables into ingredients for a warming soup.

To make Metal glisten and gain resilience, we turn our attention to the health of the Lung and Large Intestine. In Western medicine these are considered primarily as organs of elimination. And although the Lung and

Large Intestine certainly play a major role in clearing and cleansing our bodies, they also serve other functions in protecting us and providing deep meaning to our lives.

Organs: Lung/Large Intestine

Lung is the yin Organ and Large Intestine is the yang Organ.

Lung

The Lung combines the Qi of Heaven (air) with the Qi of Earth (nutrition) and the essential Qi of the Kidney, creating what is called true Qi, which nourishes our entire body. The Lung sets up boundaries and protects our inner world from harmful external influences. This is why the skin is also related to Lung health and is sometimes referred to as "the third lung." The Lung serves as mediator between the inner and outer world. This Organ is the first line of defense. The lining of the lung is made up of immune cells, and the immune system is part of what is called *Defensive Qi* or *Wei Qi*.

Large Intestine

"Drainer of Dregs" is how acupuncturist J. R. Worsley refers to the Large Intestine, leaving no doubt that its main function is to carry away the impurities of body, mind, and spirit. The role of the Large Intestine is to ensure that we let go of what no longer serves us, physically as well as emotionally.

Emotion: Grief

The Lung processes the emotion of grief. Letting go is a natural process that is intrinsic to the Metal element and the season of autumn, but it's a process that many Westerners do not understand or allow. In his teachings, Mayan elder Martín Prechtel points out that the Mayan people have 101 names for grief. He teaches that the grief of losing a child is very different than that of losing a crop, but all loss can impact us deeply. In *The Smell of Rain on Dust*, Prechtel says, "Grief expressed out loud, whether in or out of character, unchoreographed and honest, for someone we have lost, or a country or home we have lost, is in itself the greatest praise we could ever give them. Grief is praise, because it is the natural way love honors what it misses."[7]

The wailing heard at a traditional Irish wake allows the energy of grief to move. Grief is one of the most feared emotions in our culture. I feel this is because we have not been given permission to experience the range of this life-honoring response. An important teaching is to allow someone to embrace their grief and not try to make them feel better because we are uncomfortable with our own unexpressed grief.

In Chinese medicine, when a spouse dies, practitioners often treat the Metal element of the widow or widower so that the bereaved one's grief will not get stuck in the Lung and cause illness. This came home to me while I was supporting my father's end of life. My father remained healthy and vigorous even after he developed Alzheimer's disease. He lived at an assisted-living facility, which he preferred to living at home with us because he was quite a social man. But as my father's cognitive status began to decline and he needed more attention, he was moved to a setting that was more like a nursing home. While I still had breakfast with him daily and often was there at night, this move was traumatic for him, and he became very depressed. We were about to move him home, when I arrived one morning and found him still in bed, which was highly unusual for him. He had a fever and was very pale and lethargic. At the hospital emergency room, he was diagnosed with pneumonia. Once my father was settled comfortably in a hospital room, I met with the resident and asked whether it was necessary to provide treatment, or could nature be allowed to take its course. His eyes welled up with tears. He told me that if more family members understood that pneumonia is one of the most peaceful ways of passing—as the saying goes, it is "an elder's true friend"—his job would be much easier. How blessed I was to have a medical practitioner support such a difficult decision and allow my 85-year-old father to express his grief and choose his way home with peace, honor, and dignity.

Tissues: Skin and Body Hair

In alternative medicine, oftentimes skin conditions are treated as a reflection of the Liver. This relationship is significant, but it is more important to look to the health of the Metal element. The Lung brings moisture to the skin to keep it nourished and responsive to outside influences. The Large Intestine, through its eliminative capacity, cleanses the entire system and the skin also aids in ridding the body of excess wastes. Eczema and asthma can appear in the autumn and often go hand in hand. Working with healthy oils, decreasing inflammation, and supporting the Metal element can stop this seasonal pattern. The correspondence of body hair is not that clear to me, and I have had much more success working with Kidney energy in regard to changes in the health of the hair.

Taste: Pungent, Spicy

Lung energy is dispersive, so the similar energy of pungent flavors supports this. Pungent herbs and foods help clear cold from the Lung and open up the senses and sinuses. Spiciness also promotes sweating to release pathogens.

Most types of pungent herbs have a warming effect. They are powerful movers and facilitate the letting go that is so important to the health of the Metal element. Moving through stagnation and opening pores to enhance perspiration are wonderful therapies for Metal imbalances. Hot pungent herbs include cayenne (*Capsicum annuum*), chili pepper (*C. frutescens*), horseradish (*Armoracia rusticana*), garlic (*Allium sativum*), and ginger. Some examples of warm pungent herbs are basil, thyme (*Thymus vulgaris*), and rosemary. Neutral pungent herbs include coriander (*Coriandrum sativum*) and cumin (*Cuminum cyminum*).

Time of Day

Lung, 3 a.m.–5 a.m.

The Lung is at its peak performance before dawn. This is why many cultures follow a custom of rising before sunrise to do meditation and breathing practices. For those not rising early, this time is important to nourish Lung health with deep sleep, especially if there have been respiratory challenges. Defensive Qi is also a part of this Organ, so boosting immunity is supported with deep sleep at this hour.

Large Intestine, 5 a.m.–7 a.m.

The period around sunrise is a time of letting go. When we are in rhythm with our body's clock, we have a bowel movement first thing in the morning. It is best to drink water in the morning and ideally go for a walk to stimulate the Large Intestine.

Color: White

A white hue to the skin often can indicate that Metal element is out of balance. An imbalance here can be seen with a pallor around the eyes and cheeks.

Climate: Dryness

The Lung and Large Intestine are deeply challenged by dry conditions. Keeping these organs moist is so important for their healthy functioning.

Autumn Allergy Relief Tea

Begin drinking this tea in late summer to prepare the immune system and lungs for allergies of the fall season.

Goldenrod leaf	*Solidago* spp.	25%
Mullein leaf	*Verbascum thapsus*	25%
Nettle leaf	*Urtica dioica*	25%
Hyssop leaf	*Hyssopus officinalis*	15%
Elderberry flower	*Sambucus* spp.	10%

Mix the dried herbs together well. Put 1 tablespoon of the herb mixture in a cup, pour boiling water over the herbs, and allow to steep for 1 hour. Strain and drink 2–4 cups a day. Add honey if preferred for flavor.

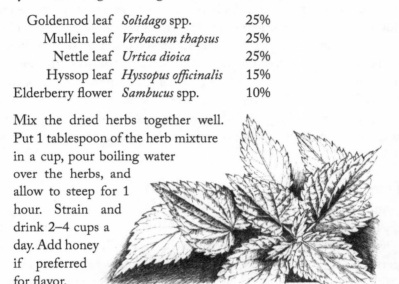

Since the most important hours for the Lung are 3 a.m. to 5 a.m., it is best to use humidifiers in the winter if the home has a dry heating system.

Sound: Weeping

The sound of weeping is ever so subtle but after practicing listening to voices you can clearly discern when there is grief woven into a person's manner of speaking. This usually is not accompanied with tears but has been described as the sound of tears.

Sense Organ: Nose

Chinese medicine says the nose is the "gateway of the Lungs" and the throat the "doorway to the Lungs." When there are repeated patterns such as loss of smell, sinus difficulties, weak voice, or chronic sore throats, look to treat this element with pungent foods and spices. Think of the effects of

Demulcent Tea for Lungs and Intestines

This tea helps to moisten dry tissues of the lungs and intestines.

Marshmallow leaf *Althaea officinalis*
Mullein leaf *Verbascum thapsus*
Plantain *Plantago major*
Violet leaf *Viola* spp.

Mix the dried herbs in equal parts.
Put 1 tablespoon of the blend
in a cup, pour boiling water
over the herbs, and allow
to steep 1 hour. Strain
and drink. Continue
drinking 2 cups a
day until tissues
feel moistened.

spicy horseradish or garlic. The eyes water and the nose runs, but afterward there is a sense of clarity.

Seasonal Medicine for the Autumn

Drink moistening, immune-enhancing teas. Both the Autumn Allergy Relief Tea and the Demulcent Tea are good choices for this time of year.

Learn pranayama. Practice deep-breathing techniques.

Try a fall cleanse. If you are prone to asthma or bronchitis at this time of year, it is important to keep the bowels moving. Although these illnesses manifest in the sinuses and lungs, they can reflect poor elimination. As the days grow colder and darker, take the preventive step of following the Master Cleanse Formula described on page 83. If you suffer from annual bouts of bronchitis at this time of the year, prepare a warming vegetable broth with pungent spices to eliminate excess mucus.

Dry brush your skin. The skin is one of the organs associated with this season, and dry brushing the skin supports the Lung and Large Intestine as well as immune function.

Clear clutter. Go through closets, basements, garages, and all the corners of your home. Don't just pass over items that you do not want to deal with: Make clear decisions, and let go of anything that no longer serves you. Recycle or give away items no longer needed, and surround yourself with what you value.

Observe an equinox ritual. Resolve not to go through another year bearing resentments, grievances, prejudices, or old patterns that need to be released. Giving death to that which no longer serves can be part of a beautiful fall equinox ceremony. Write down what needs to move on and burn it in a fire to help the Metal element shine. Honor the sensuality grief gives our lives and find courage to be comfortable with this emotion.

Winter

At this time in my life, winter is by far my favorite season. While I have lived in Virginia for decades now, I was raised in cooler, northern climes. As strange as it may sound, I find comfort in the cold days and all that winter offers. I love the vast winter sky and the way it lights up with what seems to be a million stars. This is a quieter, more reflective time of year, a time when sleep and rest are the main medicine. In some regions, snow blankets the ground, protecting the essence of life resting in the earth.

In Western culture, the frenetic holiday season contradicts what Nature intends for the season of winter. I often find myself encouraging clients, especially those dealing with chronic illnesses, to slow down after the busyness and to choose not to attend so many events or social gatherings that take their precious energy. Acupuncturist Robert Clickner is famous for this brief saying that has become my mantra: Experience consumes Qi. No matter if it is the thrills of a vacation or the stress of a late night work shift, everything we do expends vital energy. How miraculous that we have a whole season to replenish our stores of life.

Element: Water

Science and mythology tell us that life begins in the sea, and in essence we have never left it. The human body and planet Earth both consist of 70 to 80 percent water. The concentrations of salt and assorted ions in seawater are remarkably similar to those in blood plasma. The ebb and flow of our internal tides, influenced by the Moon, have profound effects on our reproductive cycle, sleeping patterns, thoughts and emotions, and more. Water is life, and even the stillest water is in motion below the surface.

Water is the most yin of all the elements, and as stated earlier, yin represents moisture, coolness, nighttime, receptivity, feminine energy, and lunar cycles. Kidney yin and Fluids are crucial for all life-supporting functions. Blood, in Chinese medicine, not only nourishes our cells in the way we understand in Western medicine, but it also carries Qi, so it plays even a larger role. Urine, saliva, tears, lymph, perspiration, and sexual fluids are all an aspect of the element of Water.

Yin is the energy of the night. Through sleep we are cooled from the active, yang daytime hours; sleep restores our reserves. If we are deficient in yin or suffer with dryness because we have been burning the candle at both ends, imbalance results. The yin that usually carries us through the night will not be sufficient to prevent the daytime yang from rising up and causing restlessness. This helps to explain why there is a preponderance of insomnia in menopausal women as well as the elderly. As we age, our bodies naturally lose fluids and moisture. Deficiency in fluids can manifest with symptoms of dizziness, low-back pain, dry eyes and mouth, tinnitus or ringing in the ears, and low libido.

Organs: Kidney/Bladder
Kidney is the yin Organ and Bladder is the yang Organ.

Kidney
This Organ serves as a storehouse of vital energy, as the Kidney preserves the Essence, that which is essential for human life. This Essence is the germ, the seed, that reaches back through ancestral origins and allows us to look back through generations, at our heritage and DNA. And because the Kidney governs reproduction and procreation, this Organ supports our instinct to look forward to the progeny that lie within. The Kidney is also the seed of our intellect and creativity, so progeny can also refer to creative endeavors.

Kidney essential Qi governs growth, development, and reproduction. Essential Qi, also called *ancestral Qi*, is the reproductive essence passed on by our parents (congenital essence) from which the fetus develops. After birth, this Qi is nourished by essence from food and water (acquired essence) and thus reaches its full maturity at puberty. Through supporting reproductive organs and activity, herbalists work with this element in supporting reproductive health, especially issues concerning fertility. As aging progresses, essential Qi begins to decline, and activities and foods should then focus on the preservation of Kidney Essence. Along with all of these functions, essential Qi is also responsible for the normal functioning of all of the other Organs. Because of this profound importance in human physiology, ancients called this Qi the "root of congenital constitution."

The complexities of the Kidney are vast, and a simple way to regard our constitutional energy is to liken it to the health of the soil we use for our garden. Those who have rock solid constitutions or good Kidney Qi are like those fortunate enough to have a garden with naturally rich soil. No amendments are needed and there is an abundance of nutrients. We all know someone like this who can eat, drink, be merry, and never seem to suffer health consequences. By contrast, others fall prey to illness easily and do not have energy to sustain simple activities. These gardens are less well endowed with nutrients or even reserves of what is needed to support and sustain good plant growth. These gardens need constant supplementation and tending, especially after a harvest.

This constitutional deficiency may be due to an early life event that depleted a person's precious store of vitality or Kidney Essence. Premature birth, pneumonia as an infant, and various other stressors early in life can affect a person's constitution for their whole life. Epigenetic trauma is initiated and intergenerational struggles are manifested in Kidney Qi. When we interview a client at the Sacred Plant Traditions clinic, we always ask about the two generations preceding their parents, the course of their mother's pregnancy with them, and the childhood illnesses they experienced. Although the genetics we inherit are something we cannot change, the beauty of energetic medicine is that it gives us the ability to identify and address these deficiencies. We can restore Kidney balance through deep nourishment. While this might take months or even years, in the long run it proves invaluable in setting the individual on a better course for the future.

This element is foundational to all human life. Kidney yin nourishes and moistens all of the Organs and Kidney yang (adrenal function) warms and activates them, supporting our vital life force. These are the root of the yin and yang of all the Organs.

Bladder

The Bladder stores and excretes urine that travels from the Kidneys. It is helpful to understand that the power of the Kidney is what governs the

Bladder's ability to hold onto urine or discharge it. This is referred to as the "opening and closing" function of the Kidney. When there is incontinence, bed-wetting, difficulty voiding completely, or frequent urination, unless there is specific Bladder disease, all of these conditions are considered under the control of Kidney. We see this with children who might be processing fear or anxiety with bed-wetting as well as elders who have diminished Kidney Essence as they age.

Emotion: Fear

Fear is the emotion processed by the Kidney. This emotion can be lifesaving—it alerts us of threats to our safety. Individuals who are fearless to a fault are said to have a Water imbalance because they are not able to provide a healthy container that can hold this emotion. At the other extreme of a Kidney imbalance are those that are constantly frightened, anxious, and unable to relax in the flow of life. In Western physiology, it is understood that the stress response arises from the adrenal glands. Our sympathetic nervous system releases adrenaline in response to a perceived threat. The Kidney governs adrenal functions. It is not surprising that adrenal exhaustion is such a common complaint these days. Aside from the personal challenges many people face, everyone must cope with fears raised by global political and environmental challenges that feel unbearably threatening to the human race. Herbs and healing foods can be wonderful ways to support this Organ that is constantly processing our fears and anxieties.

I find it fascinating that the Kidney is also seen as the seat of ambition and will. We have all heard survival stories in which, against all odds, people pushed through insurmountable challenges and lived to tell the tale. When we have little food, water, or even physical strength, the body taps into its last reserves, which are stored in the Kidney.

Fear is the tool that keeps us alive. We can say that all fears can be linked to fear of death, understanding that death can take many forms. Negative relationships and habits are draining to our Kidney Essence. If we weren't able to let go of negative habits in the Autumn, Winter is a second opportunity for doing this important work.

Tissues: Bones and Bone Marrow

The Kidney governs the bones. What this means is the Kidney stores Essence (or *Jing*), Essence builds marrow, and marrow nourishes the bones. This has huge implications for our growth, our development, and the healing of our bones. There is a traditional saying: "Teeth are the flower of the Kidney." Dental health can be a window into Kidney energy. The recent surge in popularity of bone broth has had a wonderful impact. This broth is made by boiling bones rich in marrow so that the marrow is extracted into the broth. This is pure Kidney food.

The goal of the ancient art of tai chi is to keep the bones flexible by assuring that Qi penetrates the bone marrow. Cracking joints is a sign of dryness. Practicing tai chi and keeping the bones nourished with fluids prevents brittleness and frequent fractures. After years of women taking calcium supplements to prevent osteoporosis, we are no further ahead of the game than we were thirty years ago. I help clients with bone loss by replenishing Kidney strength through tonic herbs as well as bone broth.

Taste: Salty

Salty is the flavor of the Kidney. It is a vital electrolyte that helps muscles and nerves function properly. It is also an osmotic solute, which means it assists in maintaining proper balance of fluids. Since salt nourishes the Kidney, Chinese herbalists add a bit of salt to formulas to guide the medicine to the kidneys.

Craving this essential nutrient can be a sign of Kidney deficiency, and yet this maligned nutrient has been misunderstood for decades. Current research shows that low levels of salt in the body can have damaging effects on coronary health. It can be especially dangerous for diabetics, who are often advised to follow a low-salt diet. Misinformation about salt in the diet is being perpetuated on a daily basis in clinics across the country, and it is important to correct this.

Studies on high-salt diets from the 1970s and '80s used highly processed foods, but the forms of salt in processed food products do not deliver nutrients to the kidney in the way that sea salt does. Is it any wonder elders lose their appetite when their food may be so bland as to not offer any incentive to eat? It is this very population that needs good mineral balance and Kidney support, since their reserves are on the decline.

Time of Day

Bladder, 3 p.m.–5 p.m.

The afternoon period of 3 p.m. to 5 p.m. is associated with the Bladder. This Organ governs the storage of energy, and our physical bladders are highly innervated; thus stress and anxiety can lead to loss of stored energy and cause increased urination. Many people experience low energy in the late afternoon, and they tend to reach for a pick-me-up—a cup of coffee or sugary food. But taking a break and moving or resting the body can do wonders to dispel sluggishness. The best thing to do at this time of day is be respectful of your limits.

Kidney, 5 p.m.–7 p.m.

Although the Kidney processes fear, it is also related to feelings of safety and willpower. Oftentimes people who are on a diet or restricting certain substances can maintain discipline all day with great success until about five o'clock, when their willpower gives out. This is the time of day to nourish the Kidney with herbal tonics; for those in recovery, this is a good time to go to support meetings or stay focused on tools given to maintain willpower.

Sundowner syndrome is a challenging presentation in patients suffering with Alzheimer's or dementia. In late afternoon, elders in this population present with anxiety and nervousness, and they begin wandering and exhibiting disturbing behavior. A bladder infection can be the cause of such behavior, but in many cases, elders can become very fatigued by afternoon, especially if they experience extreme confusion during the day. By late afternoon they have no root to keep them grounded. I like to teach staff at nursing facilities how to offer their patients simple warm foot soaks in the late afternoon. The warm water brings energy to the legs and to the Kidney, which calms the resident and can greatly assist in this transition of the day.

Color: Blue/Black

The colors associated with Winter are blue and black. Black beans, blackberries, and blueberries are just a few examples of Kidney-nourishing foods. How elegant are these correlations—the dark-colored berries contain high levels of antioxidants, medicines to heal the effects from stress. Antioxidant foods that contain proanthocyanidins, or blue (cyano) pigments, are key here.

If the Water element is out of balance in the body, the skin may develop a hint of blue. In classic Chinese texts, black is the color that represents the Water element. Dark circles under the eyes are called allergic shiners by many in the natural health care field. More accurately, this blue/black shading indicates low Kidney vitality, which in turn compromises one's immune system.

Climate: Cold

The Kidneys contract in the cold, so it is vital to cover our kidneys in windy conditions or when exposed to cold temperatures. That is one reason why winter is the perfect season for warm stews and broths. The traditional Japanese *haramaki*, or belly band, is worn to protect the lower back and to keep the kidneys warm and protected. In cold weather, people often suffer an increase in aching bones and joints and arthritic complaints. The ginger bath described in "Seasonal Medicine for the Winter" on page 108 is a wonderful way to send heat deep into the joints.

Sound: Groaning

The sound of the Water element is groaning and can also be described as moaning: the sound of someone who feels overwhelmed or is drowning in too much to do with little energy to spare.

Sense Organ: Ears

The sense of hearing is related to the Water element. It is thought that hearing is one of the earliest senses to come alive in utero, and it is the last sense to go when we die. The ear is shaped like an inverted embryo, and acupuncturists often use ear points to access the whole anatomy of the body. A protection against hearing loss might be to support Kidney energy while we are younger and save reserves for our elder years, as hearing can diminish with age. Winter is also the time of deep listening to our inner landscape.

Seasonal Medicine for the Winter

Rest, rest, rest. Winter is the time for going inward, self-reflection, and slowing down to conserve energy. Many people have switched from reading books to listening to audiobooks. For the winter, give your ears a rest and snuggle up to read a great book.

Do your best to live with the daylight hours. When the sun goes down earlier, have a light meal and turn electronics off. Practice hibernation.

Enjoy broths and nourishing stews. I think soups that contain a small amount of protein are the perfect winter breakfast. Along with bone broth I really like miso, a traditional Japanese food. It is produced by fermenting soybeans, salt, and koji, which is a fungus that promotes fermentation. Rice, barley, and other grains may be added. This delicious paste can be made into a wonderful vegan or vegetarian soup. It is an excellent source of protein, as it contains all twenty essential amino acids. It has a savory, meaty flavor that the Japanese call *umami*. Simply mix a teaspoon or tablespoon in water that has been boiled. You can then add the miso broth to other soups or make a vegetable soup with miso broth

Basic Congee

Serves 4

Congee is a favorite recipe for kidney health and it makes a wonderful winter breakfast. You can add a multitude of spices, herbs, and vegetables to this white rice porridge, but the basic recipe is very simple. Keep the ratio of rice to liquid between 1:6 and 1:10. Substituting other grains for the rice is fine, but rice is the easiest to digest. Use organic rice because conventionally grown rice is tainted with toxic heavy metals and pollutants.

1 cup organic white rice
7 cups chicken or vegetable stock
½ teaspoon sea salt
1-inch piece of fresh ginger root,
     peeled and sliced thin
Green onion or scallions,
     for garnish

Combine rice, stock, salt, and ginger in a large pot. Bring to a boil then let simmer for an hour. Stir occasionally to prevent the rice from clumping or sticking to the pot. When done cooking, add more salt to taste and any other herbs desired. The stew will thicken as it cools; add more stock or water if needed. Best served warm.

as the base. Never boil miso because that will destroy the nutrients. It is often served with cubed tofu and green onions, but so many variations are available.

Increase consumption of warming foods. Black beans are one of the most warming beans and a great winter addition. Beef, barley, millet, mung beans, black sesame seeds, nuts, sweet potatoes, molasses, squashes, root vegetables, winter greens, carrots, cabbages, mushrooms, and apples are other recommended foods.

Golden Milk

Golden milk is a wonderful brew for a winter evening. Turmeric (*Curcuma longa*) is antioxidant and good for bones and joint health. Be creative with your choice of milk. Sometimes I combine 1 cup whole organic coconut milk with 2 cups of nut milk; the extra fat in the winter is building and warming.

3 cups nondairy milk (or dairy if preferred)
3 teaspoons ground turmeric root
½ teaspoon ground black pepper
½ teaspoon ground cinnamon
¼ teaspoon ground ginger
Pinch ground cardamom
3 to 5 teaspoons maple syrup to your taste

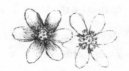

Combine all ingredients in a saucepan over low heat. Whisk for 10 minutes to blend. Serve warm. I make a blend of those spices ahead of time so it is easy to make at night.

Turn to adaptogens and Kidney tonic herbs. These are the herbs that support our health from long-term effects of stress. Examples include astragalus, eleuthero (*Eleutherococcus senticosus*), reishi mushroom, and American ginseng (*Panax quinquefolius*).

Increase warming herbs. Adding ginger, cinnamon (*Cinnamomum verum*), cloves (*Syzygium aromaticum*), coriander, anise (*Pimpinella anisum*), fennel (*Foeniculum vulgare*), and prickly ash (*Zanthoxylum* spp.) to formulas helps circulation, which keeps the low back or kidney region warm. Try adding some medicinal herbs to a chai blend, which naturally has pungent spices.

Sink into a ginger bath. A favorite restorative activity in wintertime is to make a strong fresh ginger tea and add it to bathwater. It is deeply penetrating for the muscles and allows circulation to move deeper to the organs. To make the tea, put ½ cup grated fresh ginger roots and ½ gallon of water in a saucepan. Bring to a boil and simmer lightly for an hour. Strain out the roots and add the tea to hot bathwater.

Cook with seaweeds. Honor the element of Water by using seaweeds in your cooking. Dulce, nori, hijiki, and kelp are high-protein foods and rich in essential minerals and vitamins. The strong flavors of seaweed can be hard to get used to, but this nutrient-dense food is well worth the effort. When I started using seaweeds, I toasted the nori and others, which made the strong flavor more pleasant.

Incubate dreams. Since winter is supportive of our dreamtime, learn how to incubate your dreams. Spearmint and peppermint tea can make a dream more vivid, and mimosa flower (*Albizia julibrissin*) is said to enhance color in dreams. I have found that mugwort (*Artemisia vulgaris*) is an incredibly reliable vehicle to accessing the underworld of our psyches, and while it can be profoundly healing, it can also be overwhelming, so if you are going through trauma or a particularly stressful time, you might want to start with a gentler herb.

Start a journal. If keeping a journal is something you have always aspired to, winter is the perfect time to begin this wonderful habit. Whether you journal in the evenings (now that you are engaging with less electronics) or the mornings, whether it is a diary of your experiences and thoughts or a log of your dreams, this activity is a perfect medicine for this season of reflection.

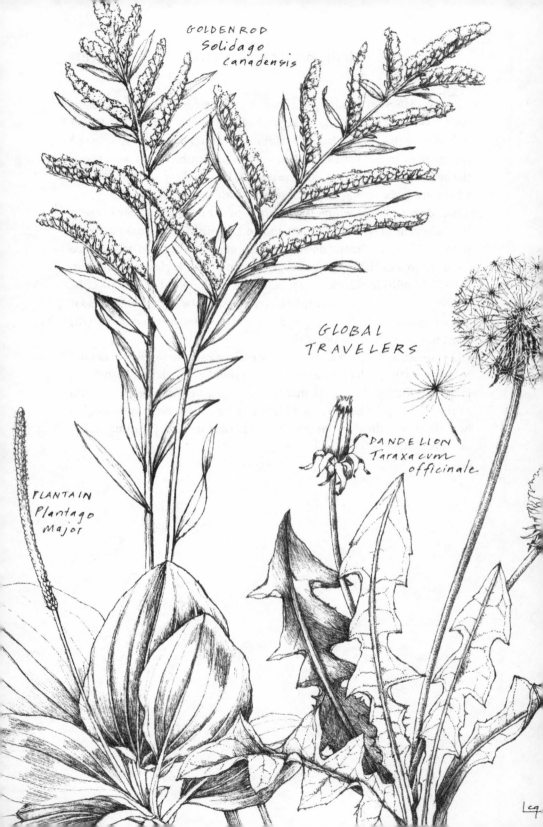

GOLDENROD
Solidago
canadensis

GLOBAL
TRAVELERS

DANDELION
Taraxacum
officinale

PLANTAIN
Plantago
Major

Lq

CHAPTER 5

Our Elemental
Selves

Ayurveda is a Sanskrit term meaning "science of life." It is said
that this system of medicine arose from the meditations of the
rishis, India's holy bards or seers of truth. For many generations,
this was an oral tradition, passed down through beautiful poems and
songs. Many of these have been lost, but one of the most ancient texts
known, the revered Vedas, survives. Of the four Vedas, the one that offers
the most wisdom on health and longevity is the *Rig Veda*. The *Charaka
Samhita*, written over 2,500 years ago, is the oldest and most important
Ayurvedic text.[1]

Ayurveda is a cosmology so vast that it literally takes a lifetime, or two,
to fully grasp. In this chapter, I cannot begin to cover the scope of this
far-reaching tradition. I present some of the very basic concepts, focusing
on those that can help in gaining greater self-awareness and understanding
of our energetic patterns. The understanding of the constitutions of this
ancient science provides a compassionate lens through which we view our
traits and tendencies. This leads to greater autonomy as we understand
how to support our well-being through food, herbal medicine, and healthy
lifestyle. As I mentioned in chapter 1, I find Ayurveda to be a very loving
system because it presents our faults and weaknesses in the terms of the
elements of Nature. It helps me understand that my fiery, pitta personality
is a gift and a challenge. Knowing that the element of Fire dominates my
actions helps me accept my nature while seeking remedies that will cool
and calm my days.

The Elements in Ayurvedic Philosophy

In Ayurvedic philosophy, the elements of Ether, Air, Fire, Water, and Earth combine in humans as three primary life forces called humors, or doshas: vata, pitta, and kapha. At the moment of conception, these energies create a person's constitution or *prakruti*. In Sanskrit *pra* means "original" and *kruti* means "creation." Thus, a person's prakruti is influenced by their parents' natures, the season of their conception, and karmic patterns. Prakruti remains unchanged throughout life and is responsible for our characteristics, personality, and strengths as well as our weaknesses. For example, someone who knows they tend toward cold in their body and temperament can learn to practice warming habits such as exercising and eating more pungent foods. To know your constitutional tendencies is to be empowered with the ultimate guide for a lifetime of self-care.

After conception, the human embryo is then influenced by external factors such as the mother's health and the environment. This state in Ayurveda is called *vikruti*, which means "after creation," or the current state of health or imbalance. (The Sanskrit root *vi* means "after.") If conditions are optimal, then vikruti and prakruti are aligned. When imbalances occur, symptoms of disease arise. When an Ayurvedic practitioner works with a client, the vikruti or current state of health is what is taken care of first; it always guides the treatment protocol. For example, if a kapha constitution, which tends to be cooler, presents with red, hot rashes, cooling remedies to clear heat, such as rose (*Rosa* spp.) or chickweed (*Stellaria media*), are indicated, despite the kapha dosha. In chapter 6, I expand on this concept of treating current health conditions in the context of the tissue states.

The Sanskrit term *dosha* can be translated as "that which has a fault," or "that which darkens, spoils, or causes things to decay." When out of balance, the doshas are the causative factors behind disease. According to the Vedas, humans are not meant to be perfect. Perfection lies in pure consciousness. It is through change that we come into our knowing self. To attain a perfect life and body is seen as burdensome because it would deplete vital energy. What is desirable and attainable is achieving balance through our doshas. While these humors mainly represent physiological imbalances, there are refined forms of the doshas. In *Evolutionary Herbalism*, Sajah Popham states, "These rarified essences of each *dosha*, called *tejas*, *prana*, and *ojas*, form a primary goal of rejuvenative therapies in Ayurveda. . . . *Pitta* is said to become rarified in the form of *tejas*, the flame of pure perception; *vata* transmutes into *prana*, the pure air of consciousness; and the essence of *kapha* is *ojas*, the refined pearl of physiological essence and rejuvenation."[2] These forms explain the elegant and sophisticated practices of many Ayurvedic cleansing and treatment protocols, which support our journey through the doshas to deeper states of being.

In Ayurvedic philosophy, all matter originates in cosmic consciousness, and this is manifest in male (Shiva) and female (Shakti) energy. The rishis perceived that consciousness is expressed through five basic elements: Ether (space), Air, Fire, Water, and Earth. From the unified consciousness, the vibration of aum (Om) gave rise to the Ether element. The movement of Ether gave rise to Air. Air breathed heat and Fire into being, which dissolved and liquified Ether into Water. This then solidified into Earth. Ayurvedic practitioner Vasant Lad, who is attributed with bringing this science to the West, described it this way: "From Earth, all organic living bodies, including those in the vegetable kingdom such as herbs and grains, and those in the animal kingdom, including man are created. . . . Thus out of the womb of the Five Elements all matter is born."[3]

Ayurvedic medicine has been influencing Western herbalism for over four decades, with many herbalists embracing its basic teachings of the three doshas. What I see happening in contemporary herbalism in relation to Ayurveda, though, is people becoming fixated on the checklist of attributes or qualities of these forces. What is lost is the intimate experience of truly getting to know the elements.

Ether

All of the spaces that exist within our bodies are manifestations of Ether: hollow channels, vessels, organs, and spaces between cells. Ether is ubiquitous—it creates the space in which the other elements reside and holds the essence of emptiness. Ether originates in the primordial space from which vibration emerges before it reaches the ear as sound, and thus hearing is the sense related to Ether. It is said that through chanting, we have access to the vastness of consciousness.

Ether's qualities are based on the absence of an opposing quality. For example, ether is light and lacks the density of Earth, it is cold as it has no warmth from Fire and is immobile as there is no force from Air. That being said, Ether is a part of every element.

Air

Air is the element of movement. As the Ether element began to create subtle movements, Air was created. This element manifests in the expansion and contraction of the lungs and with peristalsis, or actions of the bowels.

From the movement of muscles and joints, pulsations of the heart, and force of blood coursing through veins and arteries, down to the level of cellular structures that move in response to biochemical changes, all of these movements represent Air. The nervous system is greatly affected by this element because neural networks *run* throughout the body. Too much Air in the nervous system creates excitability; a deficiency leads to sluggishness. Qualities of Air are light, cold, rough, dry, dispersing, and mobile.

Air is related to the sense of touch and the skin. Through the hands we reach out, giving and receiving.

Fire

Fire evolves from Ether and Air. Ether gives Fire space in which to exist. The movement of Air gives rise to Fire, and that motion is why Fire is never still. Fire reflects the capacity for heat and light. Just as the Sun generates energy for planet Earth, Fire generates energy in our bodies through metabolism—our digestive *agni*. Fire also ignites our intellect and allows digestion of ideas.

The qualities of Fire are hot, flowing, light, dry, and soft. It is natural to think first in terms of Fire's physical nature of heat but when considering its subtler nature, we see that light is soft and revealing. To the rishis, this element also represented understanding, luster, and the power of transformation. When we shine our light on an idea or a person, they come to life and are transformed. The sense related to this element is sight. Through the eyes we receive the light of Fire in order to perceive the world around us.

Water

Through the heat of the Fire element, aspects of Ether dissolve and became liquified. Thus, Water contains Ether, Fire, and Air. Water is the protector. It represents fluidity as well as the cohesive element that contains life. Water protects against the extreme motions of Air as well as the heat of Fire. It soothes and heals inflammation and pain. Water is the great source of nourishment for the organs, tissues, and membranes. Without this element, there is no life.

Qualities of Water are cool, heavy, fluid, moist, smooth, and soft. Water is essential to stabilize the flow of neuronal impulses and protect cerebral structures through cerebrospinal fluid. It fills the bursa to help in the movement of tendons and is found in synovial fluids that maintain lubrication in joints.

The sense organ of Water is taste. We need saliva and water to keep taste buds healthy and digestive juices flowing to take in nutrients. The tongue is the sense organ of Water.

Earth

The fifth element, Earth, contains the other four, because Water materializes into Earth, and Water was precipitated by Fire, which was created by the friction of Air in Ether. Ultimately, all the elements arise from Ether and all are contained in Earth. Earth is the densest form of matter and represents the structure of the universe. All creation is born from Earth: the living bodies of plants and animals, as well as inorganic matter such as minerals.

The qualities of Earth are cool, stable, heavy, dense, dry, dull, and hard. Solid structures in the body, including bones, cartilage, muscles, nails, tendons, skin, and hair, are made of Earth. The sense related to Earth is smell and the organ is the nose.

Tridosha: The Three Humors

As noted above, everyone has a balance of the three primary energies: vata, pitta, and kapha. This balance is called tridosha, and it is the central concept of Ayurvedic medicine. These three humors, or doshas, do not exist in isolation; they are in relationship with each other and all three are necessary for all physical, spiritual, and mental processes. There are actually seven doshas, which represent the relationships of each of the doshas within an individual. In this chapter, I focus on the first three doshas. The seven doshas are vata, pitta, kapha, vata-pitta, vata-kapha, pitta-kapha, and vata-pitta-kapha. Some consider this seventh dosha, in which all three forces are in balance, as the ideal. Vata-pitta-kapha is a rare dosha.

Each of the three primary doshas is related to one of the five elements: vata to Air, pitta to Fire, and kapha to Water. However, all three doshas also relate to a second element. It is said that the second element represents the container that holds the main element. Ether holds Air for vata, Water contains the Fire for pitta, Earth gives boundaries to Water for kapha. Each dosha also has various "seats," which are the organs in which the dosha has its greatest influence. All three seats are located in the digestive tract, which indicates the absolute importance of digestion. The seat of vata is the large intestine; pitta, the small intestine; kapha, the stomach. For a summary of these three constitutions, see table 5.1 on page 116.

In the descriptions of the doshas that follow, I have included what are called the subdoshas. These are also called the five airs of vata, the five fires of pitta, and the five waters of kapha. If you are new to Ayurveda, you might want to hold off on reading about the subdoshas, and return to this part of

Table 5.1. Ayurvedic Constitutions

Aspect of constitution	Vata	Pitta	Kapha
Physiological functions governed	Breathing, muscle movement, heart pulsations	Digestion, hunger, thirst, complexion, body temperature	Form, stability, lubrication, sense of taste; provides cohesion
Mental/ emotional states governed	Adaptability, inspiration, nervousness, fear	Laughter, joy, willpower, courage, anger, judgment	Love, compassion, groundedness, attachment, greed
Qualities	Light, cold, clear, agitated	Hot, sharp, flowing, liquid, aggressive	Heavy, slow, dense, dull, cold, thick
Primary locations	Colon, hips, ears, bones, nerve tissues	Small intestine, stomach (acids), eyes, blood, sweat	Stomach, throat, chest, head, pancreas, lymph
Predominant phases	Catabolism; elder years; autumn, early winter (dry and cool)	Metabolism; adulthood; late spring and summer (hot and humid)	Anabolism; childhood; winter and early spring (damp and cold)
Frame	Tall or short but thin frame, narrow hips or shoulders, small boned	Medium, good development of muscles	Well developed, stocky, heavy bone structure, wide shoulders and hips
Weight	Tends toward leanness and weight fluctuations	Moderate	Moderate to large, gains weight easily
Hair	Scanty, dry	Moderate, soft, early to grey or bald; red hair often indicates pitta	Thick, lustrous, wavy, oily
Nails	Small, thin, dry, fissured, rough, bitten	Medium, pink	Large, firm
Teeth and gums	Thin, sometimes crooked teeth; receding gums	Medium teeth; gums bleed easily	Large teeth; pink gums

Eyes	Small, dry, light	Medium, light in color, may be tinged with red (inflame easily), radiate energy and light	Large, calm, attractive; thick eyelashes
Appetite	Erratic, small meals preferred; regular meals very important	Strong; suffers when meals are missed	Constant and steady; may eat when emotions are out of balance
Elimination/ bowels	Scanty, dry, constipation, gas	Abundant, solid but can tend toward loose, oily, yellowish	Solid, oily, sometimes mucus in stool
Menstruation	Irregular cycles with scant flow	Regular cycles, possibly longer bleeding due to heat	Regular cycles, moderate to slightly heavy bleeding
Sexual energy	Erratic, variable, good libido; fertility may be an issue	Strong drive, passionate, can be dominating	Devoted, compassionate, steady desire, slow to arouse
Physical activity	Quick, fast, nimble, erratic, low stamina	Motivated, directed, goal oriented, prone to over heating	Vigorous exercise has a positive impact and endurance is moderate
Mind	Quick, adaptable, original, erratic	Intelligent, piercing, domineering	Cautious, thoughtful, slow to express ideas
Emotional temperament	In balance: enthusiastic and visionary Out of balance: fearful, anxious	Intensity of emotions, whether joy or anger; oftentimes anger will be the first emotion when there is a challenge	Calm, dedicated, content, stubborn, complacent
Faith	Rebellious, erratic	Fanatical, passionate	Loyal, conservative
Sleep	Light, possible insomnia	Moderate, may wake up but falls easily back to sleep	Heavy, at times difficulty waking
Dreams	Moving, flying, restless	Passionate, presence of conflict	Few dreams, sentimental and water-themed

the book once you have had more experience with these concepts. I have included them because I appreciate how beautifully they express the deep understanding of this ancient system of wisdom and science. Again, these descriptions of subdoshas are intended as an aid to contemplating and comprehending how the doshas are woven throughout our entire being. For each of the doshas, I have included some limited suggestions of herbs that can be used to enhance or pacify certain conditions.

It's worth repeating that *all three* life energies need to be present in every person. Without vata (Air) our bowels would not move, without pitta (Fire) our digestion would suffer, and without kapha (Earth) we would not have a source of calm and grounding. What is determined in your dosha are the traits that are most characteristic of your prakruti. The use of a constitutional checklist to help determine your dosha can be helpful, but for me, understanding the elements is the essence of knowing who we are. There are a wide range of constitutional checklists available online, or you can ask an Ayurvedic practitioner for a recommendation of which one to work with.

Vata
ELEMENTS: AIR AND ETHER
THAT WHICH MOVES THINGS

Imagine sitting outdoors on a still, silent evening. As you allow the emptiness to settle, you begin to notice wisps of sound, or a breeze on your skin, or the sense of something moving off in the distance. The night serves as Ether in its vast emptiness, and Air is always manifest as movement, no matter how subtle. According to the Vedas, even in death there is no stillness, as our spirit rises and moves on to the next phase. From the blinking of our eyes, to the movement of our thoughts, to the nerve impulses creating our dreams, vata is responsible for all physiological functioning. Vata literally means the Air that moves things. In our bodies it is the cause of movement, sensation, and vibration and is necessary to mobilize the nervous system.

When Air is the predominant element, a person's temperament and physical form embody movement and change. The vata frame is slight with bony protuberances; there is not an abundance of flesh. Their slight build allows an agility of mind and body but often leaves them feeling vulnerable and ungrounded. There is always movement in their beings, whether foot tapping, nail biting, marathon running, thoughts racing, or imagination soaring in the composition of an orchestral suite.

Vata is aggravated in the autumn and early winter because this time of year is very similar to vata characteristics. For most locales, this is a cooler, windy, dry, erratic time. Treating vata at this time of year, no matter the dosha, prepares you for the coming winter.

The Five Airs of Vata

Prana vayu (air) is the primary air, the inspiration, including inhalation not only of oxygen, but of impressions, thoughts, and consciousness. Prana is our life force. All other airs of vata are derived from Prana. This is why the practice of pranayama, or breathing exercises, is so important, not only for vata but for all doshas. Breathing techniques provide either calming or awakening effects. All are very simple and require only five to ten minutes to perform, and they offer long-lasting results. Herbs to enhance the breath and faculties of the mind as well as meditation are gotu kola (*Centella asiatica*), ginkgo (*Ginkgo biloba*), and nervines. (See appendix 2, "Herbal Actions Glossary," page 319.) St. John's wort (*Hypericum perforatum*) is also helpful, especially as an oil applied to the back of the neck.

Udana vayu is the upward air or nervous force. It is located in the chest and centered in the throat. Udana governs exhalation, speech, and singing; when impaired it causes hiccups, belching, and emesis. Vedic scriptures write of the need to speak in gentle and loving tones because speech puts pressure on the lungs and heart due to the influence of udana. This is also why silence is sometimes encouraged during meals, so that this upward force does not prevent the downward nature of good digestion. Calming nervines such as skullcap (*Scutellaria lateriflora*) and lemon balm (*Melissa officinalis*) assist in quieting this air. Singing and chanting mantras also have a calming effect.

Samana vayu is the central air of vata; it means "equalizing air." Samana flows through the entire digestive tract as the air that fans the fire of digestion, transports enzymes, and moves wastes out of the colon. It is the movement involved in assimilation and transport of nutrients to organs and tissues. A derangement in this vayu leads to malabsorption as well as buildup of *ama* (toxins). Gently warming carminative herbs are helpful here: fennel (*Foeniculum vulgare*), cumin (*Cuminum cyminum*), and coriander (*Coriandrum sativum*), as well as the antispasmodic, wild yam root (*Dioscorea villosa*).

Vyana vayu is the distributing air; *vyana* means "diffusive." Centered in the heart, this air moves throughout the entire body. By directing the circulatory system, vyana vayu will take oxygen throughout the body, assisting in the mobilization of joints and muscles. Ginger (*Zingiber officinale*), Epsom salt bath, mimosa bark (*Albizia julibrissin*), burdock root (*Arctium lappa*), and St. John's wort are all nourishing to this air.

Apana vayu means "downward air"; it is situated in the large intestine and the organs in the pelvic cavity. This is the energy of releasing feces, urine, menstrual blood, and semen. Apana vayu supports and controls all the other vayu. Because the large intestine is the seat of vata, an imbalance of apana vayu needs to be treated before any other. In fact, no matter the dosha, treating this vayu should be a priority in any healing protocol because Air and Ether naturally tend to move up and out; effort is required to support this downward force of air that is so vital to many systems. Herbs to support downward energy are yellow dock (*Rumex crispus*), ginger, fennel, and the Ayurvedic formula of three fruits called *triphala*. A blend of three fruits, amla, haritaki, and bibhitaki, this formula is one of the greatest and most revered blends in India.

Characteristics of Vata

Qualities: light, mobile, subtle, clear, dispersing dry, hard, cold, agitated

Season: associated with autumn and early winter

Tastes: salty, sour, and sweet provide balance; bitter, astringent, and pungent aggravate imbalance

Seat of vata: large intestine, pelvic cavity, thighs, bones, skin, ears, colon, hips, nerve tissue.

Governs: nervous system, blinking, breathing, heartbeat, rhythm of bowels, movement in muscles and tissues, balance, senses, mind, consciousness

Emotions in balance: joy

Emotions out of balance: fear, anxiety, excessive worrying, panic

Physical qualities: thin frame, asymmetry in frame, prominent joints, hypermobile joints, prominent forehead, light-colored eyes, fine hair, visible veins, variable appetite

Physical qualities out of balance: emaciation, tremors, spasms, insomnia, dizziness, hyperactivity, nervous system disorders, paralysis, arthritis, cracking joints, trouble falling asleep, difficulty staying asleep, dry or chapped skin, crooked teeth, thin nails, impaired or abnormal movement, wasting away of tissues, gassiness, constipation, bloating, dry or hard stools

Mental traits: creativity, mental adaptability, comprehension of new thoughts, nervousness, spaciness, indecision, confusion

Pacifying Remedies for Vata

Pranayama. Practice Nadi Shodhana, or alternate nostril breathing, which is relaxing and calms the mind. This simple technique sharpens concentration and enhances mental clarity.

Food. Drink warm teas or fluids. Eat cooked or warm foods along with warming spices such as ginger, black pepper (*Piper nigrum*), and cinnamon (*Cinnamomum verum*). Avoid pungent, hot spices as well as raw foods. Concentrate on bringing moisture and nourishment to the diet.

Herbs. Building herbs include angelica (*Angelica archangelica*), marshmallow root (*Althaea officinalis*), ashwagandha (*Withania somnifera*), and licorice (*Glycyrrhiza glabra*). Herbs for calming vata include oatstraw (*Avena sativa*), jujube dates (*Ziziphus jujuba*), and holy basil (*Ocimum tenuiflorum*). These warmer herbs can be blended with cooler nervines such as skullcap and passionflower (*Passiflora incarnata*). Other vata-pacifying herbs are fresh ginger, hawthorn (*Crataegus* spp.), fennel, and rosehips.

Routine. Create a rhythm to the daily schedule to lessen the risk of erratic decision-making.

Warmth. Provide warmth and serenity in the environment. Dress properly to stay warm whatever the weather.

Barefoot walks. When the ground is warm, walk barefoot on the earth.

Oils and fats. Consume generous quantities of ghee (clarified butter) or a high-quality organic culinary oil.

Self-massage. Learn the Ayurvedic method called *abhyanga*, and practice it daily using warm sesame oil.

Gentle exercise. Try yin yoga or tai chi, or take walks in nature in the morning and evening.

Vata-reducing formulas. Choose warming, grounding, and nourishing herbs and use carrier oils or fats that will enhance the pacifying nature of the herbs. For example, ashwagandha can be given in ghee and honey, or add 1 tablespoon ashwagandha to warm whole milk with a pinch of cardamom and a little honey.

Pitta

ELEMENTS: FIRE AND WATER

THAT WHICH TRANSFORMS

The first light of dawn kindles a sense of hope and renewal. As the light grows stronger, the heat of the sun activates our senses and mobilizes ideas. If the sun becomes too strong, we step into a cooler space. Pitta dosha is that of light, Jyoti, or radiance. Fire is the element that digests experiences, and pitta is our digestive fire, acids, and bile, which transform food into nourishment and warmth for the body. Fire is related to vision, and this pure digestion of thoughts is what makes one's eyes shine with the truth. Located in the brain and heart, Fire marries a higher intelligence with the warmth of our compassion and shines light on our intuitive abilities, referred to as the light of awareness in Vedic texts. Fire is also the metabolic heat that transforms all that we take into our bodies.

The qualities of pitta enable someone to take charge and lead. Pitta shines light on the other senses, which gives a person the ability to perceive their environment clearly and respond appropriately to the situation. When pitta is out of balance excessive ambition can often lead to jealousy, anger, and even hatred. Fire left to rage can be very destructive. Pitta imbalance needs attention early on because of this destructive tendency. How perfect that Fire is coupled with Water in order to contain the intensity of this dosha.

Digestion and appetite are generally strong with this humor and missing a meal can easily lead to irritability. When pitta is balanced, blood will be healthy and acid secretions in the intestinal tract will be optimal for digestion. Pitta translates as "bile." This refers to the enzymatic juices needed for the digestion of food. The small intestine is the seat of pitta, the organ in which enzymes and hormones sent from the liver and pancreas transform fats, starches, and other nutrients into usable fuel for the body. It is here where agni plays one of its most vital roles. Agni is named for the Vedic god of fire. He is regarded as the protector of humankind, a great ally, and the one who safeguards the home. This protection is seen in that agni not only breaks down food so we may be nourished but also destroys harmful microbes in food we eat. Hydrochloric acid (a biochemical form of fire) is an essential acid to protect our intestines from infection and help maintain good flora.

While pitta and agni seem inseparable, pitta is the container and agni the Fire. Agni is at the heart of good health. It is the biological fire that governs metabolism. In Ayurvedic medicine, the liver is said to be the "hottest" organ in that it releases bile as well as performing many other metabolic functions.

When the agni is not metabolizing as it should, a material called ama is formed. *Ama* is a Sanskrit word that means "unripe" or "uncooked". This material is a viscous, sticky, phlegm-like substance that clogs arteries as well as the lymphatic vessels and mental clarity. This creates what traditional herbalists call "bad blood." According to many Ayurvedic physicians, ama is the root of all illness. This substance further dampens agni's transformative ability, causing a domino effect because every cell throughout the body requires agni to accomplish its tasks. As noted in the discussion of Five Phase Theory, it is recommended to fast and undertake cleanses in the spring (Liver/Gallbladder) and fall (Lungs/Large Intestine) to help clear toxins from the body and keep digestive fires burning bright.

Agni is also foundational for our immune system. While in the digestive tract, ama is relatively easy to clear, but once it reaches deeper into the tissues, it deprives cells of oxygen needed to ignite the cellular fire that transforms nutrients needed to keep immunity intact.

Late spring and summer are the seasons related to pitta. Depending on the climate, most summers arrive with some form of humidity as well. This is the time to focus on good hydration as well as cooling remedies.

Five Fires of Pitta

Pachaka pitta is the main digestive agni that resides in the stomach and small intestine. It is the first fire that needs to be tended when pitta is out of balance because it is the support of all the other fires. From this pitta comes the power of digestion in the form of bile salts, pancreatic juices, and acids that metabolize food. When this fire burns too low there is malabsorption, creation of ama, and stagnation. This is the pitta (HCl, or hydrochloric acid) responsible for destroying pathogens that afflict us via our food. When there is too much fire in the stomach, ulcers and other signs of hyperacidity can develop. In this situation, demulcents such as marshmallow, licorice, and kudzu (*Pueraria montana*) are cooling. Herbs to support this fire are the bitters such as artichoke (*Cynara scolymus*) and blue vervain (*Verbena hastata*).

Sadhaka pitta is the most subtle of fires. This is the energy of the mind, where we digest experiences and the realizations contained in those experiences. Located in the brain and the heart, sadhaka is the insight that inner and outer realities are truly connected. This fire operates through the nervous system and the senses and is the seat of discernment and discrimination. Herbs that support this fire are gotu kola and ginkgo. Fasting from media and electronics also supports sadhaka.

Alochaka pitta is located in the pupil of the eyes and governs visual perception. There is an upward motion to this energy, and this enhances our perception of light, clarity, and understanding.

Bhrajaka pitta is located in the skin and governs the luster of our complexion. Bhrajaka pitta assimilates the warmth and sunlight we absorb through the skin and disperses it throughout our body, enhancing peripheral circulation. This pitta has an outward movement, and when it is in excess, skin rashes, boils, and hot infections erupt or move outward. Cooling poultices and compresses of drawing plants such as plantain (*Plantago* spp.), chickweed, and marshmallow leaves offer relief. Other practices to support this pitta are dry brushing the skin, applying sesame oil or sunflower oil to the skin daily, and drinking alterative herb teas such as those made from burdock seed and dandelion root (*Taraxacum officinale*).

Ranjaka pitta is the fire that colors our blood, bile, and waste materials. This is the fire that is involved in many liver disorders, which is why the observation of feces and urine is helpful to discern progression or resolution of hepatic disease. Dark yellow urine can be a sign of dehydration when there is too much heat in a person's body. Cooling bitters assist this fire, as well as milk thistle (*Silybum marianum*), ghee, and taking care to stay hydrated.

Characteristics of Pitta

Qualities: oily, liquid, hot, sharp, light, mobile, penetrating

Season: associated with late spring and summer

Tastes: sweet, bitter, and astringent provide balance; sour, pungent, and salty aggravate

Seat of pitta: small intestine, stomach (as digestive acids), sweat glands, blood, lymph, eyes

Governs: digestion, heat, visual perception, hunger, thirst, luster and complexion, understanding, intelligence, courage

Emotions in balance: joy, compassion, peace, forgiveness, discernment

Emotions out of balance: excess anger, hatred, jealousy, suspicion, pride

Physical qualities: medium build; muscular; reddish complexion; soft, warm skin; freckles; little body hair; early graying; male pattern baldness; almond-shaped, hazel-green eyes; strong metabolism; good digestion; moderate sleep; excessive perspiration; low tolerance for heat and sun

Physical qualities out of balance: yellow color of stool and urine; thirst; difficulty sleeping; inflammation and infections; bloodshot eyes; skin irritations; excess hunger; burnout; tendency to sunburn; heartburn; diarrhea; bleeding gums; acne; nosebleeds; malodorous sweat, feet and armpits

Mental traits: strong powers of comprehension

Pitta-Balancing Remedies

Relaxation. Practice staying cool, calm, and collected, and make time for play.

Daily *shavasana* practice. Shavasana is a yoga pose, also called the *corpse pose*, where you lie on your back for fifteen minutes. Starting at the feet, you tense each body part, hold the tension for about ten seconds, release, and then relax until you are relaxed throughout the whole body. Daily practice allows you to drop into a relaxed state more easily any time when you feel agitated.

Emotional release. Working with a professional therapist or bodyworker or engaging in regular physical exercise to release negative emotions such as anger and jealousy is especially helpful.

Consistent moderate exercise. This dosha appreciates a challenge, but avoid exercise that aggravates heat, such as hot yoga or jogging in hot weather. Swimming, cycling, tai chi, and yoga are good choices. Most important is to spend time connecting with nature.

Bitters. Cooling bitters help pitta stay in balance while promoting digestive agni: yellow dock, dandelion root, fennel, chamomile (*Matricaria chamomilla*), and skullcap.

Cooling, building herbs. Use demulcent herbs such as astragalus (*Astragalus membranaceus*), marshmallow leaf and root, and licorice, and also astringing herbs such as plantain, red raspberry (*Rubus idaeus*), agrimony (*Agrimonia eupatoria*), and meadowsweet (*Filipendula ulmaria*).

Kapha
ELEMENTS: WATER AND EARTH

THAT WHICH HOLDS THINGS TOGETHER

When we first saw the photos of Planet Earth from space, we marveled at the blue oceans and dense landmasses. The energy of kapha is Water and Earth. Earth is home and when kapha is in right balance, we have an inner sense of security. The universal characteristic of Water is that it throbs and pulses and represents all life's movements like the ebb and flow of tides. Kapha dosha brings together all the elements and holds them with stability, structure, and love. *Cohesion* and *contentment* are the words that typify kapha.

Those with kapha constitution are solid in structure and have well-developed muscles. Often Westerners think of kapha energy as large or overweight, but this is a simplistic notion. While those who have this constitution are prone to excess weight and fluids, kapha is the quality most needed in our vata-pitta, fast-paced life. Kapha conserves, constrains, and supports the other two doshas. Without this solidity in nature, Air would dissipate and Fire would destroy. Since Water is dominant, this dosha is generally well lubricated, and so dryness in joints and digestion is not a challenge. *Kapha* also means mucus or phlegm, and this is the energy that protects all mucous membranes and is excessive when kapha is out of balance.

This dosha needs activity and Fire to keep the Water in balance. The translation of this dosha is "mucus" and although mucus is a protective and nourishing fluid, too much creates buildup or ama. This substance is sticky and tends to accumulate in places where there may have been pre-existing conditions. This accumulation leads to chronic conditions that are challenging to resolve, such as chronic fatigue, diabetes, depression, and allergies. Good digestion and elimination are key to maintaining the health of this dosha.

Just as the biological force of vata brings forward the cosmic energy of Prana and pitta gives us Jyoti, the spiritual light, kapha brings us Prema. Prema, or love, is the cosmic force that holds all of life together. Those who are predominantly kapha are blessed with qualities of kindness and loyalty. The Buddha is one of the most famous kaphas, who is blissfully available to all. What a magnificent lens that allows us to see that love is inherent in all matter and is the unifying force in our bodies and all of Nature.

Kapha is associated with winter and early spring months. Again, depending on the bioregion this is the time when there is a tendency for cold and mucus to accumulate, so treating kapha conditions promptly when they arise prevents further imbalance in this dosha during these times of the year.

The Five Kaphas

Tarpaka kapha is Sanskrit for "one that satiates and nourishes." This form of kapha influences the brain and the heart via the cerebrospinal fluid and assures emotional calm, a loving perception, and enhances memory. This is the aspect that creates contentment. Yoga has many goals but one of the primary objectives is to heighten this form of kapha. This kapha governs the nose and the sense of smell. This is why incense and perfumed oils have been utilized for thousands of years in Vedic religious practices. Gotu kola, hawthorn leaf and flower, linden (*Tilia cordata*), mimosa flower, and chamomile as well as certain essential oils are all enhancing to this kapha. Placing a drop of sandalwood oil (*Santalum album*) on your brow chakra, or between your eyebrows, is a beautiful way to support this kapha.

Bodhaka kapha relates to knowledge, in particular the subtle intelligence needed to identify tastes (see table 5.2 for more information on the tastes). This subdosha is related to the parietal lobe of the brain, which processes taste. Tongue health is necessary for proper functioning of the taste buds. Saliva also protects our mouth, gums, and teeth from infection, moistens food as it is chewed and swallowed, and begins the digestive process. Chewing on licorice root or taking prickly ash (*Zanthoxylum* spp.) tincture can increase the amount of saliva produced.

Table 5.2. The Six Tastes

Taste	Sources	Energy	Elements	Doshas*
Astringent	Herbs rich in tannins such as blackberry root	Cool	Air and Earth	P↓ K↓ V↑
Bitter	Bitter herbs such as blue vervain, goldenseal	Cool	Air and Ether	P↓ K↓ V↑
Pungent	Hot spices such as ginger or cayenne	Hot	Fire and Air	P↑ K↓ V↑
Salty	Sea salt, nettles, seaweed	Warm	Water and Fire	P↑ K↑ V↓
Sour	Fermented foods such as miso, yogurt; sour and acidic fruits	Warm	Earth and Fire	P↑ K↑ V↓
Sweet	Grains, sweet vegetables, sugars and starches	Cool/ Neutral	Earth and Water	P↓ K↑ V↓

*P = pitta, K = kapha, V = vata. ↑ indicates that the dosha is aggravated by that flavor; ↓ indicates that the dosha is balanced by that flavor

Avalambaka kapha is Sanskrit for "to hold." This is the primary center of kapha, which corresponds to the fluids distributed by the lungs and the heart. Avalambaka kapha is responsible for the support of all the other kaphas. It also supports the lubrication afforded by the pleural lining of the lungs that allows deep inhalations and exhalations to take place. The heart also has a protective covering, the pericardium, which needs fluids to nourish its tissues. To balance these fluids, warming, pungent remedies help maintain clarity. Expectorants such as elecampane (*Inula helenium*), hyssop (*Hyssopus officinalis*), and thyme (*Thymus vulgaris*) are very useful. Deep-breathing techniques such as alternate nostril breathing help move energy that can get stuck in the lungs and pericardium.

Kledaka kapha translates as "wetting" kapha. It rests in the upper part of the stomach and provides the secretions that moisten food as it enters the stomach. Kledaka kapha also protects the stomach lining from digestive acids that break down protein as well as kill harmful bacteria in the stomach. Alkaline in nature, this lining extends throughout the digestive tract. Balanced kapha here allows us to stomach issues that arise and helps to lend that overall sense of peace. When kledaka kapha is in excess, stools are loose with mucus, bloating occurs, and food is left undigested. Herbs to light digestive fire are needed to metabolize and transform the phlegm. These are pungent, warming herbs, including ginger, black pepper, coriander, and fennel.

Sleshaka kapha is the "binding or hugging" kapha that lubricates and protects the joints from wear and tear while providing stability to movement. There are over two hundred bones in the adult body, and over three hundred joints. The tendons and ligaments that hold joints in place are also fundamental to the maintenance of stability. Kapha in the form of synovial fluid not only holds joints together but offers cushioning from hard blows or excess weight. When there is not enough moisture, as occurs with excess vata, joints will pop and crack and arthritis may develop. Applying topical oils such as goldenrod (*Solidago* spp.) or St. John's wort oil nourishes the tendons and ligaments.

Characteristics of Kapha

Qualities: wet, cold, heavy, dull, soft, liquid, slow, stuck

Season: winter and early spring

Tastes: pungent, bitter, and astringent provide balance; sweet, salty, and sour aggravate

Seat of kapha: stomach, chest, throat, head, sinuses, nose, mouth, stomach, pancreas, lymph, tongue, joints, cytoplasm, liquid secretions such as mucus and cerebrospinal fluid

Governs: storage of energy, stability, lubrication, anabolism, nourishment, repair and regeneration, quality of saliva, sense of smell

Emotions in balance: love, compassion, devotion, contentment, modesty, courage

Emotions out of balance: greed, excessive attachment to outcomes, lust, possessiveness, sentimentality, dullness

Physical qualities: solid, well-built frame, pale tongue, well-formed teeth, broad chest, fair complexion, soft skin, thick hair, large eyes, heavy sleeper

Physical qualities out of balance: slow digestion, mucus in stools, stagnation, inertia, constipation, excess saliva, wet/clammy skin, wet cough, tendency to overweight

Mental traits: tolerant, peaceful, gives stability over emotional nature, and supports other two doshas

Lifestyle for Kapha

Eat warm, cooked foods. Give preference to pungent, bitter, astringent tastes. Avoid foods that are heavy, oily, or cold and those that are sweet, sour, and salty.

Brisk walks. Since kapha dosha can put on weight easily, it is important to be consistent with an exercise regimen.

Be flexible. Change up your routine either daily or weekly. Seek out the company of a person gifted with vata or pitta energy to find motivation for new and challenging activities.

Timing of meals. Lunch should be the largest meal of the day, and then enjoy a light supper.

Seek stimulation. Playing music and dancing are helpful to arouse the senses and the body.

Drink hot/warm beverages. Staying warm in cold weather helps balance the coldness of this dosha and prevents excess mucus from forming.

Craniosacral therapy. I have come to appreciate craniosacral bodywork almost as much as medicinal herbs to balance tarpaka kapha, especially when there has been significant trauma. This technique relieves compression in the bones of the head (cranium) and tailbone (sacrum). This opens up the flow of the craniosacral fluid and has profound influences on all systems, but I see it as a way to balance kapha, especially this subdosha. Trauma often creates an out-of-body experience, and craniosacral bodywork reinstates a sense of safety in the body.

Treating Constitution versus Symptoms

To illustrate how working from an Ayurvedic perspective can greatly serve us, we can look at the all-too-common case of high blood pressure. Three patients could present with elevated blood pressure: one large (kapha), one medium build (pitta), and one thin and wiry (vata). All three have different metabolisms and, more than likely, the causes for their elevated blood pressure are distinct for each person. Yet, a conventional medical approach would offer all three a diuretic medication as a first-line course of action. Lowering water volume in the body would indeed bring down blood pressure readings, but only for a limited duration because the medication does not address the root cause. When these patients return to their doctor in six months or a year with their blood pressure creeping back up, the doctor might prescribe a beta-blocker drug that slows heart rate. This would work for a while, but now they would be taking two meds and still the cause is left untreated. Next the practitioner might recommend a calcium channel blocker, and the cycle would spiral on. As the names of the drugs indicate, the treatment is defensive, intended to block effects of stress or suppress symptoms.

Conversely, energetic medicine treats the person rather than the symptoms. The mantra is "treat what you see." Diagnosis is not only by the numbers, but also determined through the patient's story, the quality of their pulse, the appearance of their tongue, the odor of their body, as well as other physical readings. We look to the individual to "tell" us how to proceed. Another factor to consider is the person's phase of life, because different doshas are dominant from childhood to adulthood to old age. This is summarized in table 5.3.

The blood pressure example I describe above is simplistic, but it does serve to illustrate the beauty of this system. Most hypertension is caused by tension, and that could be the vikruti—the current condition—underlying this example. There are different ways to treat tension in the different doshas.

A larger, more corpulent, kapha body would present with a denser, slower metabolism, and their blood pressure may be up due to vital energy being blocked or stagnant. The energetic practitioner might use stimulating

Table 5.3. Phases of Life

Dosha	Kapha	Pitta	Vata
Age range	Childhood (0 – puberty)	Adulthood (puberty – 50)	Elders (50 and beyond)
Prevalent aspect of metabolism	Anabolism	Metabolism	Catabolism
Prevalent activities	Development and building tissue	Transformation and creation	Detachment, reserves are decreasing but spiritual and creative forces are often at their peak
Prevalent conditions	Mucous conditions	Heat conditions	Bone and nervous conditions
How to support	Because children crave sweet, there is a natural tendency to build structure. Provide healthy foods and proteins.	Support digestion of food as well as experiences. Identity is forming. Care must be taken to support metabolic functions not running too hot.	Provide more oils; sweet, building foods; nourishing soups and stews made with gently warming digestive spices. Encourage enjoyment of a slower pace.

Adapted from Candis Cantin Packard, *Pocket Guide to Ayurvedic Healing* (Berkeley, CA: Crossing Press, 1996).

remedies such as prickly ash, ginger, or rosemary (*Salvia rosmarinus*) and slowly begin opening the flow and allow for a more robust circulation. These warming, moving remedies might also address depression or stagnation that prevents a person from making healthy choices. Calling in the forces of Fire and Air (pungent remedies) breathes more life and activity into the denser elements such as Earth and Water.

For the fiery pitta person with medium build, activity level is an important consideration and whether they might be too active in their lifestyle and taking on stressful activities. Adrenaline heats up the system and also constricts blood vessels, thus possibly contributing to higher blood pressure. Relaxing, cooling herbs such as motherwort (*Leonurus cardiaca*) or blue vervain would help. Acrid, antispasmodic herbs such as cramp bark (*Viburnum opulus*) or low-dose lobelia (*Lobelia inflata*) might be all that is needed to relax tension.

A case of mine is a perfect description for treating vata dosha for high blood pressure—an eighty-eight-year-old gentleman presented with high blood pressure. My client was a well-known author who traveled extensively and had a stressful teaching schedule. His physician prescribed medications for his blood pressure, which in turn caused erectile dysfunction and serious fatigue: two symptoms he found unacceptable. After listening to his story and observing his skin and tongue, I realized he was seriously dehydrated, anxious from travel, and all of that moving around was aggravating his vata constitution. This is not surprising, in that elderhood is the vata phase of life. Because his fluids were low, his blood volume was down, making the heart work harder and causing more heat. I advised him to increase fluids and suggested healthy oils and herbs to help moisten his terrain. We also looked to pacifying herbs and used a simple tea of skullcap, milky oats, and damiana (*Turnera diffusa*). Within two weeks, his blood pressure was back to normal.

When you work with a family member, friend, or client, remember that the balancing of the doshas is not simply an aid to digestion or a way to improve sleep or achieve more lustrous hair. Working with these elements is a divine act of manifesting our evolutionary nature. We understand that "faults," or doshas, are the gifts and challenges all are born with. I love how Ayurveda teaches that we are not perfect and that through our doshas we can better understand Prema, Jyoti, and Prana, or love, light, and life. This is the study of prakruti, the constitution we were born with. Working with vikruti, our day-to-day challenges, is also an important aspect of energetic herbalism, and in the next chapter we will explore that challenge using the vocabulary and concepts of Western energetics—vitalism and the tissue states.

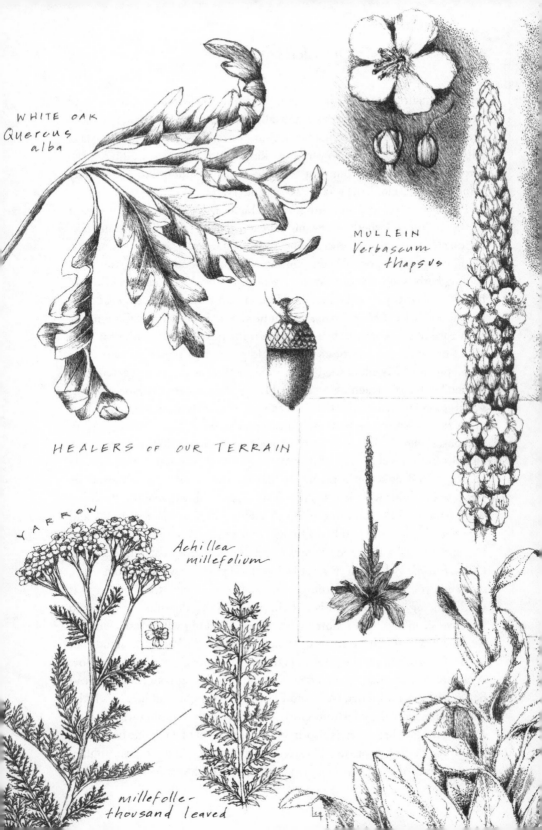

WHITE OAK
Quercus
alba

MULLEIN
Verbascum
thapsus

HEALERS OF OUR TERRAIN

YARROW

Achillea
millefolium

millefolle-
thousand leaved

CHAPTER 6

Our Inner Terrain

Western or classical vitalism has its roots in Greek and Arabic medicine, known as Unani Tibb. In some parts of the world, Arabic medicine is simply called *Tibb*, which means "medicine and healing of the physical, mental and spiritual realms."[1] *Unan* means "of the Greeks," as this form of medicine originated with the works of Hippocrates. These philosophies were based on the same energetics as Chinese and Ayurvedic theory. The four energetic qualities of hot, cold, damp, and dry correspond to the four elements in Greek philosophy of fire, air, water, and earth. These give rise to four temperaments or constitutions.

Greek humoral medicine is based on the concept of constitutional expression, as are the doshas. The four Greek humors, or vital fluids, represent the four elements of fire, water, earth, and air, and these fluids are thought to be present in the bloodstream at all times. The four temperaments—melancholic, sanguine, phlegmatic, and choleric—which rise from the elements, represent the constitutional frameworks of Greek medicine and inform diagnosis and therapy for many Western herbalists today.

Regarding the development of vitalism in North America, many histories of Western Energetic Herbalism focus narrowly on the contributions of European colonists, but theirs is only one part of the story. The diverse Indigenous peoples of North America had developed sophisticated healing traditions and knowledge for thousands of years before the arrival of European colonists. Native healers as well as enslaved African healers taught physicians and European botanists about native medicinal plants. The flora of the Southeastern states is very similar to that of West Africa and many of the enslaved were chosen specifically because of their skills in agriculture and medicine. In fact, so successful were the treatments by enslaved healers, that they became a threat to the regular physicians. Laws were enacted to suppress enslaved practitioners from providing services because white physicians felt they needed to protect their own livelihoods, but even these laws did not discourage whites from seeking the gentler medicines of African healers.

Samuel Thomson (1769–1843), a beneficiary of these teachings, was seen as the founder of the emerging American botanical system. In some ways, Thomson was the archetypal wounded healer who came to his trade and success through his own disabilities. When physicians failed to ease the severe foot and leg pain that Thomson suffered as a young boy, his father called in a local "root" doctor, the wise woman, Mrs. Benton. (Significantly, in all my research I was unable to find this woman's first name). After Mrs. Benton was able to offer Thomson relief, he became her apprentice. He already had acquired a deep interest in local flora, but when her cures were so successful, Thomson began to devote every spare moment to studying herbal medicine and the practices of the trade.

The heart of Thomson's theory was that disease arises when the internal heat of the stomach is obstructed. This would prevent the circulation of warmth and hence vitality. To Thomson, heat was life. He claimed, "after restoring the natural heat of the body by clearing the system of all obstructions, and causing a natural perspiration, the stomach would digest the food taken, by which means the whole body is nourished and invigorated and the heat of the body . . . is able to hold its supremacy."[2] Thomson's methods of cleansing, purging, and sweating all correspond to practices of traditional cultures from other parts of the world. His teachings most definitely came from local First Nations practices.

Thomson's writings are replete with his references to "canker" as an archetypal form in which disease can manifest. This comes about through cold and the body's inability to generate heat, and it manifests as stagnant blood, white discharges, or excessive mucus. This correlates to ama (Ayurveda), phlegm (TCM), and "bad blood" in the terminology of the Eclectic physicians as well as traditional healers. Today, we call it toxicity, and it is the archetype at the root of chronic metabolic diseases.

Like many folk healers of his time, Thomson was appalled that orthodox, university-trained physicians (the Regular physicians) were killing their patients with the use of toxic minerals. In 1806, Thomson made presentations in Boston and New York City demonstrating the success of his remedies with yellow fever. It was during this period that people began referring to his remedies as "Thomsonian" medicine. He traveled extensively, and it is estimated that by the 1840s, he had between four and six million followers.[3] He created the first herbal correspondence course, and the success of his business was also due to the fact that so many settlers lived far from skilled healers and the local flora was unfamiliar to them.

Despite his significant contributions to early American herbalism, Thomson's life was a series of struggles. His theories were paramount in establishing the foundation of the next wave of Western natural medicine in North America—Eclecticism and Physiomedicalism—but his obstinate and cantankerous nature led to his growing paranoia that these new practices would usurp his popularity.

The two schools of medical practice that were born from Thomsonianism, comprised physicians who wanted to create alternative treatments to the horrific practices of the day. These new physicians used "eclectic" medicines ranging from homeopathy and steam bathing to botanical formulas to serve their community. The writings of these physicians are the only written texts that capture over a hundred years of herbal medicine practice in the United States. Fortunately, many of their texts are still accessible.

With the influence of Wooster Beach (1794–1868), and his school of Reformed Medicine, Eclecticism began to be formalized through new centers of learning. There was also a new interest in pharmacy, the techniques of creating tinctures and extracts, while maintaining whole plant medicine. The Lloyd brothers of the famous Lloyd Library in Cincinnati were chemists devoted to the craft of medicine making and exploring new realms. As with all new movements, there were heated disagreements among Eclectic physicians about what their model of practice should be and how much of the older system they would retain. By the end of the Civil War, the Eclectic schools were in disarray due to such in-house quarreling, as well as the economics of the time.

Known for his compassionate ways and absolute devotion to his craft, physician John Scudder (1829–1894) revived Eclectic schools financially and provided a solid foundation for a system of treatment. Scudder introduced a new development that matured this profession and brought clarity to its tenets. This was referred to as *specific medicine*, which is similar to homeopathy in that low doses of herbal medicine would be applied and be the "specific" for a particular pattern, such as yellow dock root (*Rumex crispus*) in the treatment of skin eruptions related to bad blood. No longer were physicians treating individual symptoms, they were treating a person's overall presentation of health.

Physiomedicalism was not as heavily influenced by scientific discoveries of the day as Eclecticism was. The originator of this neo-Thomsonian movement, Alva Curtis, wanted to base his school on Thomsonian principles but with greater freedom to explore other theories. There are many other important practitioners of this movement, but a full accounting of them is beyond the scope of this book. Most notable were the contributions of Physiomedicalist physician J.M. Thurston. As stated in chapter 1, J.M. Thurston published *The Philosophy of Physiomedicalism* in which he articulated the six tissue states, but the terms he used to describe the states of imbalance were a bit archaic and derived from the theories of the time. These terms reflect the original Greek qualities of hot, cold, damp, and dry with two essential states added—*tension* and *relaxation*—to reflect the tone of the tissue.

Herbalists today share much in common with the early botanical practitioners. We, too, have been outliers and considered "quacks" judged for following Nature and trusting invisible forces called vitality. For serious students of herbalism, the history of this period of botanic medicine is not only a fascinating read but a valuable framework and appreciation of the skill many of these practitioners devoted to our craft. Equally vital to understanding where we are today and, more importantly, how we move forward as herbalists is the study of First Nations healing traditions and those of enslaved Africans.

Tissue states are a way of reading patterns of imbalance and reflect the current conditions of one's health. There are parallels between the Ayurvedic constitutional framework of prakruti (original constitution) and vikruti (the current condition or acquired constitution) and the tissue states. Vikruti guides treatment protocol because it reflects the current state of a tissue, organ, or body system. In this chapter, I present my experience with the tissue states as I have witnessed them through my practice as a community herbalist. Throughout my career, I have drawn wisdom from the work of herbalist Matthew Wood, who has made the vocabulary of the tissue states more relevant for contemporary herbalists. His excellent text *The Practice of Traditional Western Herbalism* is one of the books I return to most often as the tissue states continue to reveal themselves.

Understanding Tissue States

The six tissue states are: heat/excitation, cold/depression, damp/stagnation, dry/atrophy, tension/constriction, and relaxation (lax)/atony. These are based on the three primary energetic qualities of temperature, moisture, and tone, and they apply not only in tissues but in organs and body systems as well (see figure 6.1). Tissue states can also be thought of as patterns that describe our inner terrain when it is *out of balance*, and as explained in chapter 1, these patterns mimic the patterns of Nature. For example, constant exposure to wind (air/vata) dries out a landscape, sometimes to the point that the soil surface cracks open. In these conditions, the soil cannot retain moisture. Our bodies react similarly when there is too much movement, thought, or activity that creates "internal wind." We may experience symptoms of external dryness such as cracking skin, an inner agitation, or an inability to hold onto nutrients and present with the tissue state of dry/atrophy. Conversely, when water in a pond does not move, the pond becomes prone to overgrowth of algae. This is analogous to long-term diabetes, when boggy, swollen tissue does not receive warmth from good circulation. Infection can take hold in the tissue, leading to complications such as diabetic ulcers. This is damp/stagnation, and when understood from an energetic vantage, there are many options available for treatment.

I appreciate how Southwest herbalist and author Kiva Rose describes the tissue states as a color wheel with degrees of variation. The art of energetic

Temperature

COLD ⟷ COOL ⟷ NEUTRAL ⟷ WARM ⟷ HOT

Moisture

VERY DRY ⟷ DRY ⟷ NEUTRAL ⟷ DAMP ⟷ VERY DAMP

Tone

LAX ⟶ NEUTRAL ⟶ TENSE

Figure 6.1. The three qualities and the six tissue states.

Table 6.1. Comparison of Three Energetic Models

Qualities	Tissue States	Ayurveda	Chinese Medicine
Temperature	Heat/excitation ↕ Cold/depression	Excess pitta ↕ Excess kapha or vata	Yang excess ↕ Yang deficiency
Moisture	Damp/stagnation ↕ Dry/atrophy	Excess kapha ↕ Excess vata	Yin excess ↕ Yin deficiency
Tone	Tension/constriction ↕ Relaxation/atony	Excess vata ↕ Excess kapha	Excess ↕ Deficiency

healing is in appreciating the subtle, nuanced shifts. These are not polar opposite states but a continuum along the spectrum. Just as the yin/yang symbol at first appears to be a representation of duality, on closer study we discern that the yin and the yang, the light and dark, are actually moving, dancing, and adapting to each other's nature. So, too, with tissue states: These qualities are constantly adjusting with the intention of self-correction. When vitality has been compromised to the point where the body cannot take care of itself, we work with healing plants to remind the body of the healthful pattern or direction in which it needs to go.

Certain constitutions have a proclivity for certain tissue states, and I find it helps my students to make comparisons here between Ayurvedic constitutions and tissue states. For example, vata dosha tends toward dry, cold, and tension. Pitta constitution is prone to heat, and kapha might present with damp or cold states, as shown in table 6.1. When a person presents with a tissue state that is not typical for their dosha, deciding how long to maintain corrective measures needs to be considered. For example, if a person who is predominantly pitta has a damp, cold sinus infection, treatment would call for warming aromatics and drying remedies. However, if the illness persists for a long time, you would need to reassess and do a deeper investigation with yourself or the client. It is not advisable to treat fire types (pitta) with warming remedies for the long term. There may be a deeper deficiency that is not supporting the direction of healing you are striving to achieve.

Treating What You See

Practitioners of energetic medicine pride themselves on working to address the cause of a problem and not simply treating the surface symptoms. The tissue states represent the current state of imbalance, but a tissue state is not the same thing as a symptom. For example, a patient may be experiencing pain—that's a symptom. To treat the symptom would be to simply make the pain go away by offering painkillers or anti-inflammatory drugs. Through the lens of tissue states, the differential for pain can be a multitude of possibilities. Is it pain due to tension or due to stagnation? Is it the result of an imbalance of heat (sharp pain) or cold (dull pain)? The beauty of this approach is that oftentimes when we offer a remedy to correct an imbalance through the quality of the tissue, there are broader positive side effects. For example, if someone who presents with dry skin and eyes is offered a demulcent or oily remedy, it may also relieve constipation, a condition that at a superficial level seems entirely unrelated to dry skin.

The Whole Picture

The tissue states are intuitive—they just make sense. For example, when we see hot, inflamed tissues, we offer cooling, soothing remedies. When tissues and organs are dry, we gather moistening demulcents and make a nourishing tea. However, life is rarely straightforward, and contradictions will appear. Here's a case in point. Heat/excitation causes dryness, yet heat is caused by the tissue state of dry/atrophy. Heat can also be caused by cold and stagnant states, such as a deep-seated sinus infection. You may find a friend or client who appears to be experiencing all six states at once and have no idea where to begin to help them. I love the way Michigan herbalist jim mcdonald has described this kind of situation: "I still often see clients whose energetics perplex me: hot there, cold there, damp and dry in splotches and tense everyway 'round. It can be hard to know where to start. . . . When it comes down to it, there are lots of exceptions, just like in any system one creates to categorize nature. But exceptions and limitations don't devalue the systems they defy, they just come along for the ride."[4]

In this chapter, I describe each tissue state in detail, and I enliven the descriptions with insights gained from my own practical experiences as well as biomedical considerations. For example, I present cholesterol as a heat condition, because high cholesterol is an indicator of oxidation (heat) in the blood vessels. At the same time, elevated cholesterol can be seen as a state of ama, plaque, or a buildup of toxins—in other words, as a damp/stagnant state. Healing and Nature are not black and white, and we cannot keep these dynamic states in tidy categories.

As you read through this chapter, keep in mind that occasionally glazing over is a normal response to new concepts, especially ones that are unfamiliar, as these may be. These states and their relationships to each other take a while to contemplate. So read a bit, and then walk away and ponder. When you're ready, return to read and ponder more. When you least expect it, perhaps while walking through the woods or listening to a friend's story about a health problem, a light will come on in your mind and heart. You may even experience that feeling of aisthesis—the gasp of recognition of something inspiring, which will delight your senses as you step closer to a deep understanding of the universal patterns reflected in human nature.

For those unfamiliar with the herbal actions listed here, such as demulcents, bitters, and aromatics, you can look up their meanings in appendix 2, "Herbal Actions Glossary," on page 319. This is a wonderful way to become more familiar with the energetics of plants. Once I learned energetics, I returned to the work of David Hoffman, who is one of the best herbal authors (in my humble opinion), and looked at his formulas through new eyes, especially the formulas in his classic text *Medical Herbalism*. I was fascinated to discover that his formulas for a variety of conditions were aligned with the principles of energetic herbalism. The original, traditional definitions of herbal actions often define the energetics: astringents affect moisture, aromatics affect temperature, and demulcents affect moisture. Also, the formulas were crafted by a very skilled herbalist.

The Quality of Temperature

Temperature is a quality that relates to the level of metabolic activity. It is not the same thing as body temperature that we measure using a thermometer. Kiva Rose calls this quality *thermal dynamics*.

Heat/Excitation

This state is characterized by overactivity of the tissues, hence the term *excitation*. Excessive heat increases metabolism and can lead to oxidation, tissue breakdown, inflammation, and fever. This state is commonly seen in those who are easily reactive or irritated, such as with autoimmune disorders. These imbalances often present with redness, heat in the joints, irritation, hypermotility in digestive functions, or hyperthyroidism. Allergies are a classic example of excitation when there is oversensitivity to pollen or antigens.

While this state often presents as inflammation, heat is not the only condition to cause inflammation. Colds and chronic sinus infections will also bring on inflammation. That being said, inflamed tissues are often part of the heat/excitation tissue presentation.

Characteristics of Heat/Excitation

- Swelling, inflammation
- Associated with excess—hyperthyroidism, high blood pressure
- Hypersensitivity of immune function—allergies, autoimmunity, or systemic inflammation
- Acute conditions
- Redness of face, lips, tongue, eyes/sclera; rashes
- Irritability, agitation, anxiety, insomnia, hyperalertness, racing thoughts
- Pain: sharp and hot
- Mucus: yellow or green
- Dryness: thirst; constipation; dark, scanty urine; dry skin, hair, and eyes
- Tongue: thin, red, yellow coating, flame tipped

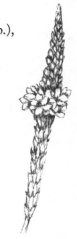

Herbal Actions for Treating Heat/Excitation

Demulcents: marshmallow (*Althaea officinalis*), chickweed (*Stellaria media*), plantain (*Plantago* spp.), self-heal (*Prunella vulgaris*)

Bitters: motherwort (*Leonurus cardiaca*), blue vervain (*Verbena hastata*), Oregon grape root (*Berberis aquifolium*)

Sour: sumac (*Rhus glabra, R. typhina*); schisandra (*Schisandra chinensis*); hawthorn leaf, flower, and berry (*Crataegus* spp.); elder (*Sambucus canadensis, S. nigra*)

Sweet tonics: nettle (*Urtica dioica*), American ginseng (*Panax quinquefolius*), borage (*Borago officinalis*)

- Pulse: rapid, bounding, or wiry
- Symptoms: worse with heat; aversion to heat
- Symptoms: improved with cool/cold

Presentations of Heat/Excitation

Oxidation. Heat is part of the oxidative process of aging or inflammation. Stress, toxins, alcohol, and many other substances create free radicals in the body by catabolizing (breaking down) oxygen molecules into reactive oxygen species, which are single atoms of oxygen that have extra "unpaired" electrons.[5] This "hungry" or excited oxygen then cleaves onto other electrons in body tissues as well as the walls of arteries, creating a micro-wound. This is the same process that causes metal to rust—aka oxidation. In order to repair damaged tissue, hormones signal the liver to release cholesterol, which is a life-saving *endogenous antioxidant*. Cholesterol repairs the wound, fulfilling one of its many vital functions. But when this type of oxidation happens day in and day out, the excessive wounding (heat/excitation) creates an immune response, which generates more tissue irritability. It also creates more cholesterol, which then builds up into plaque (stagnation). The discovery of cholesterol plaques in arteries led to a longstanding misconception that high cholesterol is the cause of heart disease, when in fact, one of the causes of heart disease is the inflammation that triggers the release of cholesterol. We have laid the blame on the messenger (high cholesterol) who runs into the streets saying the house is on fire instead of understanding that the problem is the burning house. When a person takes statins and other pharmaceuticals, it may temporarily lower their cholesterol level, but the internal fire still rages. The drugs do nothing to cool our systems, promote relaxation, and reduce inflammation.

Adrenaline's energy is heating, as its role is to increase vitality and movement. But when we fail to work off that adrenaline through physical activity, the adrenaline inflames the body's tissues, most importantly those of the circulatory and cardiovascular systems. If you sit in traffic and fume (heat/excitation response) during your daily commute, you need to release that heat through physical activity or some other method of blowing off steam or chilling out. The increase in tissue permeability that results with heat and oxidation affects our essential nature; we become more sensitive in many ways: Allergens, events of the day, and our ability to ride events out or not respond so quickly get compromised.

Cholesterol Maze

When we consider all the important functions of cholesterol in the body, we gain a better perspective of why statins or cholesterol-lowering drugs can have serious consequences, including liver damage and breakdown of muscle tissue (rhabdomyolysis). It is important to check liver enzyme levels every three to six months when someone is taking these drugs, to monitor the health of the liver; this requirement is often overlooked.

Functions of cholesterol are:

- production of sex hormones
- production of adrenal hormones including cortisol, corticosterone, and aldosterone
- production of bile
- a necessary factor for production of vitamin D by the body
- important for the metabolism of fat-soluble vitamins
- insulating material for nerve fibers
- maintenance of cell membrane permeability
- essential role in preservation of memory
- regulation of serotonin level

Food is the first medicine to turn to in addressing a cholesterol imbalance. Antioxidant foods such as berries and dark green vegetables deserve a prominent place in the diet. Red, blue, and purple berries rich in proanthocyanidins include aronia berries (*Aronia* spp.), blueberries, pomegranates, and elderberries.

Sedative sour herbs such as sumac (*Rhus* spp.) and hibiscus (*Hibiscus* spp.) are excellent medicines for clearing heat and inflammation. Roselle (*H. sabdariffa*) is easy to grow, and many clinical studies show its cooling and antioxidant effects, especially related to cholesterol.[6] Guggul (*Commiphora mukul*) is an herb traditionally used for decreasing kapha/ama and is best given to those with that dosha.

Red yeast rice extract is made from fermentation of rice with *Monascus purpureus* yeast. (This is the substance statin drugs have been produced from.) Red yeast rice is as effective as statins, but it takes longer to have an effect on cholesterol levels. It must be taken with the supplement CoQ 10. CoQ 10 is a hormone called *ubiquinone*, which is found in every cell in the body. It is stored in the mitochondria, the organelles that are the powerhouse of the cell and source of ATP (energy). CoQ 10 also acts as an antioxidant. Statins cause so much damage because they severely diminish natural production of CoQ 10. Red yeast rice does, too, but at much lower rates. Bear in mind, red yeast rice is more of a symptomatic treatment in that it simply lowers cholesterol levels. Inflammation is still an issue that needs to be addressed.

Antioxidants and bioflavonoids used to be called vitamin P—with the *P* standing for permeability. These compounds are essential in reestablishing vascular integrity and stabilizing tissues so as not to be so hyperreactive. Matthew Wood calls the cooling sour herbs "sedatives," as they quench the fire of oxidation as well as excitation. Many cooling, antioxidant herbs are polyphenols, flavonoids, and proanthocyanins, which were discussed in chapter 2. Most members of the rose family are cooling and antioxidant—blackberry (*Rubus fruticosus*); red raspberry (*R. ideaus*); and hawthorn berry, leaf, and flower (*Crataegus laevigata*). Quercetin is one of the most abundant and potent flavonoids in plants, including in onion skins (*Allium cepa*), green tea (*Camellia sinensis*), and ginkgo (*Ginkgo biloba*).

Fever. When we talk about "catching a cold," we are talking about wind heat, the outcome of outside influences (drafts, cold air, pathogens) entering our defensive system (immune system), leading to the onset of a cold or flu. This may be experienced as a sudden development of fever, muscle aches, chills, or a sore throat. To expel wind heat, it is important to stimulate the body's pores to open. Cool, acrid herbs such as yarrow leaf and flower (*Achillea millefolium*), elderberry flower (*Sambucus nigra*), peppermint leaf (*Mentha × piperita*), boneset (*Eupatorium perfoliatum*), lemon balm (*Melissa officinalis*), chamomile (*Matricaria chamomilla*), and blue vervain (*Verbena hastata*) can work well for this. Keep in mind that fever is an invaluable mechanism to help the body return to wholeness.

Fever-Reducing Formula

This classic fever-reducing formula helps the body respond appropriately to high temperature, by opening the pores to lessen damage from heat. This formula does not suppress the fever but releases the heat through diaphoresis.

Elderberry flower *Sambucus nigra,*
S. canadensis
Peppermint leaf *Mentha × piperita*
Yarrow leaf and flower *Achillea millefolium*

Combine the dried herbs in equal parts and brew a tea. Drinking this tea and then soaking in a hot bathtub can bring on a good sweat in order to complete the healing response.

Fire purifies, and in order to destroy the cell walls of most types of bacteria, body temperature has to reach at least 102°F. This is an appropriate immune response. Lowering a fever immediately by taking over-the-counter drugs dampens the intelligent response of our immune systems and their ability to perform optimally in years to come.

Secondary Causes of Heat

The presence of secondary causes of heat is an example of how boundaries can blur a bit and tissue states can overlap. This discussion thus also overlaps with the coverage of stagnation and other conditions discussed later in this chapter.

Stagnation or tension. Heat also builds up when there is stagnation or tension in the body as the flow of vital energy is blocked. This can be analogous to Liver heat rising from Five Phase Theory and to the pattern of the classic Type A personality, where tension increases heat and pressure. This is significant for cardiovascular and circulatory system health. Cooling and calming liver herbs such as motherwort (*Leonurus cardiaca*) and blue vervain are indicated.

Cooling Formulas for Conditions of Heat

The following are sample tincture formulas that address excess heat.

Hypertension Formula

Linden flower	*Tilia* spp.	30%
Motherwort	*Leonurus cardiaca*	30%
Valerian	*Valeriana officinalis*	20%
Chickweed	*Stellaria media*	10%
Dandelion root	*Taraxacum officinale*	10%

Dose depends on many factors but a simple start is ½ teaspoon three times a day. Monitor blood pressure and always work with a qualified health practitioner if you are on medications.

Anxiety Formula

Blue vervain	*Verbena hastata*
Motherwort	*Leonurus cardiaca*
Skullcap	*Scutellaria lateriflora*

Combine the herbs in equal parts. It is often best to take formulas for anxiety in small doses (15–20 drops) frequently throughout the day until heat passes and relaxation occurs.

General Stress Formula

Skullcap	*Scutellaria lateriflora*	30%
St. John's wort	*Hypericum perforatum*	30%
Motherwort	*Leonurus cardiaca*	20%
Wood betony	*Stachys officinalis*	15%
Licorice root	*Glycyrrhiza glabra*	5%

Dose depends on many factors, but a simple start is ½ teaspoon three times a day, or more often if needed.

Insomnia Formula

Passionflower	*Passiflora incarnata*	30%
Skullcap	*Scutellaria lateriflora*	30%

| Catnip *Nepeta cataria* | 20% |
| Chamomile *Matricaria chamomilla* | 20% |

This can be in a tea or tincture.

GERD/Acid Reflux/Heartburn Formula

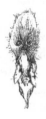

Marshmallow root	*Althaea officinalis*
Meadowsweet leaf and flower	*Filipendula ulmaria*
Plantain	*Plantago* spp.
Slippery elm bark	*Ulmus rubra*

Combine the herbs in equal parts, but note that slippery elm is on the UpS At-Risk List, so save slippery elm for hard-to-heal cases. This formula is best prepared as a tea or powder rather than tincture.

Lack of fluids and nutrition. Lack of fluids is one of the main causes of the tissue state of dry/atrophy, but it is significant with heat as well. Our bodies need cooling fluids to counter overproduction of heat. This echoes Five Phase Theory—yin (cool, fluids) is vital for tempering the effects of yang (warm, activity). Fluids include oils as well as water. Traditional cultures do not have the dietary fat phobia that developed in modern Western culture. They regard oils and fats as treasures. They know the value of saturated fats such as lard and ghee and consume these oils daily in small amounts. These fats supply cell membranes with necessary components for flexibility, which is important for proper function of hormone receptors in cell membranes. Healthy oils in the diet, such as olive and coconut, are important for good health. Another point to compare is that pitta in balance has oil or water to keep the fire in check.

Toxic heat (infections). Heat resulting from infection is often intense and, as the name suggests, can produce toxins (pus). Often this presents as sores, boils, or abscesses. It can also be caused by venomous bites. Working with snakebites as toxic heat presents an herbalist with the opportunity to help in situations where conventional medicine cannot. If someone is bitten by a copperhead and seeks help at a hospital emergency room, the advised treatment in my area of the United States is to watch and wait. This is because in recent years, many people have experienced adverse reactions to antivenom medications. I have worked with several people who have been bitten (by a copperhead), and none have been left with residual effects from the injury. The intense heat caused by a bite is logical when you think about the function of the poison. Venom is amped-up digestive enzymes that produce intense tissue destruction and swelling. The purpose of the venom is to begin digestion of the prey, and this requires a good amount of heat.

Herbs that clear heat and relieve toxicity include echinacea whole herb (*Echinacea* spp.), goldenseal whole herb (*Hydrastis canadensis*), wild indigo (*Baptisia* spp.), plantain (*Plantago major*), Baikal skullcap (*Scutellaria baicalensis*), and self-heal (*Prunella vulgaris*).

Spirit agitation. Any mental and emotional states that cause tissue excitation can be called *spirit agitation*. The manic state, in which all systems are in hyperexcited states, is an extreme example of this kind of heat. Herbs that serve to calm the restless, agitated spirit include passionflower (*Passiflora incarnata*), mimosa bark (*Albizia julibrissin*), holy basil (*Ocimum tenuiflorum*), reishi (*Ganoderma lucidum*), and skullcap (*Scutellaria lateriflora*).

Summer heat. While summer heat is not a true expression of excitation, I include it here because it is becoming more relevant as the effects of climate change intensify. Just as it sounds, summer heat results from too much exposure to sun, high temperatures, and humidity. In traditional herbalism, the foods and herbs that clear this heat also relieve thirst and are called refrigerants. These herbs can help prevent and relieve sunstroke or heat exhaustion. Roselle flowers (*Hibiscus sabdariffa*), sumac berry, lemon balm, and watermelons (*Citrullus lanatus*) are excellent choices to relieve this type of heat. Think lemonade, as lemons (*Citrus limon*) are sour, and sour foods are mostly cooling.

Cold/Depression

Cold/depression tissue state is the opposite of heat/excitation. Instead of excessive metabolism, here there is hypofunction or deficient metabolic activity. Depression of tissue function means that not enough cellular activity is taking place in order to maintain a healthy ecosystem. This low vitality leads to low immune system function. Thus, when cold/depression is allowed to persist, our tissues, organs, and systems become more vulnerable to infection. Circulation can become so impaired that tissues do not receive the necessary nutrition to support cell respiration. This lack of nutrition in turn prevents the lymphatic system from clearing debris from our tissues. Over a longer period of time this lack of cellular activity can lead to necrosis or tissue death. Deficiency of vital energy affects digestion and cognition in addition to immune function. It can be especially impactful on endocrine function and can manifest as low thyroid states.

Fortunately, many familiar herbs help to remedy cold/depression. These are the stimulants, the warming aromatics that adorn our spice racks. If tended early on, this tissue state can be brought back into balance relatively easily. It's unfortunate that in allopathic medicine this condition is rarely, if ever, acknowledged.

Characteristics of Cold/Depression
- Metabolic rate abnormally slow
- Perception of being colder than others; aversion to being cold
- Fatigue, difficulty thinking clearly, slow to retrieve information
- Conditions associated with deficiency, such as hypothyroidism
- Deficient immune responses, such as white or clear mucus
- Prone to infections
- Chronic conditions
- Paleness or blue tint to skin
- Puffiness in face, body
- Muscle tightness

Herbal Actions for Cold/Depression

Aromatics: thyme (*Thymus vulgaris*), cloves (*Syzygium aromaticum*), garlic (*Allium sativum*), elecampane (*Inula helenium*)

Pungent/Stimulants: ginger (*Zingiber officinale*), prickly ash (*Zanthoxylum americanum*), cayenne (*Capsicum annuum*), horseradish (*Armoracia rusticana*)

Adaptogens: ashwagandha (*Withania somnifera*), reishi (*Ganoderma lucidum*), holy basil (*Ocimum tenuiflorum*)

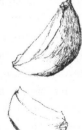

- Bloating, flatulence, diarrhea, impaired absorption, food stagnation (low agni)
- Slowness of limbs, cold hands and feet
- Pain: dull, achy
- Menstrual pain or stomach pain that improves with warmth
- Tongue: pale and bluish, possibly white coat or no coat
- Pulse: low and slow
- Symptoms: worse with cold

Presentations of Cold

Cold tissue states can arise from a variety of causes, and oftentimes they come on slowly. Early treatment yields the best results in resolving cold.

Low-grade chronic infections. With a chronic infection, it may not be clear which came first: the infection leading the body to a colder state, or the cold lowering the body's capacity to mount an immune response. Either way, low vitality compromises the immune system's function of clearing away debris that is left over from an infection. When the body is in balance, the circulatory and lymphatic systems efficiently clear the congestion. But in a state of cold/depression, these systems have less force and power to perform their task of clearing.

Hippocrates is credited with saying, "Give me the power to create a fever and I can cure every illness." This principle was the cornerstone of Thomsonian medicine. In the nineteenth century, root doctor Samuel Thomson introduced the practice of inducing a fever when treating patients because he had learned the healing power of a sweat from the Native Americans who had taught him and his teacher. Thomson believed fervently that heat was life and through sweating one could remove "canker," or cold, and phlegm from the system.

The loss of the tradition of inducing a sweat to move cold, damp conditions out of the body has had negative implications for our health. The simple action of taking diaphoretic herbs and getting into a hot bath can restore vitality, bring relief, and speed the convalescent period dramatically. Once the body is strong enough, it is important to undergo a detox process to clear stagnant lymph. This can be done by inducing sweating with cleansing herbs.

I am a proponent of bringing the practice of a sauna or steam shower into our regular health regime. Unfortunately, this practice is not readily

Medicine of the Sweat

Most ancient peoples utilized methods of sweating not only for treatment of infectious disease but also as a way to enjoy maximum health. Although traditional healers did not precisely understand the physiology of the immune system, they understood the value of raising the body's temperature to clear phlegm and ama. Artificial fever combined with the deep elimination of toxins and wastes increases overall immune system function and resistance to disease. Native American sweat lodges have been used for thousands of years for the healing of physical, mental, and spiritual ailments. The lodge is seen as sacred medicine and ceremony. In Central America, the sweat lodge (*temazcal*) is used for healing as well as a curative ceremony. In the north and west of Ireland, there are bee-hived shaped sweat houses (*teach allais* in Gaelic). These were used for the curing of maladies, most notably rheumatism. Customarily, after the sweat, people would plunge into the cool waters of a nearby stream. Finnish saunas are thought to have originated over seven thousand years ago. The South African *sifutu* is similar to other types of sweat lodges, as is the Korean *hanjeungmak*, which originally was maintained by Buddhist monks. These therapies were a way to socialize and gather as well as cure illness.

accessible, though I have found some inexpensive portable units online that make this healing technique more available.

Overconsumption of vital energy. Every activity requires vital energy, and overdoing it with experiences can leave us with little energy to keep our fires burning. Our daily lives have such an emphasis on seeing everything, being everything, and keeping up with the latest news and technology. No wonder many are running on empty and feeling deficient. This is why attending a retreat, especially a silent retreat, can be so restorative.

Poor production of vital energy. We used to say that we are what we eat, but that phrase has evolved to: We are what we assimilate. If our digestive

Hydrochloric Acid: A Misunderstood Hero

In the stomach, proteins are broken down into amino acids, which are the building blocks of hormones and many components of cells. It is very important that we have sufficient stomach acidity to achieve this task. One of the components of agni, the foundational fire of digestion, is hydrochloric acid (HCl). The presence of food in the stomach stimulates the release of the hormone gastrin, which in turn signals the release of HCl. The presence of HCl converts the hormone pepsin from an inactive form to the active form, and pepsin helps break down proteins.

When our digestive fires are low and there is insufficient HCl, undigested food can back up into the stomach and create heartburn, as there is not enough HCl to break it down and move it onward. Without sufficient HCl to kill bacteria, bacterial overgrowth can also occur in the intestines, increasing phlegm, or ama, and stagnation. Imagine trying to build a fire using wet wood. It does not burn clear and bright. Wet wood burns slowly. It is smoky and congests the air with turbidity. Over time, low digestive fires contribute to cold, damp, and sluggish systems.

While portrayed as the villain in many advertisements for antacids, hydrochloric acid is also a profound healing chemical. When we imagine the diet of ancient people before the use of fire to cook foods, we can only imagine the multitude of bacteria that were rampant in the raw meat or starchy tubers they ingested. HCl acts as a major player in our immune defense by destroying harmful microbes and preventing infection from occurring in the digestive system.

Dispelling the widespread myth that heartburn (too much fire) is caused by excess HCl can be very difficult when talking with a client who has been taking a host of antacids all their life. However, many instances of gastroesophageal reflux disease (GERD) are due to *insufficient* hydrochloric acid. This condition is called hypochlorhydria (*hypo* = cold) and can arise due to medications, stress, aging, and many other conditions. It is much more common than many people realize, and it has huge implications for our health because HCl also plays a role in absorption of such vital minerals as calcium, magnesium, and zinc.

fires are not functioning properly to break down foods into nutrients that the body can metabolize, then we will not have the requisite building blocks to make life happen. Common symptoms of this state are bloating, food stagnation, and inability to thoroughly break down food. This can be seen with undigested food in the stool and one of the possible causes is deficient hydrochloric acid.

Cold, damp foods. Many of the common foods of modern Western culture are cold in nature, and they take vitality from the body. Examples of these are dairy products and sugar. Sugar produces a cool and damp environment in the body, which is why diabetes is often presenting with this tissue state. Low digestive fire is natural in the morning, and if a person starts the day with a sugary cereal and milk, this immediately dampens the fire and puts out the pilot light needed for transforming food into usable nutrients. Starting the day with a cold smoothie has the same effect. (I can't tell you how many of my students and clients react with distress and disappointment when I say that!) It doesn't matter whether a smoothie is made with the purest spirulina, the bluest blueberries, and the highest quality of whey protein powder: Consuming cold, damp foods first thing in the morning can weaken our digestion, especially in cooler weather. Taking a shot of fire cider vinegar can also warm the digestive juices for those who know they can tolerate such stimulation on an empty stomach.

Constitutional weakness or chronic illness. Some premature infants need to draw on their constitutional reserves in order to survive, and this can lead to weaker constitutions later in life. Asking about circumstances of

Rosemary Gladstar's Traditional Fire Cider Vinegar

Fire cider vinegar contains many of the herbs and foods recommended for the cold tissue state. Not only is this tonic warming and stimulating, but in this recipe for fire cider vinegar, there is a multitude of antimicrobial herbs. This becomes the perfect remedy for the cold state in which low-grade infections may be lingering below the surface.

There are many variations of fire cider, such as the addition of black pepper, turmeric, rosemary, thyme, elderberries, and even pomegranates. Be creative! In this recipe I have added some ingredients to Rosemary's version of the recipe that she has widely shared.[7]

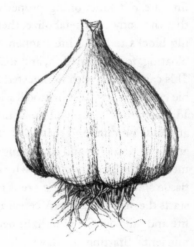

½ cup grated horseradish root
½ cup or more chopped onions
½ cup chopped thyme leaves
¼ cup or more chopped garlic
¼ cup or more grated ginger
¼ cup chopped rosemary leaves
Cayenne pepper, fresh or
    dried, to taste
4 to 6 cups apple cider
    vinegar (preferably
    raw and organic)
Honey, to taste

Place herbs in a half-gallon mason jar
and cover by three to four inches with vinegar. Seal the jar and place parchment paper against metal rim lid to prevent rusting. Shake every day for three to four weeks. Strain out the herbs, warm some honey so it will mix well, then flavor the vinegar to your preferred sweetness. Label the jar, then store in a cool pantry or refrigerator for up to several months. Take 1 teaspoon, in water, once or twice a day as a preventative, or more frequently if you feel a cold coming on.

Warming the Interior

The remedies for a cold constitution are warming and stimulating. This is not the same type of stimulation provided by caffeine or commercial energy drinks. The stimulation here comes from aromatic plants, those incredibly sensual plants whose aroma moves us to a more relaxed sense of self because we are moving vital energy. Think of the scent of ginger, rosemary, or thyme. The invigorating oils in these plants stimulate energy and bring blood to "stagnant" tissues, enlivening and relaxing them. Oxygen is the great relaxant and many herbs can help to nourish the deeper organs of the body with greater blood flow. This is called warming the interior, and here are examples of organ-specific herbs for this purpose.

Digestive system: black pepper (*Piper nigrum*), fennel seed (*Foeniculum vulgare*), anise seed (*Pimpinella anisum*), clove bud (*Syzygium aromaticum*), angelica (*Angelica archangelica*), prickly ash bark (*Zanthoxylum americanum*), fresh garlic cloves (*Allium sativum*)

Circulatory system: prickly ash bark (*Zanthoxylum americanum*), fresh or dried ginger root (*Zingiber officinale*), cayenne pepper (*Capsicum annuum*)

Respiratory system: rosemary leaf (*Salvia rosmarinus*), prickly ash bark (*Zanthoxylum americanum*), cayenne pepper (*Capsicum annuum*), fresh garlic clove (*Allium sativum*), angelica root (*Angelica archangelica*), elecampane root (*Inula helenium*)

Immune system: cinnamon twig and bark (*Cinnamomum cassia*), fresh ginger root (*Zingiber officinale*), rosemary leaf (*Salvia rosmarinus*), prickly ash bark (*Zanthoxylum americanum*), mugwort leaf (*Artemisia vulgaris*), angelica root (*Angelica archangelica*) birth is part of our intake interview of new clients, and we ask specifically whether they were born prematurely, especially if the person is running cold. Childhood illnesses and traumas can deplete a constitution, and chronic illness takes its toll on consumption of energy. Fortunately, herbal remedies have much to offer here.

If a new client tells us that they do run cold, we ask whether this has always been the case. Many times, they will say that they used to have normal body temperature, but after having pneumonia or being in a car accident or other serious incident, they noticed that they tended toward cold. The incident had taken a toll on their vitality. When I hear the phrase "never been the same since," that is when I reach for tonifying herbs or warming adaptogens.

The Quality of Moisture

Five Phase Theory helps us appreciate the value and importance of maintaining yin, Blood and fluids in our body. The quality of moisture is also a reflection of proper mineral balance because these nutrients have a direct relationship with the moisture of our tissues and organs. Herbalist Kiva Rose uses the term *fluid dynamics* for this quality.

Dry/Atrophy

Traditional healing systems treat the blood as if it were an organ system. Blood not only carries moisture but provides nourishment to every cell. In energetic medicine, lack of fluids means atrophy or lack of nutrients. Many hormones that are building to our tissues are oil/fat-soluble, as this configuration is needed to transport hormones throughout the body.

In the dry/atrophy state, the cells of the body are not producing, consuming, or holding sufficient fluids (oil or water). This state is especially important in Western culture because stress and the action of adrenaline can be very drying to our tissues. Another factor is that many popular herbs are drying. Think of herbs that are diuretics, diaphoretics, bitters, and astringents: all qualities that can have an overall drying effect because they stimulate the release of fluids. This is another reason to learn herbal energetics!

This tissue state has significant implications for the immune system as well. A layer of mucus protects the mucous membranes, from the nostrils all the way to the lungs. Mucus contains immunological components that protect the body from infection. When tissues are dry, this function is compromised.

In the digestive tract, it is critical for mucous membranes and other tissues to release sufficient digestive enzymes, HCl, and other fluids to assure proper digestion. In Ayurvedic terms, this is the oil of pitta. If there is dryness in this body system, the effects can include gas, bloating, and inability to break down food to obtain the nutrients it contains. Over time this can lead to atrophy. We can also relate this to the Chinese medicine concepts of the presentation of aging: As our yin decreases, we experience constipation, cracking joints, arterial hardening, and a loss of flexibility physically, mentally, and emotionally. Dryness contributes to the quality of being set in our ways.

Characteristics of Dry/Atrophy
- Dry skin, hair, eyes
- Bloating, gas, constipation / hard stool
- Fatigue, undernourished appearance
- Insomnia
- Skin conditions due to dryness: eczema, psoriasis, itching
- Endocrine disorders due to low oil content
- Joint stiffness and cracking
- Anxiety, emotional rigidity
- Tongue: dry, cracked, pale; red from heat if present
- Pulse: thin and weak

Presentation of Dryness
Dryness and atrophy can be caused by a multitude of factors, but the most common are deficient fluid intake, poor retention of fluids, atrophic heat, poor transformation/transportation of fluids, and prolonged stress.

Intake and retention of fluids, including oils. Many people think hydrating is only about consuming water. But our tissues, joints, organs, and cell membranes all depend on a supply of oils—long-lasting lubricants that nourish and moisten our inner terrain. Oily herbs are hemp (*Cannabis sativa*), evening primrose (*Oenothera biennis*), and borage (*Borago officinalis*). These have become very popular for working with inflammation, which is often caused by dryness.

At times hydrating with water can have an opposite effect to what's intended because water acts as a diuretic. It is best to take water with minerals and especially salt. Drinking mineral-rich teas can deeply moisten in ways that water cannot. Matthew Wood states it beautifully:

Herbal Actions for Dry/Atrophy

Demulcent herbs: marshmallow leaf and root (*Althaea officinalis*), slippery elm (*Ulmus rubra)*, chickweed (*Stellaria media*), violet (*Viola* spp.)

Mineral tonics: milky oats (*Avena sativa*), borage (*Borago officinalis*), alfalfa (*Medicago sativa*), nettle (*Urtica dioica*)

Oils: borage (*Borago officinalis*), hemp (*Cannabis sativa*), evening primrose (*Oenothera biennis*)

Sweet tonics: milky oats (*Avena sativa*), licorice (*Glycyrrhiza glabra*), astragalus (*Astragalus membranaceus*), red clover blossoms (*Trifolium pratense*)

Astringents: blackberry root (*Rubus fruticosus*), agrimony (*Agrimonia eupatoria*)

"Water without salt has no intelligence or activity. Salt attracts water and causes it to become active in the tissue."[8] This is not to say we should not drink our requisite number of glasses of water every day. The right amount to drink depends on constitution, activity level, and how well the tissues are holding onto fluids and transporting those fluids to outlying areas. Mineral-rich herbs to brew as teas are nettle (*Urtica dioica*), borage leaf, and alfalfa (*Medicago sativa*).

I have worked with many clients who drink plenty of fluids but still present with symptoms of dryness. These clients may not be able to retain water. In these cases, while it seems contradictory, astringents may actually be appropriate, even though the flavor/sensation of astringency is known for drying tissues. Astringents act by tonifying tissue: If tissue is too boggy, an astringent has a drying effect, but if tissue lacks integrity and allows fluids to be released, then astringents can actually help retain moisture. (This action is discussed further in "Lax/Atony" on page 168.) Certain herbs, such as plantain, are listed as both astringent as well as demulcent. These contradictions can be confusing to all of us, but through experience, you will come to understand and appreciate the multitude of tasks that a single potent medicinal herb can accomplish.

Atrophic heat. Because heat dries out the body, one simple way to remedy dryness is to identify signs of heat and to address those issues first. Atrophic heat is also known as yin deficiency. In menopause, hot flashes, night sweats, and other heat symptoms can produce dryness as well as irritability. Instead of chasing hormones, what women as well as men need for the aging process is good oils—foods and herbs that build tissue and kidney yin. This would be bone broth, sweet building tonic herbs, particularly plants such as burdock root (*Arctium lappa*), chickweed (*Stellaria media*), and eleuthero (*Eleutherococcus senticosus*). Sweet tonics are deeply tonifying to tissues, thus enabling them to hold on to water with greater ease. Dry tissues have tight, hard boundaries, and fluids and nutrients cannot penetrate them. Imagine trying to water a garden after years of drought. The water would simply run off the hard-baked surface of the soil—very little would be absorbed even though the soil is bone dry. Sweet tonics are like the compost we add to dry, baked soil in order to build and soften the texture of the soil.

Just as tight boundaries prevent fluids from entering tissues, they also prevent toxins from leaving. Using demulcent herbs is critical in helping dry tissues (vata imbalance) cleanse. Demulcent herbs such as marshmallow (*Althaea officinalis*), chickweed, and violet (*Viola* spp.) can cool atrophic heat through their moistening and nutritive actions.

Poor transformation/transportation of fluids and oils. When our metabolic or digestive system is functioning poorly, we don't have sufficient vitality to transform (break down) fats or transport fluids. For example, one of the most common causes of constipation is insufficient production of bile by the liver. Just as soap emulsifies or breaks down grease, bile has this same action on dietary fat. If the liver is not functioning well and digestive juices are not flowing, then fats will not be emulsified and thus will not be in the proper form to lubricate the bowels. Herbalists commonly say, "bitters, bitters, bitters," and one of the multitudes of reasons we rely on these remedies is for proper digestion of fats. Remember that many bitters are drying and cooling, so warming them up with demulcents or sweet tonic herbs can really help here.

Prolonged stress. When we perceive a threat, our adrenal glands release adrenaline. As mentioned earlier, in Chinese medicine this is a form of Kidney yang. Adrenaline warms the body, assisting in the response of fight or flight by supplying muscles, lungs, and heart with increased energy. Fear will excite the system, activating muscles needed for defense

Smooth and Moving Tonic

This constipation remedy works very well as a tea/decoction or tincture. This is a great formula to take before or during travel, as you may not be able to maintain your usual habits of consuming liquids, and also because travel itself can provoke vata or dryness. I prefer using the tincture form when traveling.

Dandelion root	*Taraxacum officinale*	30%
Burdock root	*Arctium lappa*	20%
Fennel seed	*Foeniculum vulgare*	20%
Yellow dock root	*Rumex crispus*	20%
Licorice	*Glycyrrhiza glabra*	10%

For tincture, best to start with ½ teaspoon taken with meals and increase to 1 teaspoon three times a day if needed. If making as a tea, percentages are by weight of dry herb.

from impending danger. While these are healthy responses to an injury or threat, if stress due to a threat or psychological agitation persists too long, the body's responses eventually dry tissues through excess inflammation and heat. This is the literal experience of being burned out. Your juices are consumed, and you no longer feel you can stay in the flow.

Oil is also an important nutrient for the nervous system. The myelin sheath, or insulating layer protecting nerves, is made of fat. Adding healthy oils to the diet and looking at remedies that pacify vata and increase kapha will serve in keeping the nervous system well nourished and lubricated.

Damp/Stagnant

When too many fluids build up in the tissues, this leads to stagnation. In the texts of the Physiomedicalist physicians who took inspiration from Samuel Thomson, this form of tissue state is called *torpor*. The tissues/organs/system becomes water laden and "boggy" because the water itself is inhibiting the flow of elimination. This damp condition weakens cellular health because nutrients are prevented from being taken up through the cell membrane. And when channels of elimination are not functioning, toxicity builds up, further degrading the tissue. This is kin to how water will pool after a rain if drainage is not properly devised. If the water continues to sit undisturbed over time, the supply of oxygen in the water is depleted, and the water may "ripen" into a dank and rank-smelling swamp. This is the classic "bad blood" of traditional herbalism.

A damp or stagnant tissue state is a common presentation in those who have chronic circulatory and digestive issues. This is also seen in hypothyroid cases, where vitality is too low to ignite metabolic processes and congestion builds up. Conventional medicine treats dampness with diuretics, which does drain excess water from the body but does nothing to spark the body's metabolism nor support elimination. Energetic herbalists instead work with stimulants and alteratives or "blood cleansers" to help clients with these conditions. Alterative herbs move stagnant lymph, stimulate liver and digestive function, and increase circulation. This is where herbalism shines, because there are many wonderful plants that help to clear channels of elimination.

Characteristics of Damp/Stagnation
- Swollen, weak tissues
- Dull expression—low spark of vitality
- Doughy, dull-looking skin
- Edema, swollen glands
- Green or yellow secretions in cases of active infection or heat
- Clear or white secretions in cases of cold
- "Dirty" yellowish, greenish, brownish, or black secretions indicate a chronic condition
- Lack of thirst, aversion to drink, inability to process fluids
- Cloudy head, brain fog, depression, lethargy
- Tongue: white, dirty coating; swollen or scalloped
- Pulse: slippery and slow
- Symptoms: worse in damp weather and with heavy foods or excess fluids

Presentations of Damp/Stagnation
Low digestive fire. When the digestive process is impaired, there are left over by-products that build up and cannot be easily eliminated. This creates fermentation and putrification of food, which the intestine absorbs,

Herbal Actions for Damp/Stagnation

Alteratives: red clover flower (*Trifolium pratense*), dandelion leaf and root (*Taraxacum officinale*), red root (*Ceanothus americanus*), cleavers (*Galium aparine*), burdock root (*Arctium lappa*)

Astringents: blackberry root (*Rubus fruticosus*), meadowsweet 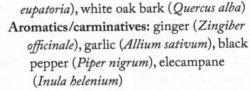 (*Filipendula ulmaria*), agrimony (*Agrimonia eupatoria*), white oak bark (*Quercus alba*)

Aromatics/carminatives: ginger (*Zingiber officinale*), garlic (*Allium sativum*), black pepper (*Piper nigrum*), elecampane (*Inula helenium*)

Bitters: wormwood (*Artemisia annua*), black walnut (*Juglans nigra*)

causing more toxicity as well as gas, bloating, and cramping. Over time, the processes of elimination and metabolic function are weakened. Aside from reigniting digestive fire (agni) to support the breakdown of food, the therapeutic goal is to spark the eliminatory functions through stimulation of hepatic function, lymphatic movement, and regular bowel movements.

Over time, digestive mucus becomes thick and very hard to move, or it has persisted long enough to create turbidity. Turbid waters are full of particles that prevent clarity. This is why those who often experience a damp condition can feel lethargic. It is also what contributes to the mental fogginess people experience when suffering from *Candida*, or yeast, overgrowth. The goal here is to warm the environment and bring the clarity of the vital spark. Dealing with the underlying processes is usually necessary for more complete resolution. This involves improving the diet to eliminate sugars, food additives, and possibly excess gluten in order to assist digestion and enhance elimination. If stagnation is chronic, it is always best to move in gently and gradually versus using strong blood cleansers or heroic fasts and cleanses.

Cold. Cold and damp often go hand in hand, and warming the body through use of warming herbs and foods can help. Try aromatics and other plants that move energy outward. Cinnamon has become very

Formulas to Clear Damp Heat

These formulas are meant to be prepared in tincture form.

Acute Sinus Clear Formula

Yarrow leaf	*Achillea millefolium*	40%
Dandelion root	*Taraxacum officinale*	30%
Ground ivy	*Glechoma hederacea*	20%
Thyme	*Thymus vulgaris*	10%

For acute infections, I tend to dose higher to clear damp conditions: ½ to 1 teaspoon three times a day for ten days.

Urinary Tract Infection Formula

Uva ursi leaf	*Arctostaphylos uva ursi*	50%
Corn silk	*Zea mays*	25%
Marshmallow root	*Althaea officinalis*	25%

One teaspoon three times a day for ten days.

popular for diabetes. One mechanism of cinnamon is increasing insulin sensitivity so glucose can more easily travel into the cells.[9] Energetically, cinnamon warms the body and moves vitality toward the core. A traditional remedy for cold, damp conditions is fire cider vinegar (see Rosemary Gladstar's Traditional Fire Cider Vinegar on page 154).

Damp heat. The presence of too much water, edema, or chronic bronchitis produces heat because the free flow of vital energy is blocked. This is a perfect setup for infections to take hold. This tissue state leads to production of yellow, green, or brown mucus. Dampness is heavy, and these infections tend to sink to lower parts of the body. That being said, dampness can also present as a classic sinus and lung infection with thick green or yellow discharge. To clear damp heat, use bitter (drying) or cold herbs, which generally have antimicrobial properties. If there is excess cold, these remedies might need to be warmed with aromatics such as thyme and rosemary. Yellow dock, barberry root (*Berberis vulgaris*), and Oregon grape root (*Berberis aquifolium*) all help with damp heat with thick, green or yellow discharge. What is important with these conditions is to work with eliminatory functions to clear metabolic waste as well as get the systems running more efficiently.

The Quality of Tone

In the vocabulary of tissue states, tone refers to the degree of tension present in muscles and tissues. This state can be difficult to conceptualize because the nature of certain organs requires a continuous shift between tension and relaxation. The beating of the heart, the peristalsis or movement of the intestines, and the pulsing of nerves all necessitate a healthy dose of tension in order to get the job done. When applied to muscles and organs, the concept of healthy tone reflects that they hold themselves with integrity as well as ease. Under too much tension, constricted vessels, nerves, or tendons prevent the free flow of energy. If the tissue is too relaxed, its flaccidity fails to provide the impetus or capacity for performing necessary tasks. In that instance, tissues and organs will not be able to hold water, and fluids are lost. Herbalist Kiva Rose uses the term *structural dynamics* to refer to the states of tension and relaxation.

Tension/Constriction/Wind

Tension has psychological as well as physiological roots. Unfortunately, for most people, this state is all too familiar. Tension restricts circulation of blood, fluids, thoughts, and creativity. Muscle spasms are a part of this picture. Some aspects of this pattern or tissue state tend to fluctuate—to come and go, or to come on suddenly. This intermittent pattern was much more common in the past, especially with the prevalence of malaria. Nowadays a common pattern is the experience of having a flu or infection and then being unable to shake off intermittent spells of wind or chills.

I advise my students that if a client presents with noticeable tension, the best course of action is to treat them with nervines, relaxants, or bitters, and ask them to return in a short time. Once the herbs begin to help the client's energy flow with greater ease, it will be easier to detect organic problems. When we are too tense, we are literally out of the flow of life. Without sufficient oxygen, our muscles spasm and we tend toward irritability and anxiety. If tension is left unchecked for too long, exhaustion sets in. I am always astounded at how much more I can accomplish when I take time to relax and open to the flow that is my vital energy.

Characteristics of Tension/Constriction/Wind

- Tension in the face, muscles, mind, or whole body
- Emotional irritability, insomnia, anxiety, spasms
- Cold extremities due to constricted circulation
- Purple hue to lips and skin
- Fatigue, exhaustion
- Tongue: red, pale, bluish
- Pulse: rapid or slow, depending on duration of the state of tension
- Symptoms: alternating or intermittent
- Symptoms: worse with stress and improve with relaxation

Presentation of Tension

Tension can be caused by a host of factors, including psychological stress, dryness and atrophy, and heat/spasms.

Psychological stress. Having inadequate shelter or food causes psychological stress as well as physical stress. And today, "perceived" stress is nearly universal. Even those who have adequate resources to meet their basic needs can tend to worry about things that are not occurring at the present moment. This can include job stress as well as worries about political upheaval or climate change. These worries manifest physiologically because fear is fear. It is the signal that releases hormones to quicken the heartbeat, constrict blood vessels, and shut down the digestive process in order to be ready to fight or run. When these hormones flood our body morning, noon, and night, they disrupt the smooth flow of thoughts and metabolic processes.

Relieving this kind of stress is one of the greatest contributions herbal medicine can make. This tissue state greatly affects the mind, the nervous system, and therefore the digestive system. There are as many personalities of relaxing herbs as there are reasons for stress. These plants have affinities for not only specific organs but also behavior patterns adopted to avoid or mask discomfort. For example, agrimony (*Agrimonia eupatoria*) relaxes tension held in the solar plexus, wood betony (*Stachys officinalis*) relaxes the anxiety that arises from not feeling grounded, and blue vervain relaxes tension in the neck that develops when we think too long and hard. For more examples, see "Herbs to Relieve Tension."

Dryness and atrophy. Because fluids ensure the smooth flow of vital energy, tension can result from insufficient nutrition through dry conditions, as

Herbal Actions for Tension/Constriction

Antispasmodics: lobelia (*Lobelia inflata*), valerian (*Valeriana officinalis*), black haw (*Viburnum prunifolium*), wild lettuce (*Lactuca virosa*)

Aromatics: chamomile (*Matricaria chamomilla*), fennel (*Foeniculum vulgare*), rosemary (*Salvia rosmarinus*)

Nervines: skullcap (*Scutellaria lateriflora*), passionflower (*Passiflora incarnata*), catnip (*Nepeta cataria*)

Demulcents: marshmallow root (*Althaea officinalis*), plantain (*Plantago* spp.), violet leaf (*Viola* spp.)

 **Bitters:** blue vervain (*Verbena hastata*), motherwort (*Leonurus cardiaca*), boneset (*Eupatorium perfoliatum*)

noted in the section on the dry/atrophy tissue state. Just as a crying baby can be soothed with feeding, so, too, our anxious minds and organs can be calmed with nutrients carried by our blood. This can be a chicken-and-egg scenario because tension blocks tissues from absorbing nutrients, and can therefore cause dryness. Constricted vessels prevent the lubricating and nourishing properties of our blood to infuse all the cells that are hungrily anticipating oxygen, calcium, magnesium, and the whole host of minerals and hormones needed for their proper functioning. Unless the digestive system is relaxed, it cannot get the job accomplished. Fortunately, as parasympathetic stimulants, bitters are both calming to our brains and relaxing to our guts, helping to break the tension cycle.

Intermittency. Intermittency is a state that alternates between tension and relaxation. The alternating fever and chills of malaria are classic symptoms of intermittency. Fever is usually what sets off this tissue state, but it can persist for years. Acupuncturist Robert Clickner has described intermittency as "usually part of a struggle with a pathogenic force or microorganism that has stalemated, with neither side succeeding."[10]

It is important to consider the possibility of intermittency, especially if a client has been diagnosed with a long-term disease such as Lyme, chronic fatigue syndrome, or fibromyalgia. These conditions usually

Herbs to Relieve Tension

Headache: St. John's wort (*Hypericum perforatum*), skullcap
(*Scutellaria lateriflora*), chamomile (*Matricaria chamomilla*),
wood betony (*Stachys betonica*)

Neck tension: blue vervain (*Verbena hastata*), dandelion root
(*Taraxacum officinale*), black cohosh root (*Actaea racemosa*),
lobelia (*Lobelia inflata*), cramp bark (*Viburnum opulus*), mullein leaf (*Verbascum thapsus*), goldenrod
oil (*Solidago* spp.)

Respiratory tension: valerian (*Valeriana officinalis*),
wild lettuce (*Lactuca virosa*), lobelia (*Lobelia
inflata*), cramp bark (*Viburnum opulus*)

Tension in solar plexus or gut: wood betony
(*Stachys officinalis*), motherwort (*Leonurus
cardiaca*), chamomile (*Matricaria chamomilla*)

Anxiety or heart palpitation: motherwort
(*Leonurus cardiaca*), skullcap (*Scutellaria lateriflora*), mimosa flower (*Albizia julibrissin*)

Muscle cramps: kava kava (*Piper methysticum*),
cramp bark (*Viburnum opulus*), valerian (*Valeriana officinalis*),
lobelia (*Lobelia inflata*)

involve depression, dampness, stagnation, and/or residual heat in some combination. Symptoms seem to come and go without obvious triggers, which can be exhausting. When working at Sacred Plant Traditions clinic, Robert Clickner has successfully worked with boneset, mugwort (*Artemisia vulgaris*), agrimony, and wormwood (*Artemisia annua*), the classic malaria remedy, to treat intermittency.

Heat/spasms. Adding relaxing herbs to a fever formula can often allow the body to respond more quickly from an immunological standpoint. These herbs can also provide needed relief from all the hard work a body needs to do to sustain a healthy fever.

Spasms create throbbing headaches, debilitating cramps, and intestinal colic. These symptoms can be the presentation of irritable bowel syndrome (IBS) or colitis, which may include intermittency between diarrhea and constipation. IBS and colic are multilayered conditions, but antispasmodics are the herbal remedy to choose when there is intense colicky pain. For intestinal spasms I have found wild yam (*Dioscorea villosa*) to be an excellent remedy. More often than not, antispasmodics are the acrid herbs. One of my favorites that Matthew Wood calls "the king of acrid" is lobelia (*Lobelia inflata*). Others are valerian root (*Valeriana officinalis*) and cramp bark (*Viburnum opulus*), as well as skunk cabbage (*Symplocarpus foetidus*), kava kava (*Piper methysticum*), and black cohosh (*Actaea racemosa*).

Wind. If left untreated, tension advances to the form called wind. This form appears as tremors, shaking, and convulsions. It can mimic the behavior of atmospheric wind—unpredictable and erratic. This is tension coupled with chronic dryness, so I always like to add demulcent herbs to these remedies. Herbs useful in this state are blue vervain, white peony root (*Paeonia lactiflora*), and prickly ash bark (*Zanthoxylum americanum*), or a calcium/magnesium supplement.

Lax/Atony

The most common definition of relaxation in contemporary life is a positive state of calm and repose. But the Physiomedicalists, as well as energetic healers back through the centuries to Hippocrates, used *relaxation* to describe a state in which the tissues are flaccid, without tone, and prolapsed. Herbalist jim mcdonald has made a substantial contribution to the understanding of the tissue states by substituting the term *lax* for *relaxation*.

Lax tissues cannot hold on to fluids because they have lost tone. They present with "free secretions," which is an overflow of fluids. These secretions or leakages can be in the form of clear and runny mucus, spontaneous sweating, diarrhea, frequent urination, and premature ejaculation. The lack of ability to hold fluids or other substances leads to loss of nutrients as well as function. Prolapse is a form of laxity. Other tissues may become spongy when they lose tone (examples are the gums or the prostate).

As stated in chapter 2, tannins are one of the significant components in astringent plants. Because of this, it's important to monitor anyone who uses astringents long term, as prolonged exposure of the gut mucosa to tannins can prevent uptake of nutrients. As mentioned in chapter 2, tanning a hide makes the skin impermeable so it is better protected and less permeable to water. Strong astringents such as white oak (*Quercus alba*) or blackberry root can be helpful in cases of acute fluid loss such as hemorrhaging, severe food poisoning, or dysentery. Over the long term, however, it's best to switch to astringents that are milder in action, such as agrimony, wild geranium (*Geranium maculatum*), or rose (*Rosa* spp.).

Characteristics of Lax/Atony

- Soft, spongy, weak tissues
- Poor muscle tone, organ collapse, tissue prolapse
- Copious, clear, runny mucus
- Clammy skin, spontaneous sweating
- Frequent, copious, clear urine
- Diarrhea; loose, runny stools
- Certain types of passive hemorrhage
- Vaginal secretions not related to infections
- Spermatorrhea and premature ejaculation (physiological not psychological)
- Habitual miscarriage
- Tongue: pale, puffy or large, moist with streamers (excess moisture) down the sides
- Pulse: soft, squishy, forceless

Presentation of Laxity

The focus when dealing with lax, atonic tissues is to hold on to fluids while improving tissue integrity.

Aging. Upward movement requires strong vitality, so as we age, there can be a tendency for downward energy to be more influential in our physiology. An elder Chinese practitioner once asked me—if all the young Americans are using ginseng as an energy tonic, what will they use when they are old? Many of the Kidney or yang tonics in Chinese medicine are reserved for the elderly or those in convalescence who may not have the stamina they need, and particularly for elders who experience urinary incontinence. Astringent herbs are useful for this state, but there are times when offering adaptogens or herbs that increase vitality, or upward energy, can assist as well. Increasing vital energy gives tissues the warmth and nutrients they need to tighten their weave and gain or regain integrity. Prolapse of organs, especially the bladder, in the elderly is not uncommon, and many elderly people are told it's a condition they simply need to get used to. Working from an energetic perspective, while

Herbal Actions for Lax/Atony

Astringents: witch hazel (*Hamamelis virginiana*), blackberry
root (*Rubus fruticosus*), sumac berries (*Rhus glabra, R. typhina*),
white oak (*Quercus alba*), sage
(*Salvia officinalis*)

Adaptogen/tonics: ashwagandha
(*Withania somnifera*), eleuthero
(*Eleutherococcus senticosus*), astragalus
(*Astragalus membranaceus*), American
ginseng (*Panax quinquefolius*)

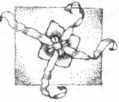

not promising great feats of magic, we can certainly help people improve
their quality of life by adding quality of tone.

Lack of tone. Many who suffer from extreme menstrual pain and excessive bleeding lack uterine tone. The astringent action of lady's mantle
(*Alchemilla vulgaris*), yarrow, red raspberry leaf, and rose has proven time
and time again to be a reliable formula to help quell excessive pain and
flooding. It might take many months to bring about results, and once
you begin to see results with astringing herbs, it's best to decrease their
use to avoid overtaxing or drying out membranes.

Inflammation. Relaxation can occur in the gut for various reasons, including infection (such as from food poisoning) as well as inflammation due
to colitis, irritable bowel, or leaky gut. Astringents can play a major role
in bringing the gut back into balance. In the instance of food poisoning,
it is best to let acute infections play out to clear the pathogen, but herbal
astringents can reduce the duration of diarrhea. The best remedies for
laxity in the digestive tract are blackberry root, meadowsweet (*Filipendula ulmaria*), plantain, and agrimony. Leaky gut syndrome describes the
condition when the mucous membrane of the large intestine has been
compromised. This condition is not a classic example of laxity, but even
so the herbs mentioned here, especially plantain, can play a key role in
restoring tissue integrity.

Organ-Specific Astringents

Sinuses: ground ivy (*Glechoma hederacea*), goldenrod (*Solidago* spp.), osha root (*Ligusticum porteri*), sumac berry (*Rhus glabra, R. typhina*)

Gums: white oak bark (*Quercus alba*)

Head (aches): feverfew (*Tanacetum parthenium*), agrimony (*Agrimonia eupatoria*)

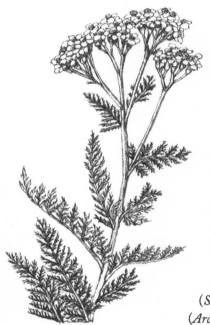

Intestines: blackberry root (*Rubus fruticosus*), meadowsweet (*Filipendula ulmaria*), plantain (*Plantago* spp.)

Uterus: lady's mantle (*Alchemilla vulgaris*), red raspberry (*Rubus idaeus*), yarrow (*Achillea millefolium*), rose (*Rosa* spp.)

Skin: witch hazel (*Hamamelis virginiana*)

Bladder: sumac berry (*Rhus glabra, R. typhina*), schisandra (*Schisandra chinensis*), uva ursi (*Arctostaphylos uva ursi*)

PART 2

The Apothecary

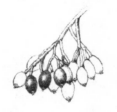

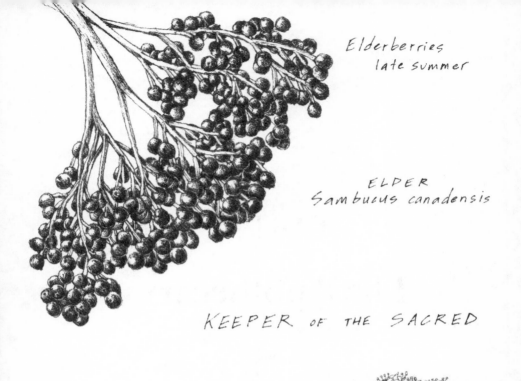

Elderberries
late summer

ELDER
Sambucus canadensis

KEEPER OF THE SACRED

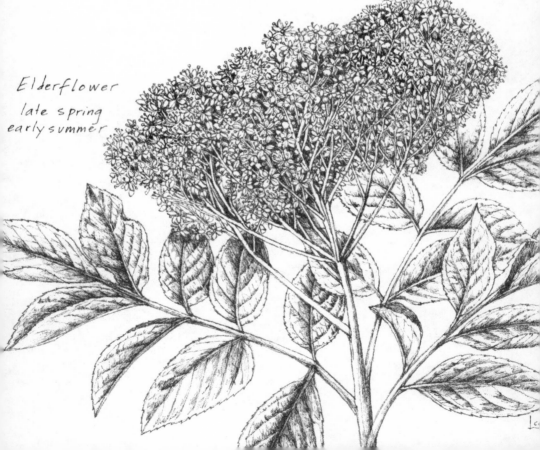

Elderflower
late spring
early summer

CHAPTER 7

The Wheel of the Year

Indigenous seasonal celebrations have been vital touchstones of community life for millennia. Some herbalists have revived such traditions as a way to incorporate ceremony into their medicine harvest and their apothecary practices. In this chapter, I focus on my European traditions, but also want to acknowledge that cultures all over the globe have celebrated their own walk through the year, following the seasons for planting, growth, and harvest. Earth-centric cultures engage organically with the environment; their lives and daily activities are defined by cycles of life and death through the planting of seeds and harvesting of foods and medicines. Cycles of nature are the cosmology that defines a culture, whether that is island life in the Pacific, or hunting season in Alaska. No matter where we live on the Earth, there is still the turning of the wheel as it is influenced by forces larger than ourselves.

The Wheel of the Year is a calendar of seasonal celebrations revived by neopaganism and contemporary Druids. Since medieval times in the British Isles, there were what were called quarter days and these reflected the agricultural calendar. Since the times were easy to remember, these became the time of year to conduct community business such as the hiring of help for planting and harvesting and tending to payments. These days fell approximately every three months and were very close to the equinoxes and solstices. It's unclear how ancient Celts celebrated these times, as their tradition was mostly told through bards and stories. What is known is the major celebrations of ancient Celts were called the four fire festivals and were of the greatest import. They were referred to as the cross-quarter holidays, as they fall midway between the quarter days. These include Samhain,

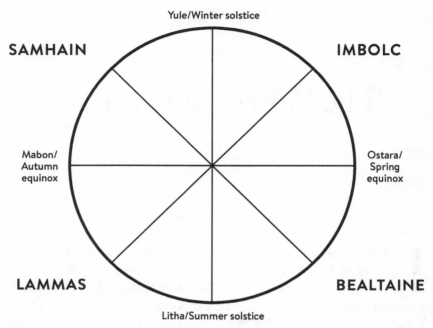

Figure 7.1. Wheel of the Year.

which takes place on November 1, Imbolc on February 1, Bealtaine on May 1, and Lammas on August 1. To the ancients these dates marked the beginning of the seasons. Contemporary practices blend these with celebrations of the solstices and equinoxes. However, we know that ancient Celtic peoples placed great importance on the quarter days, because we can see how the ancient sites at Newgrange and Stonehenge align perfectly with the rising and setting of the sun on winter solstice. In the revived Wheel of the Year, these quarter festivals include Yule/Midwinter, Ostara/Spring Equinox, Litha/Midsummer, and Mabon/Autumn Equinox.

Engaging in these seasonal rituals is a way to tap into very old energies and Earth wisdom, and in this time of ecosystem fragility, I believe that this is part of the calling for those who work with healing plants. It's also important, though, to develop your own ways of marking these celebrations in a respectful manner. As with Native American traditions, there is the risk of disrespecting Celtic and other wisdom traditions—of appropriating rather than honoring. Author Sharon Blackie, a Jungian psychiatrist and Celtic mythopoetic storyteller, writes eloquently about this dilemma and also offers a way forward. Her work focuses on exploring the mythic imagination and helping her readers understand the vitality of cultural myths and their relevance in the face of the ecological and societal challenges of today. Her writings guide readers out of the "dark forest of our forgetting."[1] I have taken inspiration from Sharon's work as I find my way, seeking guidance and always honoring those whose traditions these are. My purpose of sharing the festivals of the year here is not to pretend that we can or should recreate ancient practices, but to share the spirit of European ancestors, knowing that time-honored celebrations like these occur worldwide.

Samhain

The Celtic year traditionally begins with Samhain (SOW-in) or Hallomas on November 1. This is the time when the veils between the worlds are the thinnest, which is why this time was chosen to pray for the departed. It is no coincidence other cultures also have celebrations on this date, such as Dia de Los Muertos (Day of the Dead) in Mexico and All Saints Day in the Catholic tradition. This is a sacred time for honoring of ancestors, when altars are made and adorned with offerings for those who have departed. Ancestors are our connection to our past, and when we have had good relations or have a favored ancestor, their presence can support and encourage us. To know that we are the future ancestors allows us to cultivate wisdom and skills so that we too may serve generations to come. This celebration at this time of year serves to remind us to give thanks for those that have come before us.

In the northern hemisphere, November is the beginning of the darker months of the year, and death is a fertile offering for new beginnings that will emerge in the light of the spring. We are shedding the old and preparing for the dark of the winter. This is the time in the garden when much has been put to bed and the final tending of the land has taken place. We let go of what no longer serves, allowing us to prepare our soil for planting the seed of the winter's dreamtime. A ceremony at this time can be as simple as creating a beautiful space to display or to sit and contemplate photos or gifts bestowed to us from loved ones who have passed on.

Yule/Midwinter/Winter Solstice

Winter solstice, which occurs between December 20 and 23, is the longest night of the year and heralds the return of the light. Winter is the time to rest and dive deep into the silence of the black and starry nights. This is the time to seed the dream and nourish our dreamtime visioning: time to rest deeply, empty, and listen for the dream that is dreaming us. Our tradition at Sacred Plant Traditions is to create a beautiful nest with evergreen boughs brought by each participant from their land. With candles lit for the darkest night, we share the seeds of visions we wish to birth. We then close our school until Imbolc.

Imbolc/Candlemas

Halfway through the winter is the celebration of Imbolc, February 1. The name means "in the belly," for this was the time of ewes birthing their lambs. Ancient Celts celebrated the beginning of spring at this time, as the light is returning and there is an unmistakable stirring beneath the snow. This is the time when the sap is rising. Imbolc was also known as Saint Brigid's Day. The original goddess associated with Imbolc was Brigit (Brigid, Bridgit), the daughter of the chief Celtic deity, Dagda. They were of the Tuatha Dé Danann, the first inhabitants of Ireland. The fact that the fire for this celebration is burned inside the home (those for the other three festivals are all outdoor fires) honors Brigit's role as a goddess of hearth and fertility.

A practice at Sacred Plant Traditions on Imbolc is to gather up the boughs that have been gracing the solstice nest, recall the dream seeds planted at solstice, and rekindle our intentions. Then we burn those boughs in a fire. Dried evergreen needles make the best of tinder, as they are crisp yet still infused with volatile oils that help spark a flame. This fire is held outside; we honor our gardens as the school's hearth. Again, the medicine here is in recollecting our dreams and nourishing them with remembrance and focus. And in our apothecaries, the catalogs have arrived and the ordering of seeds has begun. The dreaming time continues.

Ostara/Spring Equinox

Spring equinox is a time of perfect balance between light and dark. This occurs between March 20 and 23. It brings to mind the spring focus in Five Phase Theory on the element of Wood, the growth and maturation of life. Partaking of early spring tonics clears the stagnancy and dampness that may have accumulated over the winter months. Internally, we shine light on the dream seeds that were planted at the winter solstice, and outwardly we begin the gardens or projects for the year to come.

Bealtaine/May Day

The Celtic word *Bealtaine* translates roughly as "bright fire." Historically, the Irish considered this date of May 1 as the beginning of summer, and the fire was a central aspect as it is held as a purifier and healer. This was the time the cows were moved out onto pastures, and the animals would be driven between twin fires as a form of protection and blessing. Another custom was the putting out of hearth fires and then relighting them from the communal Bealtaine fire. This way the community was connected through the sacred fire of this celebration. Bealtaine was a time of passion, courtship rituals, and fertility reflected in the profusion of May flowers.

For many years at Sacred Plant Traditions, we hosted a Gaia Gathering for Women on Bealtaine. We began the weekend with a fire kindled by hand with a bow drill and kept it burning for three days. Through rain and even sleet one year, the fire was tended and stayed bright. Our community of women was deeply nourished by the bright fire of this time. Sharing women-only space allowed the fertility of our ideas and projects to flourish.

Litha/Midsummer/Summer Solstice

On the longest day of the year, the sun stands still for a moment and the light is fully infusing the land. Midsummer, June 20 to 23, was a traditional time for weddings, as the work of planting had passed and the long warm nights invited the magic of a midsummer's eve. We can draw another connection to Chinese medicine here, with the element of Fire associated with the summer season. This is the season we nourish the heart and support joy in our lives.

At Sacred Plant Traditions, this is the time of year when our students travel and camp at Robbie Wooding's two-hundred-year-old family farm. This is a yang time of year; male energy is strong and we witness the accomplishments of five generations stewarding this land. St. John's wort (*Hypericum perforatum*) is in bloom and students learn about this medicinal herb as the plant that embodies the light of the sun. Midsummer is also known as St. John's Day, hence the name St. John's wort. The seasonal cycles take on deeper meaning as we learn more about the energetics of medicinal plants. St. John's wort can only be tinctured or steeped in oil when the plant material is freshly harvested, and thus our apothecary practices connect us with the meaning of ceremonies of long ago.

Lughnasadh/Lammas

Traditionally, Celtic people regarded August 1 as the day of the first harvest festival. This is the time of year when baskets are brimming with late summer berries, gardens are full of a wide range of vegetables and herbs and flowers, and grains grow heavy in the fields. This festival put the emphasis on games and matchmaking activities as the burdens of an agricultural life seemed a bit lighter once the harvest was in. Even though grocery stores and farmers' markets provide many of us with fresh produce for most, if not all, of the year, this period of summer is still a joyous and appropriate time to give thanks for the harvest.

Mabon/Autumn Equinox

At the autumnal equinox, a time of equal length of day and night, there is a last opportunity to check the stored harvest in the pantry, root cellar, and freezer to make sure all that is needed for the winter has been collected. This equinox, which takes place around September 21, is also a time when many field medicines are ripe for harvest, and herbalists begin noting root plants we wish to harvest later on. This may also be a time to gather seeds and store them for next year's planting.

In Chinese medicine, autumn is the season to honor grief. All of nature seems to be slowly returning to the earth to begin the descent into winter. When we honor grief and tend our lungs by doing fall cleansing, we prepare for the colder months ahead. Author Martín Prechtel beautifully states, "If we do not grieve what we miss, we do not praise what we love."[2] I have found that releasing grief for what we have lost is a beautiful way to honor ancestors with less sadness and more joy.

Our lives are so enriched when we step beyond the walls of our homes and routines and realize there is a rich and meaningful world the plants are calling us to engage with. No matter the region one lives, there are subtle and not-so-subtle teachings and whisperings from the tides of the seasons. The seasons are the ebb and flow created by the movement of the stars, planets, and heavens above. These celebrations may not hold resonance with you, but within us all are the stirrings of nature and the power of the transforming energies each season holds. This is our quest as plant lovers and medicine makers as we look for ways to listen to the ancestors and honor them with new and meaningful ceremonies and bring that into our apothecaries. Sharon Blackie speaks for us all, on whatever lands we may be inhabiting: "And we're finding those answers in the wisdom which all the old stories tell us can be found on the fringes, in the forest, in the wild thickets of the ancient hedge. In the rich and diverse native wisdom traditions of these islands—that deep ancestral lineage which is our inheritance. It's time to reclaim those traditions, and weave them into an authentic, grounded practice for very different times."[3]

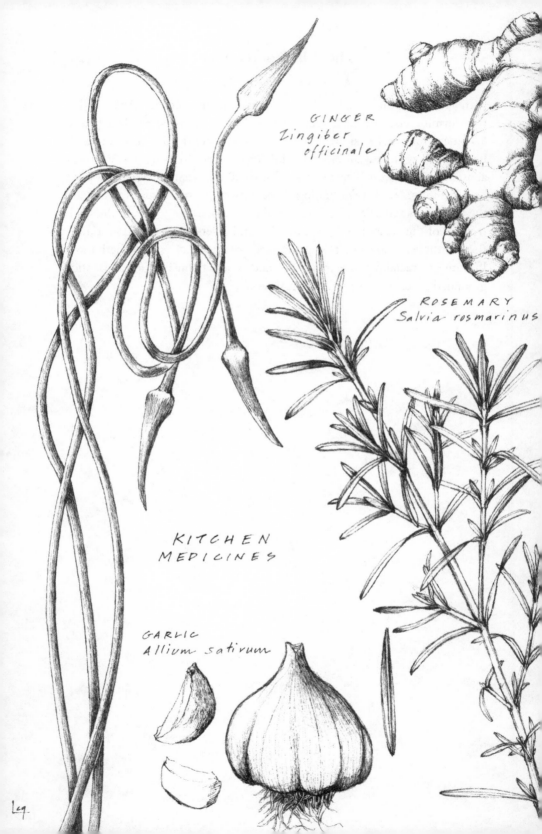

GINGER
Zingiber
officinale

ROSEMARY
Salvia rosmarinus

KITCHEN
MEDICINES

GARLIC
Allium sativum

CHAPTER 8

Kitchen Apothecary Practices

O ne of the best kept secrets is that most kitchens already have the makings of a fine home apothecary. Ordinary cooking spices such as salt, pepper, cinnamon, ginger, thyme, and garlic are the foundations of an herbal medicine cabinet. When anxious parents call me in the middle of the night to ask what to do for a child suffering from pink eye, I start by asking whether they have rosemary in their spice rack. If they say yes, I tell them to rub some of the leaves between their fingers. As long as they can smell the classic rosemary scent, then the essential oils are still present, even if the herb is several years old. These volatile oils have the power to clear heat (pink = heat) and infection. I then tell them to make a compress to gently apply over the eyes. Ginger powder is another gem that retains its potency. Even ten-year-old culinary ginger can make a paste so warming and stimulating that it brings blood to the most congested sinuses and clears the accompanying migraine. The paste is applied over the sinuses on the cheekbones.

Using what is on hand, and having on hand what is useful, is another ancestral tradition we can learn from. Previous generations needed greater self-sufficiency as there was not the availability of stores, but good medicine practices are those that prepare us to have on hand what we need for a variety of situations. Aside from herbs on your spice rack and a few healing foods in your pantry, how many herbs are needed for a well-stocked home apothecary? The answer is unique for each person and family. With the explosion of information about herbal medicines online, we are all aware of the large number of plants to choose from. My approach to medicines, though, is not quantity but quality. The words of Svevo Brooks echo in my mind: Better to know forty uses of one plant than one use of forty plants.

All medicine making is ceremony. Whether you are in a field or in your kitchen, the more grateful and focused you are as you work, the more the plant will gift you its medicine. My first teacher of medicine making was Susun Weed. Her Wise Woman tradition was perfect for me because I had just graduated from my allopathic medical training and I was conditioned to follow long lists of rules and regulations and to put limits on what one could expect with healing. Susun provided a teaching that miracles can and do happen when we deeply nourish. Allopathic medicine has so little to offer depleted and exhausted patients. From Susun, I learned the art of simpling—working with one herb at a time rather than a blend of plants. This approach makes herbal medicine so accessible.

In most cases, medicine making involves creating extractions, which simply means a preparation that pulls out the plant's medicinal components into a liquid medium called the *menstruum*. A tea is a water extraction, a tincture is an alcohol or vinegar extraction, and an herbal oil is an oil extraction. Each plant has a preferred menstruum depending on its constituents as well as energetics. After a plant has soaked in a menstruum and the liquid is strained off, the plant material left behind is called the *marc*.

One important practical note about making medicines. For any medicine you plan to store, even for a short time, label the container with the date on which the medicine was made, the source of plant material (wholesale/retail company or location harvested), and the type of menstruum (including the percent alcohol for alcohol-based tinctures).

Kitchen Herbs

Common kitchen herbs such as rosemary and ginger have been some of my most loved and used herbal allies. Every kitchen apothecary deserves these tried and true medicines. These are some of the first herbs I go to when I need an herbal hand. I mention them here, rather than including them in the materia medica in chapter 9, because so much wonderful information is easily available about these herbs. All of the kitchen herbs discussed below (except cinnamon) can be grown in most locales, even in containers on an apartment windowsill or patio. While garlic might prefer to grow in a garden bed, I have known folks who grow it in containers on a city balcony with success.

Cayenne ❋ *Capsicum frutescens, C. annuum*

This red-hot spice needs no introduction, but there are so many medicinal uses of cayenne that it deserves our attention. A South American native that was taken to Europe, its use spread rapidly, as its qualities were immediately appreciated. It has earned a reputation as a cure-all—its ability to enhance blood flow addresses so many issues. When used in hot, tropical climes, this stimulant moves blood so well that it actually cools the body as it brings blood to the surface. Dr. John R. Christopher, founder of The School of Natural Healing, used it quite successfully for cases of angina. Although angina is a very serious condition, in an emergency situation, this herb taken directly in powder form in water or tincture directly under the tongue, can stimulate circulation while medical help is being sought. It can stanch bleeding if used topically but it will create a burning sensation. This is one of the easiest garden plants to grow and you will be stringing them or giving them away before you know it.

Chamomile ❋ *Matricaria chamomilla, M. recutita*

While not generally considered a culinary herb, chamomile offers so many benefits that every kitchen should have a supply on hand. As a digestive bitter, chamomile is excellent for all types of digestive complaints. It is calming and soothing for inflammation. It contains antioxidants, and thus a cup of chamomile tea is a general healthful beverage. Applying a tea bag on a sty or inflamed wound is a great antimicrobial as well as astringent. *Matricaria chamomilla* (also called *Matricaria recutita*) is the preferred medicinal species rather than Roman chamomile (*Chamaemelum nobile*).

Cinnamon ❋ *Cinnamomum cassia, C. verum*

This warm, pungent, aromatic bark is a wonderful stimulant for digestion as well as circulation. Traditionally, the cooler months were greeted with the aroma of cinnamon added to cooked fruits or added to milk as a warming, relaxing sleep tonic. Such a common kitchen spice, yet a complex and revered medicine. There are actually two types of cinnamon to consider. *Cinnamomum cassia*, or Cassia cinnamon, is the most common one we find in commercial spices and is pungent and spicier. *C. verum* (also known as *C. zeylanicum*) is considered the preferred cinnamon and has the common name of Ceylon cinnamon. This variety is sweeter. Research shows that consumption of either bark increases the production of insulin by the pancreas, thus lowering blood sugar for type 2 diabetes. If you plan to take larger quantities, such as ½ teaspoon of bark powder two to three times a day for medicinal purposes, it is best to work with Ceylon cinnamon. No matter which species, though, sprinkling cinnamon into tea blends, coffee, and rice dishes is a healthy way to spice up our lives. This spice is wonderful in savory dishes as well, especially winter soups.

Garlic ✳ *Allium sativum*

Garlic is a veritable apothecary in itself. Best known for its antimicrobial action, garlic has been seen to clear deep-seated infections. *Allium* is warming, pungent, and drying, so it is perfect for damp, cold congestion. To get the benefit of its antimicrobial actions, though, it's necessary to eat garlic raw or very close to raw. A favorite method is to mince a clove (if you have never eaten raw garlic, start with a small amount and work your way up) and add that to a teaspoon of honey. The honey also is a medicine and it protects the stomach if the heat of garlic is too upsetting. While the odor of garlic on the breath can be bothersome to others, it is evidence that the volatile oil has reached the lungs and the medicine is doing its work. This food strongly transforms and expels damp stagnation from the lungs and digestive tract.

As a cooking spice, garlic is wonderful for digestion; it even contains inulin, a prebiotic that is necessary for good intestinal flora. The myth that eating too much garlic can wipe out gut flora is just that—a myth. Unless, of course, you consume several entire bulbs in one session! Garlic works as an amphoteric for balancing high and low blood pressure. Aged garlic capsules can be effective for treating this condition, but the preferred form for most other applications is as a food, preferably fresh.

Ginger ✳ *Zingiber officinale*

This is usually the first herb I reach for when I feel a cold or flu coming on. Fresh ginger is one of the most important herbs in Chinese medicine for treatment of wind cold in patients with tissue depression or weak defensive energy (feeling run down). Dried ginger is hotter and more intense, so I freeze organic fresh ginger. It keeps well frozen for at least six months, so it's a good method for ensuring you always have some fresh herb available. If the root is large, break it into smaller pieces and place in a well-sealed container. Ginger root is very easy to peel and grate when it is frozen. (Peeling is not necessary if it is organic.) Many healing herbs are cool in nature, and adding ginger to a blend warms up the formula. The addition of fresh or dried ginger to a formula keeps the herbs in the system longer as well, helping to be sure the medicine permeates to the extremities. Dried ginger powder makes an excellent paste to apply to sinuses or areas of the body you want to warm. Be mindful that it will bring blood quickly (desired action) and that you may need to take off the paste in 10 to 20 minutes. To make a paste simply add a small amount of warm water slowly to powder, mix well, and when the consistency is right, apply to the face near the cheekbones.

Ginger is possibly best known for reducing nausea of morning sickness, motion sickness, or nausea arising after consuming a heavy meal. Ginger works by warming the stomach, which settles queasy feelings. As an acrid herb, it reduces spasms internally and externally. There is nothing so divine as a fresh ginger bath. Make a very strong ginger tea by grating half a fresh ginger root into a two-quart pan, add cool water, bring to a boil, then simmer for an hour. Strain this, add to bathwater, then slip into a warm, relaxing realm. Ginger deeply penetrates tense muscles.

Rosemary ※ *Salvia rosmarinus*

Rosemary is one of my favorite herbs for stimulating circulation and carrying other herbs to the sites where they are needed. Rosmarinic acid is the compound that makes this revered Mediterranean spice a powerful antioxidant and anti-inflammatory. (Rosmarinic acid is also found in many other plants.) Rosemary is a wonderful stimulating tea for enhancing memory, alertness, and for clearing headaches. It is a strong-tasting herb, so blend well with other herbs, or you can make a tea rather than a strong infusion. It is my go-to remedy to clear pink eye as well as skin infections. It works particularly well for thrush and fungal infections. *Rosmarinus*, rose of the sea, makes a beautiful, aromatic topical oil for chest congestion. Its antioxidant properties are seen in the way this wonderful ally lasts and keeps its potency in our spice racks.

Sage ※ *Salvia officinalis*

Sage is an unsung heroine of our spice cabinets. This lack of favor might be due to its astringent taste, but this plant held center stage in ancient times. Its power is evident even in its name—*salvia* means "to save" in Greek. This culinary herb is so drying that nursing mothers are advised to use this tea if they want to cease milk production. This same astringing power makes this my number one remedy in working with sore, swollen throats. I use it in a throat spray, a gargle, or a tea with honey and lemon. Used as a mouth rinse, sage is wonderful for all inflammation of gums and the mouth. Highly aromatic, sage contains antioxidants and other compounds that support immune function when working against microbes. As the name implies, it has been used for centuries with elders to promote memory and cognitive health.

Thyme ❋ *Thymus vulgaris*

One of the easiest culinary plants to cultivate, this humble, low-growing herb is one of the hottest and most penetrating of spices. Thyme is a very powerful medicine for all kinds of infections but especially those in the respiratory and digestive systems. Due to its intensity, it is the perfect remedy for cold, thick, phlegmatic bronchial conditions. As a specific for whooping cough, this medicine is coming back into the limelight in a time when antibiotic-resistant strains are challenging our immune systems. As a topical, thyme is wonderful for clearing fungal infections as well as wet, oozing skin conditions. A favorite steam inhalation is a blend of thyme, sage, and rosemary.

Harvesting and Drying Herbs

When deciding the best season for harvesting a particular herb, simply think about where the energy resides in the plant. In the winter, roots are dormant, which actually means they are storing energy for new growth. In the spring as leaves unfurl, energy rises skyward to increase surface area of foliage for optimal photosynthesis. Flower formation requires a tremendous amount of energy; flowers express sexuality and reproduction and are the creators of the seeds that will ensure proliferation of the species.

Although timing of harvesting varies somewhat by region, here are some general guidelines:

- If you want to harvest leaf medicine, it is best to gather before the plant flowers.
- When harvesting flowers, gather blossoms just before or at full flower.
- Gather seeds after they have turned from green to maturity, but do not wait too long because the oils and medicine in them can dissipate.
- For roots, harvest after the second frost. The first frost alerts all above-ground parts of the plant to drop into the root for winter storage. After the second frost most of the plant energy has moved into the

root. If you live in a region where temperatures do not drop below freezing, harvest the root when the plant is in its most dormant state.

For all aboveground plant parts, it is best to wait to harvest until after 10 a.m., or after the dew has evaporated and before the intense heat of the day wilts the plant. Harvesting after a series of sunny days is ideal because it makes drying the harvested plant parts that much easier.

Drying herbs is an art and a wonderful skill to learn. Start simple and with small quantities. Hanging herbs in bundles is the traditional method. It is important to provide good airflow; on humid days, set up a fan to keep air moving. One method I've used is to throw a sheet on the floor of a spare room and lay out the herbs on the sheet. Once a day, I shake the sheet to turn over the stems, flowers, or leaves. Plants that contain a lot of water, such as comfrey, are the most challenging to dry. If you see black spots on leaves or tell-tale fuzzy growth, those are signs of mold. Simply break off those parts of the leaves, as the rest is still good for use.

A warm attic is ideal for drying herbs. Be mindful, though, that too much heat will crisp the material, which speeds up deterioration of constituents. Using a food dehydrator to dry herbs works well, as does using an oven (the very low heat provided by the pilot light serves well for drying herbs).

There's nothing sadder than losing a harvest because you moved herbs into storage too soon. You want the leaves to crumble when you rub them between your fingers, but you don't want them too crisp. A tried-and-true test of whether herbs are ready to be stored is to put a small amount of the dried herb in a mason jar and screw the lid on tight. If there is still moisture in the herb, condensate will form on the wall of the jar in a day or two. If this happens, continue drying and test again.

Those fortunate enough to have a greenhouse can try this very rapid method of drying described by seasoned herb farmers Andrea and Matthias Reisen from Healing Spirits Herb Farm in New York State: "The high shelves we use for the herbs that have less water in them, Nettle, Red Raspberry, Alfalfa then the lower shelves that have more shade from the upper shelves, for Comfrey, Mints, Lemon Balm, also Roses and Calendula so they don't lose any of their color. We turn the herbs during the day so the underside also gets dry faster. Drying this way, we can usually move herbs through in twenty-four to thirty-six hours. Roots take longer of course. Because we are in Western New York we do not use a shade cloth, like you would in an area that gets hotter sun."[1]

Water Extractions:
Teas, Infusions, Syrups

Even before the discovery of fire, people made herbal teas. This form of medicine is universal and is still the most commonly employed and enjoyed form of herbal remedy today. The beauty of this method is that it costs nothing to prepare. All you need is a container, water, a source of plants, and heat (and heat is not always required). Always best to drink teas at room temperature unless you are trying to warm up from a chill or from being out in the cold. Water has the ability to extract nutrients and constituents that are not soluble in oil or alcohol. It is also a great medium for extracting chlorophyll from plant tissues, and chlorophyll has blood building and cleansing properties. Mucopolysaccharides give up their medicine best in water, so a water-based remedy is the best way to prepare most mucilaginous plants. Minerals such as calcium for nerve and bone health are also more available when extracted in water. For many minerals, though, extracting in herbal vinegars can be the best method.

Teas or Tisanes

Technically speaking, *tea* refers to a beverage made from the tea plant, *Camellia sinensis*. This includes white, green, black, and oolong teas. *Tisanes* are what are better known in the herb world as herbal teas. These serve as a beverage for enjoyable consumption and are not used for deep healing, but are medicinal nonetheless. In this chapter, and throughout this book, whenever I use the word *tea*, I am usually referring to an herbal infusion.

Everyone knows how to make a cup of tea, don't they? But just to be thorough, here's how I brew herbal tea.

1. Place 1 tea bag or 1 teaspoon loose tea in a cup or mug.
2. Add 1 cup boiling water.
3. Steep 10 to 15 minutes covered.
4. Strain, if loose tea is used, and drink and enjoy.

Infusions

Infusions are strong medicinal brews that call for using more plant material and a longer steeping time than for beverage teas. I usually prepare infusions in a pint or quart-size glass jar; the dose is commonly two to four cups a day. Some herbs will produce an infusion that is too bitter

Teas: Pros and Cons

Advantages

- Prime source of nutrients and minerals
- Affordable and materials are easily attainable
- Preferable for children, those with sensitivity to alcohol, and those who choose not to use vodka or other liquors
- Can be drunk daily
- Can be delicious, unless the called-for medicine is bitter (and you can even learn to love a bitter tea)

Disadvantages

- Takes time to brew and strain
- Difficult to make while traveling
- Short window of use; most teas should be consumed within twenty-four hours of brewing; if refrigerated, most remain good for forty-eight hours
- May not be palatable, especially if dosage is high

or sour for drinking if steeped longer than an hour. Chamomile and sage are more palatable with shorter (fifteen to twenty minutes) brew times. While the taste of an infusion is definitely part of the medicine, when drinking nourishing brews such as borage (*Borago officinalis*), nettle (*Urtica dioica*), and oats (*Avena sativa*), it is fine to add your preferred flavor such as mint (*Mentha* spp.), lemongrass (*Cymbopogon citratus*), or roselle (*Hibiscus sabdariffa*). It is always important to cover a steeping infusion so the volatile oils are not lost when hot water is added to the plant material. When working with fresh plant material it is important to chop very well and to let sit longer than dried since the cell walls are still intact and the medicine is not as easily accessible.

Hot Water Infusions

Some herbalists call for an ounce of plant material per quart of water to make an infusion. I find that quantity to be more than what is needed, and oftentimes requiring this amount can make infusions' cost prohibitive. As a rule of thumb, when making infusions, use 1 tablespoon dried plant material per cup water; for fresh plant material, use 3 tablespoons per cup water. Here are basic instructions for making an infusion:

1. Add plant material to a wide mouth glass jar.
2. Add boiling water.
3. Cap with lid and steep 1 hour for flowers and leaves, 4 hours for roots, barks, and seeds.
4. Decant (pour off) the liquid from the plant material. Squeeze the plant material with your hands or with muslin cloth to remove as much liquid as possible.
5. Compost the marc (herb matter that has been steeped). If desired, rewarm the liquid and then add honey to taste if so desired.

Cold Water Infusions

Cold water infusions are useful when working with highly mucilaginous herbs such as comfrey (*Symphytum officinale*) and marshmallow (*Althaea officinalis*) because the mucopolysaccharides are more soluble in water. Using cold water with herbs high in tannins such as uva ursi (*Arctostaphylos uva ursi*) is also a good strategy because it allows for extraction of arbutin, which is good medicine for bladder infections.

Follow the same steps as when making a hot infusion, but allow the plant material to steep overnight. After straining off the liquid in the morning, it can be rewarmed if the demulcent tea is more palatable to you warm, or these teas can be drunk at room temperature. One of the most effective cold infusions is fenugreek seed tea (*Trigonella foenum-graecum*), which helps to ease hot flashes or increase mother's milk flow.

Decoctions

An herbal decoction is made by boiling herbs, and this method works well for plant material that is dense and fibrous, such as with roots, seeds, and barks. Because of the hardness of the material, more energy (heat) is required to extract its constituents. Decoctions, along with infusions, are possibly the most traditional forms of herbal medicine. Decoctions are also the method used for making syrups. It is always best to start with cold water. In *The Herbal Medicine-Maker's Handbook*, herbalist James Green explains why: "If the herb is immersed in boiling water, the albumin contained in cells will possibly coagulate at once and can interfere significantly with the extraction of the other constituents."[2]

1. Place 8 heaping tablespoons of dried herbs into a stainless steel or glass cooking pot.
2. Add 1 quart of water.
3. Bring to a low boil then reduce heat and simmer for 20 minutes.
4. Decant plant material and drink recommended dosage. Decoctions are usually stronger than infusions so it is recommended that only 1 or 2 cups be drunk per day. Store any remaining decoction in the refrigerator for up to 2 days.

Syrups

A syrup, or electuary, is essentially a (strong or reduced) decoction preserved with a sweetener. Before the days of refrigeration, making syrups was a way to extend the shelf life of water-based medicines. The ratio of sugar to decoction is one cup sugar to one cup liquid. This is the amount needed to prevent spoilage. Today, herbalists use honey and maple syrup as well as raw sugar when making syrup. Syrups are a wonderful preparation method to use with bitter-tasting herbs such as horehound (*Marrubium vulgare*) and boneset (*Eupatorium perfoliatum*), and honey serves to soothe inflamed throats.

Even when I use honey, I find most syrup recipes too sweet because I love the tartness of berries and I want to be able to taste the herbs. To make up for the lost preservation power when I use less sweetener, I add a bit more alcohol, which is standard for preserving syrups. I prefer brandy for this purpose when making a cough syrup because brandy also has a relaxing effect. Syrups can be stored on the counter for one week and in the refrigerator for up to three months. I include instructions below for a few syrups made using common healing foods. These syrups can serve not only as medicines but as condiments to be used daily for health as well as prevention of colds, flu, and other common ailments. The recipes for elderberry elixir and garlic elixir are from herbalist Suzanna Stone, a staff member at Sacred Plant Traditions who specializes in teaching ferments, oxymels, and fermented beverages.

Elderberry Syrup

There are many possible variations of elderberry syrup (*Sambucus canadensis, S. nigra*), so be creative!

1. Place 2 cups dried elderberries and 1 quart cold water in a pot and bring to a low boil. Use a chopstick as a "dipstick" to measure the level of the liquid in the pan.
2. Turn down heat to simmer and add other herbs, such as ginger, cinnamon, or cloves (*Syzygium aromaticum*), as desired for flavor as well as to add a warming quality.
3. As the liquid simmers, recheck the level occasionally with the chopstick.
4. When the liquid has been reduced by half, remove from heat, and decant the liquid from the marc.
5. Let cool slightly, and add ¼ to ½ cup honey to sweeten, as well as brandy (1 teaspoon per 3–4 ounces syrup) as a preservative if desired. Cap tightly and label.

Simple Onion Syrup

Onion syrup is excellent taken by the teaspoon to soothe respiratory infections and ease congestion. It also makes a great addition to salad dressings and winter dishes.

1. Place 1 cup roughly chopped fresh onion in a pint jar with a small handful of fresh or dried sage, rosemary, or thyme. If desired, you can also add the juice from half a lemon or 1 teaspoon freshly grated ginger root.
2. Add enough honey to cover the onion and herbs.
3. Cap tightly and label.
4. Let sit overnight. The honey will very effectively absorb all the juice out of the onion.

The syrup will be ready for use in the morning. Some people like to eat the onion bits along with the honey, others prefer to strain out the solids. All I know is this syrup does not last long around my house!

Elderberry Elixir

This flavorful elixir can be added to other tinctures or teas or taken by itself. A preventative dose is 1 tablespoon per day.

1. Fill a glass jar half full with equal parts dried elderberries and honey.
2. Add 80 proof brandy to fill the jar to the brim.
3. Use a chopstick or similar implement to release any air bubbles trapped in the liquid.
4. Cap tightly, label, and let sit in a cool dark place for 6 to 8 weeks.

Basic Herbal Honey for Fresh Aromatic Plants

This is an excellent food/medicine for sore, inflamed throats and irritating coughs. Fresh plant aromatics are beautifully released into the honey. Some great choices for flavoring a honey are ginger, rosemary, sage, holy basil (*Ocimum tenuiflorum*), bee balm (*Monarda* spp.), mints, and garlic. Have fun experimenting! Honey is antimicrobial but if you use fresh plant material, that will introduce water and possibly a range of microbes into the honey. Surprisingly, in my experience this has not negatively impacted the honey or made it turn bad, but if you are concerned about spoilage, simply store the herbal honey in the refrigerator.

1. Fill a dry glass jar with coarsely chopped fresh herbs.
2. Cover herbs with honey.
3. Stir with chopstick to be sure all plant material is coated with honey.
4. Fill jar to the top with honey.
5. Use a chopstick or similar implement to release air bubbles trapped in the honey.
6. Cap tightly and label. Let sit for 2 to 4 weeks.
7. Strain out the herb material. You can use the herbs to make a delicious tea with honey-soaked herbs. Or, do not strain, and simply eat the honey with the herbs included.

If you want to make garlic honey, follow the instructions above, using whole unpeeled cloves. The sitting time for this honey is much shorter—it will be ready for use after 24 hours, and the leftover cloves will be delicious, too. You can eat them raw as they will be tempered by the extraction process or you can cook with them as usual.

Garlic Elixir

1. Fill a glass jar one-third full with equal parts chopped garlic and honey.
2. Fill up the jar with apple cider vinegar.
3. Use a chopstick or similar implement to release air bubbles trapped in the vinegar.
4. Cap tightly with a plastic lid, or use wax paper or plastic wrap under a metal lid to prevent corrosion.
5. Label the jar, and shake the jar to dissolve the honey in the vinegar.
6. Let sit in a cool, dark place for 2 to 4 weeks.

Flower Essences

Flower essences are infusions of flowers in water, preserved with brandy or vinegar, and they are vibrational medicines to treat our subtler energetics: our emotional selves. These remedies are profound medicines that treat on a vibrational level, much as homeopathic remedies do. While flower medicine has been used for centuries, the modern form originates with the work in the 1930s of the extraordinary British physician Dr. Edward Bach. Trained as a medical physician and homeopath, Dr. Bach came to see that the physical complaints of his patients were deeply rooted in their emotional and mental health. He left medical practice and devoted his life to developing thirty-eight Bach Flower Remedies, of which Rescue Remedy, used for shock and trauma, may be the most well-known. These essences help shift patterns of emotional, mental, and spiritual challenges.

According to Patricia Kaminski and Richard Katz, owners of Flower Essence Services in the foothills of Nevada City, California, "The fresh, dew-filled blossoms are gathered in the early morning of a clear, sunny day. Floating on the surface of a bowl of water, they are irradiated by the warmth and light of the sun for several hours. This process creates an energetic imprint of the etheric energy pattern of the flower in the water, embodying the healing archetype of that plant. This 'mother essence' is preserved with organic grape alcohol and then further diluted and potentized to form the 'stock' which is sold in stores and to practitioners."[3] Flowers that bloom at night or have special relationships to lunar aspects of healing can be left to infuse in the light of the full moon if possible. Some flower essence companies use vinegar as a preservative for those who do not wish to take alcohol. You can substitute apple cider vinegar for brandy in this recipe.

Here are basic instructions for making a flower essence:

1. Find a container for preparing the essence. It's best to use a clear bowl without writing or any images because flower essences are vibrational. Everything that comes into contact with the infusion will have an effect upon the preparation.
2. Gather the flower in the early morning as stated above. I use scissors and tweezers to do this because even touching the flower with the hand will impact the quality of the essence. Some folks gather a few flowers or fill the bowl with many flowers, but I usually feel that one is sufficient.

3. Fill the bowl with either distilled water or water that is as pure as is available. Carefully place the flower(s) in the water.

4. Allow the infusion to sit 4 to 6 hours in the sunlight. If the flower is a night-blooming species, leave it out in light of the full moon if possible (rather than in sunlight).

5. Pour the infused water into a bottle that will hold twice the amount of water you used. Add half the amount of brandy to the flower infused water. This is called the mother tincture.

6. In another bottle, usually an unused dropper bottle, add 80 percent water and 20 percent brandy. Then add 10 drops of the mother tincture. This can be further diluted in yet another bottle or used as is. Keep in mind that this is vibrational medicine—diluting the remedy will not make it weaker. The "imprint" of the flower will remain intact no matter the amount of the original preparation.

The recommended dosage for most flower essences is three to five drops as needed. Since flower essences are working with our subtle energetics and emotions, I recommend taking them first thing upon rising and last thing before going to sleep. It is also fine to take them at other times during the day if needed.

Alcohol Extractions: Tinctures

Many people are introduced to herbalism through the use of tinctures, those small amber bottles sold in health food stores. Tinctures are made by steeping (macerating) fresh or dried plant material in alcohol. From sacred ferments such as the ancient Mayan balche to Appalachian moonshine, herbs have been steeped and preserved in alcohol for centuries.

For most home apothecaries, vodka and brandy are the alcohols of choice, as these are generally easy to acquire. The percentage of alcohol needed to extract medicinal constituents varies by plant species. For example, marsh-mallow root and other demulcent, mucilaginous herbs are mostly water soluble, so these can be extracted using 20 to 30 percent alcohol (70 to 80 percent water): Most plants that are used in a home apothecary require a 40 to 65 percent alcohol to make an effective tincture. Gums and resins such as myrrh (*Commiphora myrrha*), or local propolis, must be extracted using grain alcohol or another high percentage alcohol. Milk thistle (*Silybum marianum*) seed also requires high-strength alcohol to break down the hard seed coat. Most commercial herbal product companies simply start with grain alcohol,

95 percent, then add water to dilute to the prescribed solubility. Susun Weed teaches that if you use 100 proof vodka, (which is a blend of 50 percent water and 50 percent ethanol), it will work well for the majority of herbs tinctured in home apothecaries. This makes life much simpler, and I have used 100 proof vodka for years with excellent results. (The percentage alcohol in a liquor is always half the proof. Subtract the percentage alcohol from 100 and that tells you the percent of water in the liquid.) Another popular menstruum is brandy, which is 80 proof or 40 percent alcohol and 60 percent water. Alcohol itself is an "herb" in that it has energetic qualities. Alcohol quickens the blood and slightly warms the interior in small doses and is dispersive, or moving.

Fresh plant material often requires 95 percent alcohol for satisfactory extraction results because of the high volume of water in the plant material itself. That said, I have made potent fresh-plant tinctures using 100 proof (50 percent alcohol) vodka as well as brandy. Usually if I do not have grain alcohol on hand, I will let the plant material sit and wilt for a day or two before extracting; that allows a lot of the water to evaporate. Skullcap (*Scutellaria lateriflora*) and St. John's wort flower (*Hypericum perforatum*) can only be tinctured fresh, so if I am traveling when I come upon this medicine, I make do with whatever alcohol is available.

Many home herbalists now work with higher percentage grain alcohols. The brand most commonly available is Everclear, but if you make a group order with friends for a large volume, you can purchase organic grape or cane alcohol for the same price as Everclear. The flavor of these alcohols is smoother than that of Everclear and seems to allow the essence of the herbs to come through. Some states require that you procure a license to buy grain alcohol, but others allow sales of grain alcohol directly to the public at liquor stores. There are some wonderful companies that offer organically produced spirits. Two of our favorites at Sacred Plant Traditions clinic are Alchemical Solutions and Glacial Grain Spirits. If there's a local distillery in your area, check with them to see what they offer and what you think of the quality of their products. You may be able to buy local!

The Folk Method—Keeping It Simple

This is a simple way to make a tincture that doesn't require precise measuring.

Tincturing Fresh Plant Material

As noted above, I recommend using 95 percent alcohol when extracting fresh plant material if possible, due to the high water content of fresh plants.

1. Fill a glass container to an inch below the rim with chopped fresh flowers or leaves. For fresh roots, barks, and seeds, chop well and fill jar half full with alcohol.
2. Cover the herb with alcohol.
3. If a blender is available, transfer herb/alcohol mixture to a blender and blend until all plant material is saturated with alcohol.
4. If blender is not available, use a chopstick or similar implement to release air bubbles trapped in the alcohol. Top off if needed.
5. Cap tightly and shake.
6. The next day, top off the container with more alcohol if needed. (Sometimes the plant material will absorb alcohol.) To prevent spoilage, it is important that there be no air in the container.
7. Let the container sit out on the counter, out of direct sunlight, for 4 to 6 weeks, and shake the container every other day.
8. Decant or pour off liquid through a strainer lined with cheesecloth. When all the liquid has dripped through, take up the cheesecloth with the plant material in it and wring it to get the last of the liquid. This is some of the best medicine, as it was in very close contact with the plant tissues.
9. Label the container, cap it tightly, and store it in a cool, dark place.

Tincturing Dried Plant Material

If you need tincture in a hurry, you can use powdered herbs and follow the instructions below, but allow the herbs to steep for only 2 weeks.

1. Add dried plant material to a glass jar. For dried leaves, fill the jar one-half to two-thirds full. For fluffy leaves, three-quarters full. For dried roots, barks, and seeds, fill the jar one-third full.
2. Completely fill the jar with alcohol.
3. Cap the jar tightly and shake.
4. Use a chopstick or similar implement to release air bubbles trapped in alcohol. Top off if needed.
5. The following morning, top off with more alcohol as needed. Completely cover the plant material with alcohol to prevent spoilage; it is important that there be no air in the container.
6. Let the container sit out on the counter, out of direct sunlight, for 4 to 6 weeks, and shake the container every other day.
7. Decant or pour off liquid through a strainer lined with cheesecloth. When all the liquid has dripped through, take up the cheesecloth with

the plant material in it and wring it to get the last of the medicine. If working with powdered herb, it's best to run it through a coffee filter.

8. Cap the container, label it, and store it in a cool, dark place.

Weight-to-Volume Tincturing

In clinic, we use a tincturing method called the weight-to-volume method. Most dry herbs are tinctured at a 1:5 ratio: one part of herb by weight steeped in five parts of menstruum or alcohol by volume. Each ounce of herb is extracted into 5 fluid ounces of menstruum. For example, 2 ounces of dried echinacea root would be steeped in 10 fluid ounces of 60 percent alcohol.

The ratio is important because it governs the strength of the tincture. Most tinctures prepared in clinics and in some home apothecaries are made using a ratio of 1:3, up to 1:5. A 1:1 tincture, the strongest extract one can make, is called a fluid extract. It is much more concentrated than a typical dry plant tincture. Because there is a large amount of plant material relative to menstruum, a different kind of extraction process is required. Percolation is an effective method; this method is described well in *The Modern Herbal Dispensatory*.[4]

If you buy a commercially prepared tincture, be sure to read the label in order to know how to dose. The stronger the medicine (e.g., 1:1), the smaller the dose. Most professional and commercial companies use grain alcohol or 95 percent then dilute to the proper level, usually 1:3 or 1:5.

Lorna Mauney-Brodek teaches medicine making at our clinic and serves as a mentor at our free Botanica Mobile Clinic. Lorna is founder of Herbalista, a nonprofit located in the Atlanta area that educates on all aspects of plant medicine, from urban farming to Pay-It-Forward Medicine-Making classes. The Herbalista Foot Clinic at the Harriet Tubman Center has served as a model of foot clinics around the world. Lorna believes that for the unhoused, their feet are their home. Her offerings of recipes, instructions, and guidelines to herbalists through the Herbalista website are vast. She has graciously shared her instructions for preparing tinctures using the weight-to-volume method. (See "Weight-to-Volume Method.")

A note of caution if you are working with people who are in recovery or have issues with alcohol. Some sources recommend adding boiling water to a tincture and letting it sit for 20 minutes to burn off the alcohol. For those who simply prefer to not be able to taste the alcohol, that practice is fine. But for those with allergies to alcohol or those struggling with alcoholism,

(continued on page 203)

Weight-to-Volume Method

by Lorna Mauney-Brodek

This is a standardized method that takes at least one of the variables out of plant medicines. And how many lovely variables still remain (growing conditions such as sun, rain, and soil, etc.). To do this method you will need both a scale (preferably measuring to the tenth of an ounce) and a measuring cup (at least 16-ounce size). This method utilizes a ratio where the left side represents the amount of herb by weight and the right side shows the menstruum by liquid volume. Commonly used ratios are 1:2 when working with fresh herbs and 1:5 when working with dried herbs. Whatever the weight of your herb, you will multiply that by the right side of the ratio to determine how much menstruum to use. See examples below.

Dry herbs, 1:5. 1 part dry herb by weight to 5 parts menstruum by volume. For example: I have 2 ounces dried chamomile. 2 × 5 = 10. I will need 10 fluid ounces of menstruum.

Fresh herbs, 1:2. 1 part fresh herb by weight to 2 parts menstruum by volume. For example: I have 4 ounces fresh *Pedicularis canadensis*. 4 × 2 = 8. I will need 8 fluid ounces of menstruum.

If you find that the menstruum does not cover the herb, you will need to add more. Be sure to measure out the menstruum you add and change your ratio to reflect the additional menstruum. It is helpful to add your additional menstruum in "parts."

For example, in the chamomile scenario above, if you needed more fluid to cover the herb, you would add 2 fluid ounces at a time (whatever the weight of your herb was). Each time you poured in 2 more fluid ounces; you would increase the right side 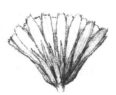 of your ratio by 1. The first additional 2 fluid ounces would take the ratio from 1:5 to 1:6. If you added 2 additional parts, then it would become 1:7, and so on. You do have the option of adding in half parts as well.

Fresh Plant

This method for extracting fresh plant macerations using undiluted alcohol (95 percent) is based on the guidelines established in 1902 at the "Conference Internationale pour l'Unification de la Formule des Medicaments Heroiques" that took place in Brussels, Belgium. The protocol agreed upon at this conference was made official in the *US Pharmacopoeia VIII* in 1906. In order to extract plant constituents through a still functional plant cellular wall you need absolute alcohol. If your menstruum percentage is lower than that, it lacks the pulling power.

- Tincture fresh plant at a ratio of 1:2 with undiluted (190 proof / 95 percent) alcohol.
- No shaking is necessary, as extraction is based on the principle of dehydration.
- Packing style: Since no room to shake is needed, you can pack the jar to the brim. This method allows the cap to act as a barrier holding the plant material down in the menstruum, saving you from adding more menstruum (further diluting your preparation) to ensure your herb is fully submerged during extraction.
- How do you know how much herb and menstruum will fit into a jar? Add your parts together and divide the size of your jar by that number (i.e., if doing a 1:2 ratio, add 1 + 2 = 3; divide the size of your jar by 3) to determine the amount of herb to use. Here is an example for fresh sage (1:2, 95 percent) with a 16-ounce jar:

Herb. $16 \div 3 \approx 5.3$. Weigh out 5.3 ounces fresh sage.
Menstruum. $5.3 \times 2 = 10.6$. Measure 10.6 fluid ounces 95 percent alcohol.

- When using leafy material, don't pack in all of the herb at once. First, pack half into the jar, then add half of the alcohol. Press and poke out the air bubbles. Continue to add herb and alcohol until filled to the brim. Cap and label. After 2 weeks, strain and compost the marc.

Tinctures: Pros and Cons

Advantages

- Easy and convenient
- Longest shelf life of any extraction
- Effective for acute situations
- Excellent for more potent botanicals because you can control dosing more effectively
- Superior extraction for alkaloids, resins, and oils
- Good for elders, who may have weaker digestion
- Efficient extraction for bitter, warm, aromatic, and blood-moving herbs

Disadvantages

- Not as nutritive because minerals and immune constituents are more soluble in water than in alcohol
- Not safe for those who have issues with or sensitivity to alcohol
- Can be cost prohibitive if using long term, unless made for oneself or purchased in bulk

this technique is not recommended. Alcohol addiction can be a chemical sensitivity that has nothing to do with willpower. In these circumstances, the boiling water method is not reliable enough to remove all traces of alcohol from a tincture. It is simply not worth the risk when there are so many other forms of plant medicines available.

Glycerin Extracts

Glycerin is a sweet, syrupy, odorless liquid derived from plants through hydrolysis of various plant oils. Glycerin does not extract herbs as deeply as alcohol, but there are benefits to its use. Glycerites (medicinal preparations made using glycerin as the menstruum) are wonderful for children who are just getting used to herbal tastes and do not need strong medicines. For those who are sensitive or unable to use alcohol, glycerites can be very helpful, especially when there is not time to prepare infusions. From my work with street medics, I have learned they may not have time to gather information from patients about alcohol use during a crisis situation; in such settings, glycerites are a safe and gentle choice. Because glycerin is not a sugar, it does not affect blood sugar negatively. The late herbalist Michael Moore taught that adding glycerin to a tincture (5 to 10 percent glycerin by volume) would reduce precipitation (separation) of alkaloids and tannins from the solution.

I find that for the best extraction it is necessary to use heat. My experience with glycerites is limited but the instructions in *The Modern Herbal Dispensatory* are very easy to follow and several wonderful instructional videos are available online. The shelf life of glycerites is up to three years if stored in a cool, dark environment.

Vinegar Extracts

A bottle of organic apple cider vinegar (ACV) can be a medicine cabinet in and of itself. Vinegar is derived from the French phrase *vin aigre* which means "sour wine." At the bottom of a bottle of organic ACV rests what is called the "mother." This substance, which contains enzymes, proteins, and beneficial bacteria, is considered a prebiotic. The mother gives quality ACV its cloudy appearance.

Here are some of the benefits of ACV.

Antimicrobial. With a history as a natural disinfectant and preservative, acetic acid is effective in controlling spread of microbes.[5]

Topical anti-inflammatory. Applying diluted vinegar (1:3 vinegar to water ratio) to the skin is very cooling and astringing. A cloth soaked in diluted ACV is an excellent compress for sprains and strains.

Blood sugar reduction. ACV has been shown to raise insulin sensitivity and to assist in balancing blood sugar.[6] Drinking a glass of water with 2 tablespoons of ACV added shortly before sleep may assist in better sleep as it reduces fasting blood sugar levels.

Weight loss. I first learned about the health benefits of ACV from the classic book *Folk Medicine* by D. C. Jarvis, MD, a rural Vermont physician who inspired a whole generation of herbalists. Weight loss was a major topic in his book. There are no definitive studies on the relationship of ACV to weight loss, but it is hypothesized that ACV creates a greater sense of satiation, which encourages eating less.[7] Consumption of ACV has also been linked to improved metabolism.

Muscle cramps. Because it is high in potassium and helps with calcium absorption, ACV is helpful for muscle cramps, especially after workouts.
Clear sinuses and phlegm. Vinegar has the ability to thin mucus and help with sinus congestion and sore throats as well as digestive stagnation. The most effective recipe for clearing phlegm is fire cider vinegar (see the recipe on page 154).

Herbal vinegars are used mostly for cooking and dressings, but are also very effective medicinal extracts. Lobelia (*Lobelia inflata*) is one medicine that prefers to be tinctured in vinegar because it is high in alkaloids, and vinegars excel at extracting these constituents. Vinegar also enhances extraction of calcium and minerals from plants.

Our bodies need an acidic environment in the stomach in order to absorb calcium. Adding herbal vinegars to your daily diet is a wonderful practice for supporting digestive health and enhancing absorption of minerals. Here are instructions for making herbal vinegar. My favorite herbs to put in an herbal vinegar are nettle, chickweed (*Stellaria media*), rosemary, violet (*Viola* spp.), sage, and oregano (*Origanum vulgare*).

1. Fill a glass jar halfway with coarsely chopped fresh plant material. (You can use dried but fresh is preferable.)
2. Add organic apple cider vinegar to fill the jar to the brim.
3. Use a chopstick or similar implement to release air bubbles trapped in the vinegar.
4. Cap tightly with a plastic lid. If you don't have a plastic lid available, place parchment or wax paper up against the inner rim of a metal lid to prevent corrosion.
5. Label the container.
6. Shake daily for 2 to 4 weeks.

It is best to decant herbs from vinegar as you would other extracts if you do not plan to use the vinegar quickly. Many people like to replace the marc with a few sprigs of herbs for aesthetic purposes. If the taste of the fresh herbs is not strong enough you can repeat the extraction process with more fresh material.

Oxymel

Oxymels are wonderful tonics that are made simply by adding equal parts of honey and vinegar to herbs of your choice. These have been used for centuries as digestive tonics as well as elixirs to boost the immune system. Honey is very soothing to mucous membranes and vinegar helps break up phlegm, making oxymels especially useful for respiratory diseases.

1. Fill a glass jar one-quarter to one-third full of dried herbs.
2. Cover with equal parts honey and vinegar and mix well. It is best to first heat the honey slightly, which will make the mixture easier to blend.
3. Close tightly with a plastic lid. If you don't have a plastic lid available, place parchment or wax paper up against the inner rim of a metal lid to prevent corrosion.
4. Leave the jar in a cool dark place but not completely out of sight because it should be shaken every other day for 2 weeks.
5. Decant or strain liquid through a strainer lined with cheesecloth. When all the liquid has been pressed through, take up the cheesecloth with the plant material in it and wring it to get the last of the liquid. Compost marc.
6. Label and store oxymel in a cool, dark place. These preparations keep well for at least 6 months.

Powders

Making a powder is a simple process that does not require the steeping time that an extract does—you can have a finished product the same day. The only work is in powdering the herb. You can use a coffee mill to powder herbs, but mills often do not thoroughly powder material, especially if it is woody such as barks and roots. A Vitamix or similar high-speed blender is the optimum tool but also a very expensive one if you are not processing herbs often.

This method of preparing herbs is very convenient as long as the client doesn't mind the texture and flavor. Powders are generally mixed into some type of food that readily accepts a powder, such as peanut butter or other nut butter, yogurt, or applesauce. Some people just stir the powder into a glass of water and drink it down.

One drawback is that powders degrade in quality more quickly than tinctures, extracts, or any other type of herbal preparation. This is because so much surface area is exposed to air in a powder. The loss of quality is not rapid enough to be a concern when providing a small batch of a freshly made powder to a client, but it is a concern for clinical settings in terms of how much of a powdered herb to keep in stock at any given time. Another drawback is that powders are the hardest type of preparation to digest, especially powdered forms of roots, twigs, barks, and other woody material. This is because the powdering process does not remove any of the indigestible material. With powders, all of the "extraction" of medicinal components happens in the digestive tract. Adding ginger powder to a blend of powders can stimulate digestion and help with breakdown.

Capsules

Capsules are a convenient way to take herbs that avoids any issues with unpleasant taste, presence of alcohol, or the need to fiddle with liquids. There are two ways to make capsules. The simplest way is to powder the herb(s) and encapsulate them, and this is something that can be done fairly simply in a home kitchen or small clinic. The other method, which is usually carried out only by commercial herb product companies, is to extract the herb into a liquid, concentrate the liquid, and then dry it into a powder, which is then encapsulated. Capsules prepared in this way will have a higher concentration of medicinal components. This is important to remember when you are taking any herbal products in capsule form. Simple capsules prepared with hand-powdered herbs only are often only a fraction of what is considered the appropriate dose for many herbs and often this is not enough to be effective, especially if there are multiple herbs in the capsule. Dosage can be increased by increasing the number of capsules taken, but this can be discouraging because powders are difficult to digest. Encapsulated herbs can also be expensive, especially if you need to take several capsules per day.

Standardized Extracts

Making a standardized extract is not a kitchen apothecary practice. The process for making standardized extracts requires sophisticated techniques such as thin-layer chromatography (TLC) and high-performance liquid chromatography (HPLC), which essentially isolate pure compounds. These techniques bring about the chemical standardization of marker compounds (active ingredients) in botanicals and herbal preparations. The advantage of using standardized extracts is that you can monitor dosage with more precision, and thus anticipate a response with greater certainty. This is not foolproof. In some cases, studies of some medicinal herbs reveal that the desired therapeutic effect is not due solely to one constituent, but rather to a combination of compounds that work together to create an effect.

When taking standardized extracts it is best to work with a qualified practitioner who is familiar with botanical therapies because some of these have been found to have negative consequences. There are no long-term studies on the effects on the human body of ingesting isolated compounds in this form. While there can be immense benefit from taking these supplements, our goal as community practitioners is to ensure safety.

I have deeply appreciated working with the standardized extract of one of my favorite herbs, milk thistle. The seed of this superb liver herb requires a high percentage of alcohol for extraction, and I do not think daily use of grain alcohol is beneficial for the liver. Using a standardized extract allows me to offer clients the benefits of milk thistle without the alcohol. Milk thistle is also one of the most benign herbs; to my knowledge to date, there are no contraindications for its use, even for infants. Aside from this one herb, however, I am an ardent supporter of whole-plant medicine. I feel that it is the synergy and complementary actions of plant constituents as well as the plant spirit that makes a medicine effective.

External Applications

Poultices, compresses, and other methods for supplying medicines through external application to the body is where herbalism truly shines. Conventional modern medicine offers very few options to effectively treat injuries topically.

Simple Poultices

Poultices are applications of thickly packed herbs that are used to soothe inflammation, draw out toxins, or calm inflammation. A poultice is the most potent form of topical application because it allows for use of a large amount of herb to be placed directly on the skin. Examples are a plantain poultice for bee stings and a mullein leaf poultice for moving lymph. A traditional way to make a poultice was to thoroughly chew a wad of fresh plant material and then apply it directly to the skin over the area requiring treatment. Another way to make a poultice is to mix fresh plant material (or a powder of roots, branches, or bark) with some type of liquid to make a thick paste or slurry and heat the mixture long enough to "release" the herb. Here are the basic instructions:

1. Chop, grate, or mash fresh plant material.
2. Add enough hot water to rupture the cell walls of the plant material and make a paste. For dried herb or powders, add enough hot water to make a paste or plaster.

3. Apply the paste directly on the skin or fold it into a thin piece of cotton fabric and then place over the affected area.

4. Secure the poultice by covering it with a bandana or piece of gauze, or wrap with an ace bandage.

5. In most instances (except for mustard, onion, or other respiratory poultices—see below), leave the poultice in place until it dries. After a poultice dries, remove it and reapply a fresh one. Continue applications for 1 hour. Afterward, unwrap the area and compost the plant material.

Hot Poultices and Mustard Plasters

Onion and mustard plaster poultices are time-tested traditional recipes to bring circulation to the lungs. Enhanced blood flow brings immune components to the site of application and clears mucus. A beneficial side effect is that these poultices are deeply relaxing and help promote a good night's sleep. Onion poultices were used by practitioners in the United States and Europe to treat people suffering from COVID-19 with great success. The great relief brought about by this poultice is due to its ability to break up stagnation through its warmth and penetrating power.

Caution: Onion poultices and mustard plasters can be irritating to the skin, so the skin must be covered with a thin cloth before applying the poultice to prevent burning. It is not advisable to leave these remedies on for more than about 10 minutes without checking their effect on the skin underneath. For children and those with sensitive skin, be especially vigilant about checking the skin for increasing redness. If applying a poultice or plaster to yourself, make sure you set a loud timer in case you fall asleep. Even after all those warnings, the therapeutic value is impressive.

Raw Onion Poultice

Here are the steps in making a raw onion poultice:

1. Cut half a medium-sized onion into small pieces or mash it a bit with a pestle or large wooden spoon.

2. Place the onion mash in the middle of a tea towel. Gather and tie the corners of the towel to make a bundle.

3. Place the tea towel directly on the skin of the affected area.

4. Leave the poultice in place for 10 minutes, check the skin, then continue monitoring every 10 minutes, leaving poultice on for a total of 30 minutes.

Cooked Onion Poultice

Here are the steps for making a cooked onion poultice:

1. Peel two onions and cut into thin pieces.
2. Place the onion pieces in a pot containing a small amount of water or in a steamer. Gently cook or steam the onions for 4 to 5 minutes.
3. Scoop the onion pieces out of the water or steamer onto a tea towel or thin cotton cloth. Gather and tie the corners of the towel or cloth to make a bundle.
4. When the poultice is cool enough, apply it to the chest or back in the lung area. You can cover the poultice with a hot water bottle to hold in the heat, or allow it to naturally cool.
5. Check condition of the skin under the poultice every 10 minutes. Remove immediately if skin irritation is apparent. Otherwise, continue monitoring every 10 minutes and remove after 30 minutes.

Mustard Plaster

This time-honored plaster has been used for generations for serious lung congestion. It is deeply penetrating and must be checked every 5 minutes and not left on for more than 20 minutes. If you are applying this to yourself, set an alarm for every 5 minutes to check on skin and make sure you do not fall asleep. Despite this apparent drawback of mustard plasters, they are extremely effective in breaking up lung congestion by enhancing circulation and bringing immune components to infected tissues.

1. Mix 4 tablespoons flour or flax meal and 2 tablespoons dry mustard with enough lukewarm water to form a paste. The paste should be spreadable onto a cloth but not too runny, as this might stain bedsheets and linens.
2. Apply to half of a tea towel or cotton cloth. Fold over the other half to cover the paste.
3. Place the folded tea towel or cloth on the chest or back and cover it with a towel. Also pull up any blankets that are covering the person to promote warmth.
4. Every 5 minutes, check the skin underneath the tea towel. If the skin is becoming red or the person complains of a burning sensation, remove the plaster. In any case, remove the plaster after 20 minutes.
5. Wash off the skin with warm water.

A mustard plaster treatment can be repeated every 6 to 8 hours, making a fresh plaster each time.

Compresses or Fomentations

A compress or fomentation is very easy to use. Cloth material is dipped in an herbal infusion and applied to the body. Compresses can be applied cool or hot.

Hot Compress

A hot compress can also be covered with a hot water bottle. The heat will bring blood to the affected area, opening the pores and allowing the medicated compress to have a greater effect. Here are basic preparation instructions.

1. Prepare a strong herbal infusion, making sure the volume of tea is sufficient for soaking a cloth large enough to cover the affected area of the body.
2. Dip the cloth in the hot/warm infusion, and then wring out the excess liquid. If using a large towel, simply dip a part of it into the infusion.
3. After wringing out the cloth, test for temperature, then apply it to the affected area.
4. If it is a hot (rather than simply warm) compress, cover the compress with a dry towel and place a hot water bottle over the towel. Leave the compress in place until it cools and then repeat.

Cool Compress

Cool compresses are more astringing than hot compresses, and they serve well to decrease inflammation. A vinegar compress or a compress made with vinegar added to an astringing tea is an excellent application for strains and sprains. Here are basic instructions:

1. Prepare a strong herbal infusion, making sure the volume of tea is sufficient for soaking a cloth large enough to cover the affected area of the body. Allow the infusion to cool, and add vinegar in a 1:4 ratio of vinegar to infusion.
2. Dip the cloth into the vinegar-infusion mixture, and then wring out the excess liquid. If using a large towel, simply dip a part of it into the infusion. (Or, you can skip making an infusion, and simply dip the cloth in diluted vinegar.)
3. Apply the compress to the affected area.

Castor Oil Compress

Castor oil packs or compresses are remarkably effective at breaking up congestion or stagnation. The oil has a dispersing quality. I have observed that when applied consistently, castor oil compresses can work miracles to break up scar tissue and adhesions and to clear up breast cysts and uterine fibroids. This treatment is extremely helpful for endometriosis. Take care not to ingest the oil. All parts of castor plants are toxic.

1. Warm castor oil in a non-aluminum pan.
2. Place a flannel or cotton cloth in the oil until it is saturated and place it on affected area.
3. Cover saturated cloth with a towel that will be used only for this purpose (over time the oil will discolor the cloth).
4. Leave the compress in place for 30 minutes minimum and optimally for 1 hour. Wash the skin with soap and water or a dilute solution of baking soda (1 teaspoon baking soda per pint of water). All cloth materials can be washed separately in a washing machine with no harm done to the machine. Best to reuse cotton/flannel cloths.

Oils

Herbal oils are excellent for treating sprains, strains, muscular tension, arthritis, and other musculoskeletal issues. The oil chosen will depend on budget as well as preference. Cold-pressed extra virgin olive oil has been the mainstay as a base oil, but other high-grade vegetable oils can be employed. Those who raise their own livestock can render lard and tallow.

A student taught me a great technique when using plantain oil for mosquito bites. She placed the oil in a roller used for applying perfume or deodorant. These rollers are easily found at most stores that sell herbal wares. The roller makes applications easy and practical, and plantain oil works immediately to relieve the itch of annoying insect bites.

When working with fresh plant material, it is best to wilt the herb for a day or so because mold formation in an herbal oil can be an issue. The warm infusion method below greatly reduces the chances of spoilage and provides an effective technique when you need an oil quickly. Herbal or medicated oils can be used directly or for making a salve.

Dried-Plant Oil

When using dried plant material to make an herbal oil, a 1:5 ratio of plant material to oil is best.

1. Grind dried herb into a coarse powder with a coffee mill or break it down more roughly with mortar and pestle.
2. Put the plant material in a glass jar and cover it with an appropriate amount of oil. For example, 1 ounce of dried plantain leaf would require 5 fluid ounces of oil.
3. Shake gently every other day for 2 weeks, then decant oil through a cheesecloth or strainer.

To preserve the oil longer, add vitamin E oil or store the herbal oil in a refrigerator.

Warm Oil Infusion

This is a quick method to make an oil using fresh plant material.

1. Harvest plants after the dew has evaporated, preferably following a couple of sunny days. Let the plant material wilt for a day or two to expire excess fluid.
2. Place the plant material in a slow cooker or double boiler.
3. Cover the plant material with oil.
4. Heat the oil and plant material gently for 48 hours; this allows water to evaporate from the plant tissues. Oil should not be heated at temperatures higher than 110°F. Another option is to use a yogurt maker, leaving the heat on for 1 week (yogurt maker temperature is 110°F).
5. Press fresh plant material through a cheesecloth or a strainer.
6. Allow the oil to sit in a closed container for a couple of days. Any water that is still present will separate to the bottom of the container.
7. Carefully pour off the oil into a separate container, leaving the water behind. Store the oil in a cool, dry place. Oils will keep for approximately 1 year and can be refrigerated for safekeeping.

Herbal Salves

Salves are herbal oils thickened by the addition of beeswax. Salves are more convenient to transport than oils are. The beeswax also serves as a preservative and has a soothing medicinal quality. Salves are wonderful for moistening the lips and for treating insect bites, eczema, and burns, as well as any applications listed for oils.

While many suppliers offer beeswax in small pellets and convenient forms, we have worked with local beekeepers to procure blocks of local wax. This is a bit more labor intensive but a block of wax can last a long time in our apothecary. The process of melting the wax into the oil happens very quickly, so be sure to mind the stove at all times when making salves.

1. Gather your ingredients. The folk method of making salves calls for 1 tablespoon grated wax per fluid ounce of oil.
2. Warm the oil slowly in a pot on a stove top and add beeswax.
3. Watch the pot closely, because beeswax melts relatively quickly. When all the wax has liquified, give the pan a gentle stir to make sure wax and oil have mixed, then remove the pot from the heat.
4. Test the consistency by dipping a teaspoon into the mixture and allow it to dry on the spoon. If too runny, add more wax; if too solid, add more oil.
5. When a sample of salve dries to the right consistency, pour the warm oil into salve tins or small wide-mouth jars.
6. When the salve has cooled completely, put lids on the tins or jars. If salves are covered while still warm, condensate will form on the salve surface, leading to spoilage.
7. Label then store salves in a cool dark place.

Alcohol-Based Liniments

Since alcohol quickens the blood, alcohol-based liniments are generally used when there is blood stagnation and poor circulation. These liniments are useful for bruising after sports injuries or chronic musculoskeletal complaints in the elderly. They also make great training liniments for cold, tight limbs and muscles. **Caution:** Liniments are made with rubbing alcohol and are undrinkable. Liniments should always be labeled *for external use only*.

One of the most famous liniments is that of herbalist Jethro Kloss, author of the renowned *Back to Eden*. Here is the method for making Kloss's linament:

1. Combine the following herbs:
   • 1 ounce echinacea powder
   • 1 ounce goldenseal powder, or substitute Oregon grape root powder
   • 1 ounce myrrh powder
   • ¼ ounce cayenne powder
2. Put the herbs in a quart glass jar and cover them with 1 pint rubbing alcohol. Leave a 2-inch margin between the surface of the alcohol and the rim of the jar.

3. Cover the jar tightly. Shake every other day for 2 weeks.

4. Strain and label *for external use only.*

5. The liniment can then be added to a spray bottle. While it will sting initially upon application, it is an excellent antiseptic for wound care.

Essential Oils

Most essential oils are commercially distilled, although a few herbalists do obtain the equipment and develop the skills needed to distill their own. These are very concentrated products, and they have markedly different energetics than other types of herbal preparations. Distilling is very effective in capturing volatile compounds that are easily lost during a hot-water extraction process. Essential oils can penetrate body tissues, so they are often used on parts of the body where circulation is poor, such as the sinuses (inhalation) or the joints. Many essential oils can be very irritating to the skin, especially in those with sensitive skin. Distilling essential oils requires enormous amounts of plant material. This is a major reason why essential oils should be extracted only from the leaves and flowers of plant species that can be sustainably harvested.

No essential oils should be used internally unless under the supervision of a licensed medical provider. Essential oils are highly antimicrobial, to the degree that even excessive external use can disrupt healthy gut flora. Hydrosols are a very popular method of working with the essential oils of plants but in a much safer form and can be made easily at home. These are the aromatic waters that are created during steam distillation of fresh plants that are high in essential oils. There is a wide range of wonderful websites with simple instructions on how to make hydrosols, and they are a beautiful way to work with oils in an ecologically minded fashion while still gracing your home and life with magical aromatic mists from plants.

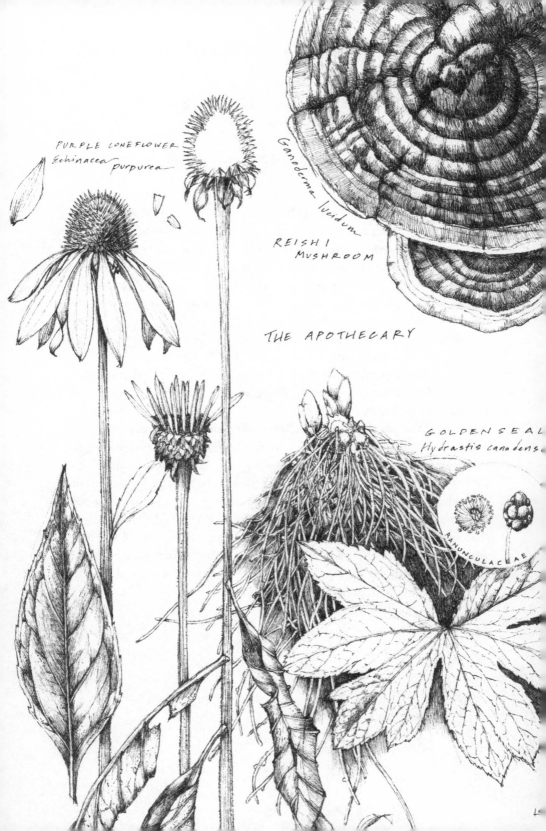

PURPLE CONEFLOWER
Echinacea purpurea

Ganoderma lucidum

REISHI
MUSHROOM

THE APOTHECARY

GOLDEN SEAL
Hydrastis canadens.

RANUNCULACEAE

CHAPTER 9

The Plants:
Materia Medica

As you have read throughout this book, I am honored to be a story-teller and steward of these amazing medicines. Given the plight of the environment and how threatened plants are becoming, my goal in preparing a materia medica was to select those medicinal plants that thrive in most locales and that provide sufficient resources for a home and even a clinic apothecary. In Traditional Chinese Medicine, there is a famous list called the Fifty Fundamental Herbs, which is the list recommended for starting a Chinese medicine apothecary. When I started writing this book, I gave myself the challenge of presenting only twenty-five plants in this materia medica chapter. I knew that the selection process would be difficult, and indeed it was. When we slow down and understand the multitude of actions and forces, and the spirit of a medicinal plant, we can certainly make do with less. I am not naive enough to think that modern societies will revert to relying on goods and services only from local sources. Nor am I discounting the important medicine that comes from other parts of the world. I am indebted to the many herbal product companies that work tirelessly trying to understand what sustainable harvest and methods mean and how to implement those methods at scale. But I can dream, and maybe that is the dream dreaming us—that we will learn to develop deep and sufficient relations with the natural world within our own bioregions.

Depending on the region where you live, there are local herbs growing close to your favorite haunts and hollows, dunes, and desert ravines that I have not chosen. Certainly, those plants have a place in your materia medica and they may become your twenty-five plants. I have chosen to highlight the weedy herbs and the pollinators. Weedy plants tend to be those that can grow well in a range of conditions and climates. The need to help support plant pollination is becoming a crucial aspect of maintaining intact ecosystems. The plants we choose to grow in our home and clinic gardens can have a vital impact on species support for monarch butterflies, native bees, and the myriad of beneficial insects. There are twenty-five waiting in line behind these that are equally valuable, so know that I left many a favorite off the list.

Seeing with the Energetic Lens

I have arranged the applications and actions of the following herbs according to their energetics. I must admit this was challenging, as these medicines do not fall neatly into one category or another. My intention is to offer a way of practicing how to recognize patterns and energetics. The information about energetics in the plant entries in this chapter reflects *my relationship* with the plants, and it is helpful that you also develop your own knowledge of plant energetics. The plants I present here are safe, reliable, and have broad applications. How I categorize them is simply an offering and not a rigorous laying down of any laws. **Note:** I have included hot presentations under the category of Heat/Excitation that may not classically present as a hypermetabolic condition but do present infection or heat, which calls for a need to work with cooling, cleansing herbs.

When looking to choose a particular plant for yourself or someone else there are a few considerations. First consider the constitution of the person and their energetics, then that of the plant. Think about which organ or special tissue you would like to affect, as different plants have specific indications for different systems.

An example of how to choose remedies is the herbal action of expectorant. There are many herbs that act as respiratory expectorants. Their action is to expel phlegm, but there are so many variations of lung congestion to consider when deciding which plant to use. We begin by asking simple questions. Is the cough dry and hacking? If so, we need to moisten the lungs and relax the muscles to ease the tension. Possibly marshmallow (*Althaea officinalis*) as a demulcent and cramp bark (*Viburnum opulus*) as a muscle relaxant. Is there a lot of phlegm and mucus? If so we want expectorants that dry mucosa as well as have a bit of an antimicrobial action because damp terrain can turn quickly into infection. Here we would look to osha root (*Ligusticum porteri*) or poplar bark (*Populus* × *candicans*, *P. tremuloides*). With all conditions, we consider the person's temperature, moisture, and tonal quality. Keep in mind that an herb rarely sits in a single category. Just as a woman can be a sister, daughter, mother, artist, and scientist, herbs can serve many roles. That is why intimacy with your apothecary will allow you to accomplish so very much with one or two medicines.

Building Formulas

There are a great variety of styles when it comes to the craft of blending herbs—it is an artistic endeavor as well as a practical one. Native Americans were known to combine only a few plants at a time, and European colonists thought this was due to their lack of knowledge. In fact, it had to do with Native Americans' deep relationships with plants—they needed only a few to produce excellent healing results.

In the 1800s, the great Eclectic physician John Scudder revived Eclectic medical schools financially, and he also provided a clear and solid foundation for a system of treatment that was very similar to homeopathy. Scudder introduced a new development in herbal medicine that matured the profession and brought clarity to its tenets. Referred to as *specific medicine*, this is an approach in which low doses of herbal medicine are applied as the "specific" for a particular symptom picture. No longer were physicians treating solely symptoms, they were treating the individual person. Herbalist David Winston says, "In this system small doses of high-quality single herbs replaced large quantities of often nauseating polyherbal preparations. Each herb was carefully studied to find its 'specific indications' in clinical practice."[1]

At the same time, elaborate and elegant formulations are a component of global traditions such as Unani Tibb and Chinese medicine. Again, from David Winston: "With classic traditional formulas there are clear strategies to create a mixture that is more than the sum of its parts."[2] The art of complex formulation varies depending on the culture and system of healing.

When I am not working with one or two herbs at a time, the simplest formulation method that I enjoy using is the triangle model. This is a tool that Rosemary Gladstar and other herbalists use in teaching the art of formulation. It is based on an incredibly elegant yet complicated system of formulation called the Triune System of Formulation developed by herbalist and acupuncturist William LeSassier. William was known as the teachers' teacher. Rosemary learned this technique from William many

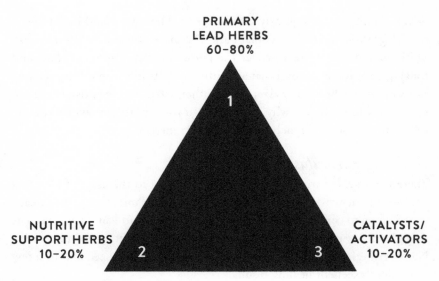

Figure 9.1. The triangle model of formulation.

years ago and simplified the concept to make it accessible for those just starting out in herbalism.

Figure 9.1 provides a visual representation of the triangle model. At the top of the triangle, point 1, are the primary herbs, which represent at least 60 percent and as much as 80 percent of the formula. These are the herbs that directly address the primary complaint and are the focus of the formula. They have been called the lead or chief herbs. Point 2 is the support herbs. These are the herbs that build and nourish the organ or system being worked with or enhance the effects of the lead herbs. Support herbs comprise 10 to 20 percent of the blend. Point 3 is the catalysts or activators. These herbs lend a specific energy to the formula. This can be organ specific, as well, and may provide a particular action, such as diuretic, diaphoretic, expectorant, or stimulant. When we work with herbs energetically, oftentimes there is no need for a catalyst because we consider how the primary and support herbs will affect the energy of the blend.

For example, if you were helping someone with hypertension, the primary action might be relaxation. Motherwort (*Leonurus cardiaca*) and valerian (*Valeriana officinalis*) would be suitable choices as the primary herbs, as shown in figure 9.2. To support the cardiovascular system, you could add nutritive herbs such as hawthorn (*Crataegus* spp.) and linden (*Tilia cordata*), which also lend a relaxing tone to the formula. Overall, these choices make

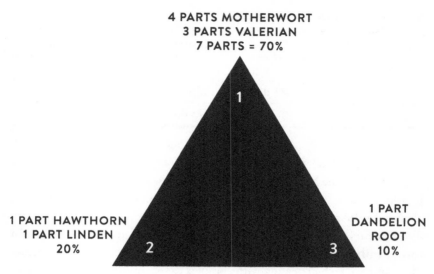

4 PARTS MOTHERWORT
3 PARTS VALERIAN
7 PARTS = 70%

1

1 PART HAWTHORN
1 PART LINDEN
20%

2

1 PART
DANDELION
ROOT
10%

3

Figure 9.2. Sample hypertension formula.

for a cooler formula, so if the person runs cooler, you could add another herb that would warm it up, or you could add dandelion root (*Taraxacum officinale*) to activate eliminatory functions.

This formula should be prepared as a tincture because a variety of plant parts need to be combined in the formula. Generally, when making teas, it is recommended to use similar plant parts. This is a practical consideration. For example, if a tea blend includes both roots and leaves, the roots may fall to the bottom of the blend because they are heavier than the leaves, making it difficult to keep the blend well mixed in storage over time. Also, when making teas, it's important to consider how the blend is going to taste. With tinctures you can use the less palatable herbs with greater ease.

Dosing

How much of an herbal medicine to take and how often are two of the most frequently discussed questions in herbal medicine. In the plant entries in this chapter, I sometimes suggest dosages, but for the most part, dosage depends on the individual and their situation. Body type, age, metabolism, list of medications, history, sensitivities, and so forth all come into play when deciding proper amounts.

In general, for nourishing infusions to be effective it is helpful to drink a pint to a quart of the infusion a day. When working with tinctures,

Table 9.1. Tincture Dosage Equivalents

Teaspoon Measure	Dropper Measure	Milliliter Measure
¼ teaspoon	1 dropperful (35 drops)	1 ml
½ teaspoon	2½ dropperfuls (88 drops)	2.5 ml
1 teaspoon	5 dropperfuls (175 drops)	5 ml

oftentimes 20 to 30 drops, or ½ teaspoon, taken three times a day will gradually allow the herbs to move the body in the right direction. For acute situations, 1 teaspoon, or 5 milliliters, may be required and may need to be taken more frequently throughout the day (table 9.1 provides a summary of equivalents for teaspoon, dropperful, and milliliter measures). For years, I worked with physiologic dosing, which is a standard 1 teaspoon three times a day. And even when dealing with complex cases, this dosing brought good results in many instances. As I began working with plant energetics and reckoning with the need to protect plant populations, I shifted to working with drop doses. These are also called spirit or energetic doses. This is the beauty of developing relations with the plant teachers. When we understand their specific medicine and energetics, we will need less of a material dose (large dose). That being said, if I am helping someone who has a urinary tract infection starting to develop, I may recommend a dosage of 1 teaspoon of a blend every three to four hours to get ahead of the infection before it takes hold. Trust your intuition and intelligence and you will find your way.

Young's rule is a classic formula for children's dosing that calculates dose by age. The rule is to add twelve to the child's age and then divide the child's age by this total. For example, to calculate the dose for a six-year-old child:

$$6 \text{ (child's age)} + 12 = 18; \text{ then}$$
$$6 \text{ (child's age)} \div 18 \text{ (total from above)} = \frac{1}{3}$$

From this we can see that a six-year-old child should receive one-third of the adult dose.

Inclusive Language

At long last, we are acknowledging the diversity of our one human race with regard to color, sexuality, gender, ability, and the spectrum of choice that is not the dominant culture's norm. The terminology of the LGBTQIA community is dynamic and evolving, and as health care providers our use of this language demonstrates our respect for all. Inclusive language is a way of acknowledging and respecting the diversity of bodies, genders, and relationships. I offer the information in this materia medica with the hope that these herbs are applicable to all. Instead of discussing reproduction systems based on gender, I focus on the organs associated with the herb and the ways in which the plant will support that tissue state or organ system.

Herbal Actions

In the plant entries that follow here, I use many terms that describe herbal actions—the ways in which the herbs work. There can be a tendency to gloss over terms such as *cholagogue* and *hepatic*. They may seem a bit incomprehensible, especially if you are new to herbal medicine. Yet these are the terms of the herbalist and are foundational concepts that reveal the nature of our medicines. If you are new to this terminology, be sure to refer to appendix 2, "Herbal Actions Glossary," page 319, which provides definitions of all of the herbal action terms that appear in the plant entries below.

Agrimony

Agrimonia eupatoria, A. gryposepala
Cocklebur, Sticklewort, Church steeples

Family	Rosaceae
Parts Used	aerial parts
Energetics	drying, relaxing, cooling
Tissue States	tension, atrophy, relaxation
Taste	sweet, astringent, acrid
Actions	anti-inflammatory, tonic, bitter, diuretic, vulnerary, antispasmodic

Agrimonia is an edge dweller, as it thrives along fire roads and is found on the edges of woodlands throughout North America. The plant bears slender spikes of small, yellow, five-petaled flowers (rose family) that bloom from June to September. The seed capsules are sticky—these are the small burrs you may find stuck to your dog's fur or your clothes after a hike through the fields; hence the common names of cocklebur and sticklewort. This effective mode of seed transportation is why agrimony can be found in such a variety of locales.

Uses

Agrimony is a superb tonic for the digestive tract because it blends astringency and bitter tonic properties. While it is gentle acting, it has a focus for mucous membranes of intestinal tissue so it is very effective for colitis and irritable bowel and for issues with weakness of tone in elders or nervous children who suffer with repeated "belly aches." It is an important plant for treating tension. Often times the word tortured will come up as a description of the colic, spasms, and sharp shooting pains. I rarely prepare a formula for gallstone or kidney stones without adding agrimony. In TCM, the presence of constricted Liver Qi is seen as hypertension, anxiety, anger, and frustration. Agrimony has a wonderful specificity for this presentation, and its yellow flowers are a signature for the liver. Dr. Edward Bach, famed physician who developed Bach Flower Remedies, used agrimony for the person who hides their tension behind a cheery façade.

I am so grateful that Matthew Wood has taught us of the magical use of this plant. He has stated, "I have to say that if there is one plant I know from over a decade of clinical experience to have had an effect which is magical—that is, it will change the environment around the person using it—Agrimony is the one. This remedy also prevents meddling and interference."[3] The application of this seems best in situations of discord with neighbors or in the workplace. It releases tension from the environment, and story after story from students and clients has proved this so. It does not matter what form the plant is in, it simply needs to be placed in the area of conflict. For example, many nurses experience very stressful work situations due to the hierarchical nature of the medical profession. Some nurses have either brought in some dried herb and left it close to their station or they have brought in a potted agrimony plant. Following that, something happens that relaxes the tension of the environment. A problem boss has been relocated or has shifted their behavior. Such resolutions to tension have manifested in ways that can only be described as magical and amazingly reliable!

Indications

Tension/Constriction (Relaxation)

Mental health. For the person who experiences tension and anguish hidden behind a cheery façade or inappropriate use of humor.

Head. Drop doses of the tincture for tension headaches with pressure at the temples, which may indicate Liver/Gallbladder tension. This is manifested with irritability, tension, and frustration.

Gallbladder. For sharp and shooting pain related to gallbladder spasms or colic, especially when passing stones.

Digestive system. Relaxant for irritable bowel, colitis, and other digestive complaints with colic and spasms. Works well for gripping pains and cramps from food poisoning.

Respiratory system. Excellent addition to formulas where the breath is held in tension or there is gasping due to pain elsewhere in the body.[4] Works well for asthma.

Kidney. For cystitis, nephritis, and cases of irritation or inflammation of the urinary organs. The pain of passing a kidney stone is sharp, intense, and spasmodic, and agrimony can play a role in easing the spasm that occurs from passing a stone.

Uterine health. In Chinese medicine, Liver governs flow and "stores the blood." Agrimony added to a formula can greatly ease menstrual pain and regain rhythm of flow.

Relaxation/Atony

Digestive system. Useful for all GI complaints arising from inflammation, including mouth ulcerations and gum disease. This plant is especially useful in lower bowel inflammation such as colitis, IBS, and Crohn's disease. Because it is tonic to mucous membranes as well as a relaxant, agrimony helps reduce diarrhea from spasm as well as excess mucus. Specific indication is for elders and those with weak digestive tone.

Skin. Use as a wash or compress for skin ulcerations and irritations.

Urinary system. Excellent mucous membrane tonic in chronic urinary tract infections. Very helpful for elderly with incontinence as well as children troubled with bed-wetting.

Habitat & Harvest

Agrimony grows with abandon in fields, meadows, and along the edges of woodlands. For the sweetest flavor, harvest leaves before plants flower. Leaves harvested after flowering are more astringing due to higher tannin content. I prefer these leaves for skin eruptions and wound healing.

Preparations

Infusion: 1 cup two to three times a day.

Tincture: Fresh leaf (1:2, 95% alcohol) or dried leaf (1:5, 40–60% alcohol). Drop doses (3 to 10 drops as needed) for emotional support;

½ to 1 teaspoon three times a day for bowel inflammation; 1 teaspoon as needed for acute pain in passing stones.

Poultice/compress: Apply as needed to relieve skin irritation and inflammation.

Contraindications

Care must be taken if using with persons with dry or cold constitutions. For those individuals, use agrimony for short periods only or add moistening and or warming herbs to the formula.

Ashwagandha

Withania somnifera
Indian ginseng, Indian winter cherry

Family	Solanaceae
Parts Used	root and leaf
Energetics	nutritive, warm, drying
Tissue States	atrophy, depression/deficiency, tension
Taste	bitter, sweet, pungent
Actions	adaptogen, nervine, tonic, aphrodisiac, alterative, anti-inflammatory, antispasmodic, anxiolytic, bitter, immunomodulator, sedative

If you can grow tomatoes, you can grow this highly revered tonic native to India, Africa, and the Mediterranean. I am including this medicine in this limited sustainable apothecary because it is one of the rare potent adaptogens that can be grown in such a wide variety of soil and climate conditions and it takes only a year to reach maturity. Plant the seeds early in spring and the root can be harvested by fall. The beautiful lantern-like pod that holds the fruit resembles a tomatillo. After the first frost, or when the lantern (the calyx) turns brown, it is time to harvest. This herb from Ayurvedic practice is truly a gift for our stressful and depleting times.

Ashwagandha is a Sanskrit name that means "smell of a horse." The root has a strong, earthy, pungent scent. It is also said that this plant imparts a vigor and vitality as strong as that of a horse. Another name is winter cherry because the red or orange fruits resemble cherries, albeit small ones. The fruits are loaded with seeds that can easily be dried and saved for planting the following year. The yellow flower is an exquisite nightshade beauty. The species name *somnifera* indicates that this herb is indeed helpful for relaxation and promoting sound sleep.

Uses

In India, ashwagandha is held in the highest esteem as a *rasayana*, which is the term in Ayurvedic medicine for a restorative tonic that promotes youthful vitality and clear cognition and is said to expand happiness. Ashwagandha is a household remedy in India given to small children prone to weakness and taken throughout life as a longevity elixir and aphrodisiac. It is purported to be one of the favored nervine tonics in Ayurveda.[5]

Ashwagandha is a welcome addition to the Western herbal apothecary because it is so deeply restorative to the nervous system and endocrine system.[6] While most adaptogens are stimulating, *Withania* brings a calming force that settles the spirit while nourishing the body. I have found that ashwagandha does a remarkable job for conditions that I used to rely on American ginseng (*Panax quinquefolium*) to treat. Because American ginseng is threatened by overharvesting, I now limit myself to using only ginseng that I have grown myself. As an immune amphoteric, ashwagandha treats low, deficient immune systems of those struggling with conditions such as Lyme or cancer. It also addresses excessive immune responses such as autoimmune conditions.

Withania belongs to a subgroup of the rasayanas termed *medhyarasayanas*. These have a specificity for the mind, enhancing the mental and intellectual capabilities. Safe for all ages, ashwagandha is used to promote memory, cognition, and convalescence from head injuries, as well as to help those with depression, children who have learning challenges, and those experiencing a decline in mental functioning as they age.

Ashwagandha is appropriate for many deficient conditions due to stress and overwork—it is incredibly useful for those experiencing chronic fatigue, fibromyalgia, and exhaustion from cancer treatments. It works so beautifully with the endocrine system that it seems to enhance all hormonal profiles. I have seen ashwagandha work consistently to improve those with hypothyroid conditions, especially when working with the deficiency even before blood levels of thyroid hormones are off balance. Even in clinical cases, this root medicine has tremendous value because it is thought to assist in conversion of the inactive (T4) form of thyroid hormone into the active (T3) form. It is also helpful for balancing mood swings due to hormonal fluctuations as well as being a key player in recipes for balancing blood sugar. *Withania* enhances sexual performance as well as libido that is lessened due to stress and is well understood as a sexual/reproductive tonic in many African nations. All of the conditions named are treated using *Withania* root; the leaves of the plant can be applied topically for infections, abscesses, and eruptive skin issues.

While this tonic needs to be taken over the course of one month or six weeks for effects to truly take hold, I have had the experience myself of taking ashwagandha tincture and feeling its calming effects within the hour.

Indications

Cold/Depression (Warming/Nutritive)

Mental health. Especially useful for anxiety due to deficiency and for those who are easily excited or fearful.

Joints. Decreases inflammation of autoimmune conditions, such as lupus and rheumatoid arthritis, via its nutritive qualities.

Nervous system. A supreme nerve tonic, useful for insomnia, depression, nervous exhaustion, neurasthenia, and long-term damage from herpes lesions.

Libido. Treating low libido due to stress or aging is a traditional use.

Immune system. Specific for hypoimmunity, and many autoimmune diseases arise from deficient immune function. Most of these diseases present with dry tissues, and ashwagandha also nourishes mucous membranes. Ashwagandha is warming; it moves blood to help with nourishment of tissues and organs.

Thyroid. Thought to increase conversion of inactive thyroid hormone to the active form of the hormone (T4 to T3).[7]

Aging. As noted in the discussion of tissue states in chapter 6, aging decreases yin (fluids) as well as yang (energy, function). Ashwagandha deeply nourishes both of these vital energies, which is why it is a famous longevity elixir.

Adrenals. Specific for adrenal exhaustion from overwork or chronic illness.

Blood. Excellent absorbable source of iron. Best made into a syrup with molasses instead of the usual honey, because molasses is blood building.

Testes. Enhances sperm count as well as motility.

Tension/Constriction (Relaxant)

Musculoskeletal system. Excellent relaxant for spasms such as nighttime muscle cramps or the tremors of Parkinson's.

Habitat & Harvest

As stated above, ashwagandha can be grown in the garden just like tomatoes, and it does not even need special training or staking. It does best in
areas with strong summer heat. Ashwagandha root will be ready for harvest
after the first or second frost. For topical applications, it is best to harvest
leaves before plants flower.

Preparations

Tincture and powder are my preferred methods.

Tincture: Dried root (1:5, 50% alcohol), 30–40 drops three times a day, or
  in drop doses.
Powder: 1 to 2 tablespoons or 3 to 6 grams a day. The powder can be mixed
  into nut butter, ghee, or honey or stirred into warm milk. It is important
  to find a source who can guarantee that the powder of ashwagandha root
  is not more than a year old, and it is best freshly ground at time of use.
Decoction: 1 cup a day. This is a strong-tasting brew.

Contraindications

Although Ayurvedic practitioners recommend ashwagandha as a pregnancy
tonic,[8] it is best to avoid use during pregnancy as there are contradictory
findings on the safety during this time. The use by Ayurvedic practitioners
shows their preference for dried root because fresh root has more toxicity.
Ashwagandha is not recommended for those with hyperthyroidism, hemo-
chromatosis (excess iron), or a nightshade sensitivity. For those who run
hot constitutionally, combine this herb in a formula with herbs that have a
cooling effect.

Blue Vervain

Verbena hastata

Swamp verbena, Wild hyssop, Blue verbena, Simpler's joy

Family	Verbenaceae
Parts Used	aerial parts
Energetics	relaxing, cooling, drying
Tissue States	tension, atrophy, heat
Taste	bitter, slightly acrid
Actions	bitter, nervine, antispasmodic, tonic, mild sedative, emetic, febrifuge, diaphoretic, relaxing expectorant, moderate hypotensive

A lover of moist soil, blue vervain has found a welcome home among the low-lying plants that surround the lily pond at Sacred Plant Traditions school. Its tall, stately stalks appeared on their own there a couple of years ago, and it shows no sign of leaving. We take its presence as a daily reminder to slow down and relax. Blue vervain is a three- to five-foot-tall, proudly upright perennial. The stunning flower spikes are described as branching like a candelabra. The rings of purple blooms open first at the bottom of each spike, and by late summer, blooms reach the top. The leaves are simple in shape and opposite. The flowers are great pollinators and the seeds are a favorite food for song birds, so it is best not to deadhead the plants until winter's end. In its natural habitat, blue vervain often grows among other tall medicinals such as ironweed (*Vernonia* spp.) and Joe Pye weed (*Eutrochium purpureum*), where it stretches even taller than it does as a solitary volunteer.

Some confuse blue vervain with tasty lemon verbena (*Aloysia citrodora*) or the European vervain species *Verbena officinalis*. There are over 250 species of verbenas and it is written that many are interchangeable. *Verbena bonariensis* is a showy, leggy perennial that self-seeds easily in our garden. In cooler climes it is an annual It is used interchangeably with *V. hastata* according to Southern herbalist Phyllis Light, who also uses the very similar *V. brasiliensis*.

Uses

There is a fair amount of magic surrounding this plant. It seems that its ancient folklore relates not only to common verbena (*V. officinalis*), which is the species native to Europe, but also to *V. hastata*. *Verbena* was the classical

Roman name for "altar plants." It is written that the wounds of Christ were washed with vervain as his body was prepared for burial. The Druids employed verbena in their lustral waters, a holy water used for blessings and special prayers. The word *vervain* is derived from the Celtic *ferfaen*, from *fer* (to drive away) and *faen* (a stone), and this herb helps clear calculus or stones from the kidneys and bladder. Vervain was thought to be a panacea, and Hippocrates recommended pairing it with red clover (*Trifolium pratense*) for a perfect blend in easing all discomforts.

Today the plant is beloved for its relaxing and tonifying effect on the nervous system. It has specificity for the pitta, Type A personality that has a great need to control events. Ithaca, New York, herbalist 7Song says that verbena is for those folks who have contingency plans for their contingency plans and maybe one more plan after that. You can see why we welcome this magician into our courtyard where we pass by it frequently as we walk to the classroom, to the garden, or to the office. It is a beautiful reminder of how to walk with presence. Herbalist jim mcdonald describes the person in need of vervain as the one who walks headlong, head down, moving fast even when there is no reason to rush.

The vervain Bach Flower Remedy is made with *V. officinalis*. The vervain type is a person who holds very strong opinions and ideas that they hardly ever change and that they wish to impose on others. The rigid, erect, and proud stem of this plant suggests an imposing force.

Blue vervain is bitter, and it has a wonderful relaxing influence on tension from Liver heat, which can be influenced by strong emotions such as anger and irritability. Liver is influenced by wind, and when there is dryness, strong fiery emotions can rise upward, increasing blood pressure or headaches. When this is the case, add blue vervain to the formula to help ease that tension. It blends beautifully with other nervines, but it works just as well alone in drop doses (which is my preferred method). The key with blue vervain, though, is to take it over a period of time in small and frequent doses because it is a tonifying, trophorestorative nervine. This is probably the mechanism that makes it an effective aphrodisiac—it restores normal functioning, and healthy libido is the norm.

Indications
Heat/Excitation (Cooling/Sedating)
Digestive system. As a bitter, blue vervain is cooling and sedating to an overactive digestive tract.

Cold/Depression (Bitter Stimulant)

Mental health. Chronic stress can lead to what the Greeks termed *melancholy* (*melanos*—black, *chole*—bile), and this can lead to exhaustion of the nervous system, which presents as depression. Anxiety is a frequent escort to depression and blue vervain is an excellent remedy. Also effective for those recovering from trauma and adrenal exhaustion.

Lymphatic system. Eclectic physician John Scudder listed blue vervain for its use in colds, coughs, and respiratory issues as well as for "obstructions of the glandular system."[9] I am certain its tension-releasing qualities aid in this function.

Dry/Atrophy (Bitter Stimulant)

Liver. As a hepatic, blue vervain stimulates the liver, and since the liver governs flow, our bodies are moistened. This is a wonderful galactagogue or herb to increase breast milk.

Tension/Constriction (Relaxant)

Mental health. Excessive thought, worry, and a tendency to overwhelm (which can lead to insomnia) are indications for blue vervain.

Head. Useful for Liver tension headaches that are focused on the temples or headaches due to neck tension.

Neck. This herb is a specific for neck and shoulder tension that can lead to tension headache. Good for the person who feels they need to shoulder the cares of the world because those around them do not live up to their expectations or standards.

Liver. "Liver heat rising" often presents as high blood pressure, irritability, quickness to anger, pitta aggravation. Since Liver governs flow, *V. hastata* aids with flow of digestive juices, menses, thought, and ideas, especially for those hemmed in by rigid thinking.

Uterine health. *V. hastata* is an excellent choice for premenstrual syndrome (PMS) symptoms—especially anxiety, irritability, and extreme mood swings. It is a relaxing tonic for menstrual cramps as well as mittelschmerz pain; *mittelschmerz* is a German word for "middle pain" and is experienced midcycle, at ovulation. As a uterine tonic (nervous system influencing reproductive organs), blue vervain helps to bring on menses when delayed due to pelvic congestion or uterine weakness. Blends beautifully with motherwort for this purpose.

Habitat & Harvest

Blue vervain grows readily from seed and does best in moist soil. It takes two years to reach full flowering potential. Gather the plants just before or close to the height of flowering; the medicine is found in the leaves and flowers.

Preparations

Infusion: Although bitter, this tea can be improved by adding a pleasant-tasting herb such as alfalfa (*Medicago sativa*) or lemon balm (*Melissa officinalis*). Take ½ cup two to three times a day.

Tincture: Fresh plant (1:3, 95% alcohol) or dried (1:4, 70% alcohol). Best taken frequently in small doses. For chronic neck pain, ½ teaspoon three to four times a day.

Poultice/compress: Make a fresh plant poultice for healing wounds, cooling burns, and moving blood to clear old bruises.

Contraindications

Not to be used during pregnancy.

 # Burdock

Arctium lappa, A. minus
Gobo, Bur seed, Cocklebur

Family	Asteraceae
Parts Used	leaf, seed, root
Energetics	nutritive, cooling, moistening
Tissue States	heat, dry/atrophic, stagnation
Taste	leaf and seed—bitter; root—sweet, very slightly bitter
Actions	alterative, lymphatic, bitter, hepatic, diuretic (seed), nutritive tonic

When given space and sunlight, the mighty burdock grows six feet tall and almost as wide. This biennial produces a basal rosette in its first year, with heart-shaped leaves growing more than a foot in length. You can distinguish burdock from other kinds of dock by the fine gray down on the underside of the leaves. In the second year, a stalk rises skyward and upper branches are spotted with purple flowers. Flowers turn to seed or fruit that gives this plant such a notorious reputation among farmers, hikers, and pet lovers. The tenacious bur (seed head) is extremely difficult to wrangle out of clothing and animal fur.

To my mind, you cannot claim the title of herbalist until you have dug an entire burdock root. Burrowing straight down for up to two feet, you work with a tamping bar to patiently loosen soil, then remove it, then loosen more and remove it, continuing until the root tip releases you from your hard day's work. This experience shows you the signature in this deep-acting medicine for chronic conditions. This root, which burrows through years of built-up accumulation, can, with patience, help a chronically ill person attain a deeper sense of wellness. Early American botanist Thomas Bartram wrote that burdock is "one of the most powerful and reliable of blood tonics of herbalism." He also noted that "persistence with low doses is more favorable than larger." Bartram lauded burdock's success for treating arthritis, gout, rheumatism, boils, cystitis, and many skin diseases.[10]

Herbalist David Hoffman attested that burdock will "move the body to a state of integration and health, improving indicators of systemic imbalance."[11] This is also what burdock accomplishes with the Earth herself. Burdock is usually the first to take up residence in newly developed or disrupted soils. It is highly revered here in Virginia where the clay soils give way to nothing save the roots of this plant. Burdock breaks up the compacted earth, pulls nutrients to the topsoil, and with its abundance of leaf matter, gives generously of rich compost back to the soil. Almost 50 percent of the root mass is comprised of inulin, a polysaccharide that acts as a prebiotic for humans and is a massive storehouse of energy to sustain the plant's aboveground structure. A mighty plant indeed.

Uses

Burdock root and seed are known for their deep action when working with the skin. This plant has an interesting energetic profile, with seemingly contradictory actions. Burdock is used to moisten and nourish dry, scaly skin conditions but also to clear oily, "stuck" eruptions such as acne and boils. The confusion abates when we realize that *Arctium* is the archetypal alterative, that action of plants that is also termed "blood cleanser." Alteratives are invaluable because these plants enhance the elimination of waste through natural metabolic processes, including those of the lymphatic, digestive, hepatic, and renal systems. Clearing the waste material is about keeping our waters moving. When backup occurs in the body's detoxification processes over a period of time, our endocrine system struggles. The body's hormonal messaging systems depend on healthy blood flow to carry those messages and communicate the body's needs. When the blood is thick with excess debris of platelets and plaque buildup (ama in Ayurveda), these communication systems are challenged. Burdock root is appropriate for long-term liver support. The seed has a stronger action so is best used with acute conditions or specific indications for skin complaints. If digging burdock root gains certification as an herbalist, harvesting and processing the seed is graduate school.

Gobo is a Japanese name for burdock root and is sold as a fresh root in many farmers' markets and Asian food stores. Burdock root is a wonderfully nutritive wild food.

Indications
Heat/Excitation (Cooling)
Skin. A poultice of fresh leaves, or one large leaf (and they do get very large) wrapped completely around injury, is excellent for burns or red rashes presenting as heat. Excellent to relieve sting from nettle.

Dry/Atrophy (Moistening/Nutritive)
Skin. Through enhancement of production and processing of oils, burdock moistens dry, itchy skin afflictions. Improves function of sebaceous glands in skin responsible for production of healthy oils. Seed especially useful for this purpose.

Digestive system. As a hepatic, burdock stimulates release of bile, which breaks down fats so they can be utilized by the body. Useful in constipation, dry stools, and wind (gas).

Blood sugar balance. With a high inulin content, which can comprise up to 50 percent of the root's mass, burdock acts as a prebiotic. Inulin is a polysaccharide that feeds healthy gut bacteria, improves digestion, and facilitates in balancing the blood.

Stagnation (Alterative)
Lymphatic system. Burdock root is a deep-acting lymphatic alterative. Best to combine with other alteratives to help move toxins through other eliminatory channels.

Liver. As a hepatic, it stimulates bile, which enhances digestion and elimination.

Kidneys. Seeds are diuretic. Root can alleviate edema in chronic conditions such as diabetes and lymphedema.

Habitat & Harvest

Burdock is prevalent in fields and recently disrupted landscapes. When looking to harvest roots of wild plants, it is best to do so from sites where the soil is not compacted. Oftentimes, herb growers create double-dug mounds to plant burdock in, which makes the eventual digging of the roots much easier. Since burdock is a biennial, roots are harvested at the end of the first year. Seeds are harvested in the fall of the second year.

Preparations

Decoction: 1 cup a day.
Tincture: Dried seed (1:4, 75% alcohol); fresh root (1:2, 75% alcohol); dried root (1:5, 50% alcohol).
Poultice: Steamed fresh leaf preferred.

Contraindications

As when using any alterative, symptoms may get worse before they begin to improve. Drink plenty of water and use other cleansing herbs to support the clearing process.

Burdock is a wonderful wild food to add to stir fries and soups. For some though, burdock can prove difficult to digest and creates a lot of gas. Start slow and work your way up if you wish to include burdock in your diet with frequency.

Caution: Rhubarb (*Rheum rhabarbarum*) is not very common in the wild, but it looks a lot like burdock and has toxic properties. Be sure you can tell the difference between these two plants.

Calendula

Calendula officinalis
Marigold, Pot marigold, Golds

Family	Asteraceae
Part Used	flower
Energetics	slightly warming, drying
Tissue States	depression, atrophy, stagnation
Taste	aromatic, bitter, pungent
Actions	lymphatic, stimulant, vulnerary, emmenagogue, antifungal, antibacterial, anti-inflammatory, cholagogue, alterative, astringent, relaxant, hepatic

As one of our greatest wound healers, the radiant yellow flowers of calendula are a required presence in any herb garden. It is one of the easiest plants to grow from seed and is not fussy when it comes to garden requirements. Supply plenty of sunshine and good drainage and this plant will regale you with a multitude of flowers for three seasons. The fuzzy leaves range between three to eight inches long, and the plant can grow as tall as three feet. The flowers are either bright yellow, deep gold, or vibrant orange. The characteristic medicinal resin is found at the base of the flowers as well as on the stems.

The name calendula comes from the Latin *calendae*, a reference to the fact that it enjoys a long blooming season—every month of the year in some regions.

Uses

Down through the ages, calendula was revered as a wound healer both internally and externally. It is employed to bring out eruptive diseases such as measles and chicken pox, and it can work miracles on gangrenous wounds. A yellow resin called calendulin is the constituent that serves to make this herb so effective in treating fungal diseases such as thrush.[12] Calendula has traditionally been used as a food, and it was said the yellow petals of calendula would be "dried and kept throughout Dutchland against winter to put into broths."[13] In Italy, especially in the olive groves, field marigolds, *C. arvensis* (a wild species), are harvested and dried, then the petals are removed from the resinous green bases (though this is a major source of the immune enhancing medicine). As with *C. officinalis*, the more that are picked, the more robust is the flowering. Due to its warm orange color and slightly bitter taste, field marigold (*C. arvensis*) has earned the name of "poor man's saffron," and both the dried and fresh petals are added to many soups, broths, and cooked dishes. The nutrient-rich petals are filled with flavonoids, carotenoids, and other antioxidants.

While many authors have reflected on this plant as "herbal sunshine," its use in working with trauma and deep wounds from past experiences cannot be underestimated. I use calendula similarly to St. John's wort, when a presence of light and a sense of the sacred needs to be reinstated in a person's life.

Indications
Heat/Excitation (Sedating)
Fevers. A hot infusion serves as a mild diaphoretic in releasing internal heat.

Skin. Use as an external wash and infusion to shorten the duration of eruptive diseases. Combine with chickweed in a soothing wash for diaper rash. Specific for fungal infections on the skin and for thrush.[14] "It is especially applicable to severe burns, to promote healing and to prevent the formation of a contracting scar," according to Eclectic physician Finley Ellingwood.[15]

Cold/Depression (Warming/Nutritive)
Sinuses. Excellent infusion to clear sinuses.

Digestive system. Calendula works beautifully for healing ulcers, inflammatory bowel disease, and any heat from toxicity or infection. Calendula's antibacterial action helps clear *Helicobacter pylori* (a bacterium that causes gastric ulcers).

Immune system. The mucopolysaccharides in calendula stimulate immune function.[16] For those who have depressed immune function, the addition of calendula flowers brings valuable flavonoids into the diet.

Vaginal/cervical health. Superb wash or douche for vaginitis, whether bacterial or fungal. Calendula is also part of a naturopathic protocol for cervical dysplasia.

Trauma. When there has been sexual abuse, this wound healer can shine light where there has been trauma and shame. Offer in tea, tincture, or salve form, where applicable.

Damp/Stagnation (Warming Stimulant)
Breasts. Excellent topically as well as internally for mastitis.

Lymphatic system. This is where calendula really shines—moving stagnant lymph material. Useful for most infections where there are swollen nodes, especially in the groin and under the armpit (places not often exposed to light).

Wounds. Calendula is antifungal and thus specific for moist, purulent wounds. Consistent application prevents putrification.[17]

Tension/Constriction (Relaxation)

Liver. As a hepatic, calendula relaxes liver tension, which can benefit a painful menstrual cycle or one that is delayed.

Laxity/Atony (Astringent)

Digestive system. For chronic diarrhea caused by gut dysbiosis or pathogens. Calendula dries excess mucus, checks diarrhea, and can be hemostatic when there is bleeding due to irritation and inflammation.

Habitat & Harvest

You can direct-seed calendula or start seedlings in a greenhouse or on a sunny windowsill indoors. To promote continued flower production, harvest blossoms often and deadhead flowers that have begun to go to seed. Wait to harvest until all the morning dew has evaporated from plant surfaces, because calendula needs special attention when drying. Harvest with the green bases of the flowers intact because the flower base is where the resinous medicine resides. Lay each flower face down on a screen or cloth and make sure there is good ventilation. The resin will hold on to moisture so make sure flowers are completely dry.

Preparations

Infusion: This is the most nutritious form to prepare; useful for long-term convalescent protocol.

Tincture: Fresh flower (1:2, 95% alcohol) or dried flower (1:6, 70% alcohol). Blends well with other immune herbs, or take ½ teaspoon three times a day for two weeks to move stagnant lymph.

Oil: I prefer using the heat method due to the high resin content. The oil can then be made into a healing salve. Remember to use washes rather than an oil when there is heat in a wound, because oil can trap the heat and prolong or even aggravate the situation.

Sitz bath / wound wash / douche: Make a strong infusion and apply as needed. This can be spritzed on tender vaginal tissue or used for traveling when constant application is needed and a wash is impractical.

Contraindications

Not safe for internal use during pregnancy. As a member of the Aster family, it might cause allergic reactions.

Chickweed

Stellaria media
Chicken wort, Starweed

Family	Carophyllaceae
Parts Used	aerial parts
Energetics	cooling, moistening, nutritive
Tissue States	heat, dry/atrophy, stagnation
Taste	sweet, salty
Action	antimicrobial, nutritive tonic, anti-inflammatory

Early on in my practice, a young couple brought their infant to me for help with impetigo, which is a serious skin infection caused by *Streptococcus* bacteria. The rash on the infant's neck was red and hot, oozing infectious material. The couple were from a strict Mennonite order so conventional medicine was not an option. Herbs were their only recourse. I led them to my garden and showed them what chickweed looked like. We harvested handfuls, and I instructed them how to apply a compress. I asked them to bring the child back the following day. The baby's skin changed dramatically overnight. It was still slightly red but the oozing, angry nature of the infection had passed. The parents were greatly relieved.

This is the mighty, yet tender, chickweed, who is among the most prolific of weeds. Most gardeners are very familiar with *Stellaria media*, as she is an indicator of rich, moist soils. Just as we have spring and fall plantings for kale or mesclun greens, so too does chickweed flourish in both seasons. In summer, the plants decline and go to seed.

The leaves of young chickweed are oval. As the plant matures, the smooth leaf edges begin to ruffle slightly. One distinctive characteristic is a single line of hairs that run the length of the stem. The beautiful white starlike flower has five petals but appears to have more because each petal is deeply notched. This gives the flower the look of gentle yet penetrating rays of light; this is a signature of the plant's essence—chickweed helps dissolve boundaries.

Uses

Chickweed's succulent nature is cooling and moistening. Yet one of its most useful actions is to clear damp heat such as boils or the impetigo noted above. Dr. John Bastyr, founder of Bastyr University of Naturopathic Medicine, is noted to have said that his mother saved his life applying a chickweed poultice to his pustulent wound after his appendectomy.[18]

How does a plant such as chickweed clear fluid from various sites while moistening tissue at the same time? One explanation is that chickweed stimulates metabolism. Thus, it promotes the breakdown of fats, fluids, and lymph material, which helps the body move them and stay fluid. By its very nature, chickweed is soothing because of the demulcent or mucilaginous sugars present in its leaves. When eaten raw, it adds sweetness to bitter spring greens. Sweet is the flavor of building and nourishing, and this beautiful little star child is loaded with nutrients. Chickweed is high in chlorophyll as well as minerals such as magnesium, calcium, zinc, manganese, potassium, and iron. Carotenes present in the plant yield vitamins A and C.

A major use of this plant is to dissolve boundaries, on the emotional and psychic levels as well as the physical level. I have worked with chickweed tincture or tea to shrink benign tumors, cysts, or boils that were hard to dissolve. It is excellent for treating benign breast lumps. This is the spirit medicine of chickweed: dissolution of boundaries and clearing away of toxic energies.

Early on in my relationship with chickweed, I was given an indication to use this plant with children who had lung issues and did not laugh readily or much at all. I made the connection that chickweed helped those constricted by their tight boundaries. Drop doses used over a period of time can help dissolve the tight weave of self-protection that some people feel caught in. As with many medicinal plants, we can talk about actions and energetics, but sometimes we simply have to acknowledge the superpowers that lie within the seeds and stamens.

Indications

Heat/Excitation (Cooling/Moistening)

Head. As a tea or a compress, chickweed can clear a headache due to fever or too much sun on a summer day. Also soothes inflamed throat.

Eyes. Compresses or poultices clear pink eye remarkably quickly. Keep in mind that pink eye is highly contagious: dip one corner of a washcloth into chickweed infusion, place over eye for 5 to 10 minutes. Next, dip a second corner into the infusion and place over eye. This keeps the tea from becoming contaminated. Continue until all four corners are used and then place used washcloth in the laundry.

Skin. A wash or salve will cool hot, angry, itchy skin conditions such as eczema, impetigo, poison ivy, heat rashes, and burns.

Bladder. Soothing for hot bladder infections and inflammation from interstitial cystitis.

Liver/gallbladder. As a wild food or freshly juiced, chickweed can cool livers that are "hot" due to too much alcohol consumption or for those taking pharmaceuticals that tend to overwork the liver and stimulate liver energy.

Menopause. Excellent remedy to clear heat from menopausal hot flashes. As a moistening plant, it addresses dryness from aging.

Damp/Stagnation (Stimulant/Nutritive)

Respiratory system. Useful for bronchitis, asthma, and bronchial infections, especially in children, as it breaks up congestion.

Thyroid. By stimulating metabolism, chickweed counters the effects of a slow or hypo-functioning thyroid, including conditions such as water retention, weight gain, and sluggish digestion.

Lymphatic system. This herb contains minerals and is high in salt. Thus, it acts to move water out of lymph tissue. Also softens hard lymphatic nodules.

Breasts/uterus. Chickweed tincture has been most effective in moving stagnation in breast tissue, benign cysts, or fibroids when combined with other lymphatic decongestants such as violet (*Viola* spp.) or poke root (*Phytolacca americana*).

Habitat & Harvest

Plant a vegetable garden and you will have more chickweed than you will ever need. Another favorite place to harvest this nourishing medicine is in a greenhouse during the winter. Chickweed sprawls along the ground. When you harvest, it is easiest to gather the stems as a bundle, then snip the bounty at the base as one intact mat. Chickweed prefers moist, damp places and prefers shade.

Preparations

Infusion: Fresh or freshly dried preferred.

Tincture: Fresh plant (1:2, 60% alcohol) or freshly dried (1:5, 40% alcohol). To break up stagnation, may need up to 1 teaspoon three times a day.

Oil: Best extracted from freshly dried plants because there is so much water in fresh material.

Poultice/compress: Use fresh plant material for a poultice, or a strong infusion for a compress.

Contraindications

Chickweed is safe for general consumption.

Dandelion

Taraxacum officinale

Blow-ball, Lion's tooth, Piss-a-bed

Family	Asteraceae
Parts Used	flower, root, leaf
Energetics	leaf—cooling, drying; root—cooling, building
Tissue States	damp stagnation, depression, heat
Taste	bitter, sweet, salty
Actions	flower—emollient, vulnerary, nutritive; root—hepatic, cholagogue, nutritive, galactagogue, antibacterial, aperient, laxative; leaf—tonic, diuretic, cholagogue, nutritive

The ubiquitous dandelion is recorded to have been used for thousands of years in China as well as in ancient Egypt and Greece. The genus name *Taraxacum* comes from the Greek words *taraxos*, "disorder," and *akos*, "remedy." Dandelion was held in the greatest esteem as it was considered the remedy of all disorders. The species name *officinale* refers to the fact that this plant was used as the official medicine in the marketplace or apothecary. Indeed, it was a highly revered tonic for all. How interesting that this great healer is now the bane of many a manicured lawn. And how ironic that dandelion is one of the best medicines to help our bodies clear toxins and pollutants, including the chemical herbicides and fungicides that many lawns are laden with.

In medieval times, this plant was called *dente-de-lion*, which is French for "lion's tooth," referring to the deeply toothed edges of the leaves. While able to grow in most conditions, dandelion prefers full sun and well-drained soil. Interestingly, the flower head is actually a bunch of florets—each is an individual flower. This flower has a single ovule, which becomes one seed in the magnificent seed ball.

Most herbals say *Taraxacum* is native to Eurasia and arrived in America in the time of early European settlement. Indigenous scholar Valerie Goodness, who is of Ojibwe and Tsalagi lineage, has reported that *Taraxacum* (though a different species) has been in use by First Nation people for over a thousand years. Sean Sherman, Oglala Lakota, founder of The Sioux Chef, also supports the use of dandelion by Indigenous peoples long before colonists arrived.

Uses

Dandelion's main action is moving stagnation. By increasing elimination, dandelion enhances metabolic functioning on many levels. As a diuretic it stimulates and enhances kidney function. The leaf is a source of potassium so it is nutritive rather than depleting. Dandelion is a superb remedy for conditions of metabolic imbalance such as diabetes, heart disease, and endocrine disorders. So many of these conditions are rooted in years of toxic buildup and poor liver function. I often counsel my clients that they may need to take a month of herbs for each year they have experienced a health condition (although I have seen people enjoy good results in a much shorter timeframe, too). This allows them to realize that herbs work on a deep cellular level to truly open channels of elimination and restore a healthy ecosystem. I have also worked with dandelion for clients who struggle with joint and muscle pain after a year or two of taking statins. Those who take these cholesterol-reducing drugs are advised to have liver function tests every six months due to their toxic effect.

Indications for Root
Heat/Excitation (Cooling)
Skin. Roots can be used to treat boils, abscesses, and acne.

Damp/Stagnation (Alterative/Stimulant)
Sinuses. Dandelion cools and clears sinuses. Good for use with infections.
Mental health. The spring root is more stimulating than one harvested in the fall and is wonderful for lethargy and foggy thinking.
Digestive system. One of the few herbs that directly increases hydrochloric acid in the stomach, so it is helpful for relief of bloating, gas, and

heartburn due to insufficient stomach acid (hypochlorhydria). Especially helpful for elders with weak digestion.

Liver. For liver congestion, gall stones, and jaundice. I have used drop doses of root tincture with newborns with jaundice.

Cardiovascular system. As an alterative, dandelion enhances metabolic functioning, which helps make blood vessels healthier.

Uterine health. This is a great ally when working with menstrual irregularities due to its support of liver function. For the same reason it is a menopausal remedy for excessive hot flashes and stagnation.

Breast. Relieves congestion and pain from fibrocystic breasts, cysts, or benign swelling. Root oil blends well with violet oil for breast massage.

Indications for Leaf

Cooling. Leaves make a compress to clear heat.

Diuretic. *Taraxacum officinale* leaf is one of the most powerful yet gentle diuretics. It is mineral-rich and is known for its high potassium content. This makes it safe to use as a diuretic because it balances the sodium–potassium exchange that happens in the kidneys.

Nutritive. The leaves are very high in minerals such as potassium, calcium, manganese, magnesium, and silica. Vitamins include A, D, C, and even B.

Indications for Flower

Vulnerary. The tea makes an excellent wash for sunburns, acne, insect bites, or age spots. Spray infusion on face and leave overnight.

Habitat & Harvest

Cultivation of dandelions is clearly not a challenge, but if you are intent on harvesting large quantities, it is best to do so in well-tended, loose soil where the roots are easy to lift out.

Harvest leaves in early spring before flowering to avoid excess bitter flavor. Flowers are best harvested late spring, early summer. While the roots can be harvested early spring as well, I prefer late autumn after the frost. I find the roots are juiciest and most nutritious at that time of year.

Preparations

Infusion: Leaf and flower.

Decoction: Fresh or dried roots.

Tincture: Fresh plant (1:2, 75% alcohol) or dried root (1:5, 50% alcohol).

Fresh greens: Best eaten in spring and early summer, then again in early fall.

Contraindications

Since dandelion stimulates HCL production, do not use in cases of heartburn due to excess hydrochloric acid. Also avoid with damp, cold digestive system.

Echinacea

Echinacea angustifolia, E. purpurea
Purple coneflower, Kansas snakeroot, Black Sampson

Family	Asteraceae
Parts Used	leaf, flower, seed head, root
Energetics	cooling, drying, stimulating
Tissue States	depression/deficiency, heat, stagnation
Taste	acrid, bitter, sweet, pungent (tingling)
Actions	alterative, diffusive, immunostimulant, antimicrobial, febrifuge, lymphagogue, vulnerary, stimulant

Echinacea is a national treasure. Native to our prairies, this plant is extolled by Plains Indians and other First Nations for its profound medicine and breadth of applications. The lists of applications reveal how echinacea was most likely one of the most revered plants of Native Americans.

Of the nine species native to North America, the three that are most prevalent in herbal medicine are *Echinacea angustifolia*, narrow (*angus*) leaved (*folia*) coneflower; *E. purpurea*, purple coneflower; and the pale purple-flowered *E. pallida*. The term for the genus is derived from the Greek word *ekhinos*, which refers to the prickly seed head.

E. angustifolia is the species that first caught the notice of the early Eclectic practitioners. It was introduced to them by H. C. F. Meyer, a German folk doctor from Nebraska. In the late 1800s, Meyer learned from the Sioux and the Pawnee of echinacea's prowess as a remedy for snakebites. He spent sixteen years perfecting his infamous "Meyer's Blood Purifier," a blend of *E. angustifolia*, wormwood (*Artemisia annua*), hops (*Humulus lupulus*), and other herbs. He tried numerous times to introduce this remedy to the leading Eclectic medical practitioners physician John King and pharmacist John Uri Lloyd. They eventually listened and King lamented at waiting so long, because the success of this medicine was far-reaching. In the end, echinacea was the only relief from the severe pain of cancer that King could offer to his wife. It is said that she could not be without the herb until the day she died.

Echinacea became one of the most popular remedies and reigned supreme in the Eclectic practice until the 1930s. At that time, since it did not have the backing of the American Medical Association, its popularity with white Americans dwindled. Herbalists took it to Germany, where it was taken up with great fervor. The *E. angustifolia* species is difficult to germinate and grow, so early German research was conducted on the popular garden species *E. purpurea*. While this species has wonderful medicinal qualities, in my experience, the deeper medicine resides with *E. angustifolia*. That being said, *E. angustifolia* is on the At-Risk List, as explained below, and I prefer recommending *E. purpurea*. However, since we deal with a lot of snakebites here in the Shenandoah Valley, I always grow *E. angustifolia* and keep a supply of it on hand.

It is said that Eastern Nations were not very familiar with *E. purpurea* until it gained notoriety as a snakebite remedy by a slave doctor in North Carolina named Sampson, hence one of the plant's common names, Black Sampson. This doctor was given his freedom because of his far-reaching success with *E. purpurea*. Remember this was a time when serious infections, including tuberculosis and many venereal diseases, were prolific, and *Echinacea* had profound effects in clearing these challenging, purulent diseases.[19]

Uses

In addition to its renowned benefits for treating snakebites and clearing venom, echinacea is also used topically and internally for throat infections, septic infections, boils, and all known pestilent eruptions. Energetically it is cooling, but it is also diffusive and stimulating, which is why it moves toxicity. Chemically, echinacea works by inhibiting hyaluronidase, the enzyme in venom that breaks down hyaluronic acid (a component of the intracellular matrix). This enzyme effectively digests tissue, allowing the attacking animal to draw sustenance from its prey. Tissue destruction from enzymes occurs with other microbial toxic reactions and this is why echinacea is such a superb wound healer. Preparations of good-quality echinacea root and seed heads produce an immediate tingling effect, which is due to the presence of immunostimulating compounds called alkylamides. It is also antiviral because it increases production of interferon, the chemical messenger that identifies the genetic material of the virus to neighboring cells. The seeds of all species are equally potent. Harvesting some of the seed from *E. angustifolia*, instead of the root, is an excellent way to conserve this endangered plant.

Indications
Heat/Excitation (Clears Heat)
Venomous bites. Having worked with many people who have experienced copperhead snakebites and intense spider bites, I find it difficult to imagine rural life without this medicine.

Damp/Stagnation (Clears Heat/Alterative)
Throat. Excellent for strep throat and bacterial infections that include the lymph nodes. An echinacea throat spray is an excellent and effective topical application and is soothing and even numbing to painful tonsils. Simply switch out the dropper top on a tincture bottle with a spray nozzle and spritz tincture directly onto throat.

Breasts. In cases of mastitis, use large and frequent doses the first day.

Uterine health. Higher and more frequent doses are also recommended for infections from retained tissue after birth or miscarriage.

Septic fevers / eruptive diseases. Helpful to complete process for clearing toxins following mumps, chickenpox, measles, mononucleosis.

Cold/Depression (Stimulant)
Immune system. Stimulates immune system function. At the first sign of a cold or flu, echinacea can be effective for staving off the illness or shortening its duration. Best taken with ginger if condition is cold. The leaves and flowers are more of a tonic, building herb.

Lymphatic system. Echinacea moves stagnant, cold conditions resulting from buildup of excess phlegm. It promotes the flow of lymph to address swollen lymphatic glands and even stimulates saliva.

General health. This herb's acrid taste is numbing on the throat and tongue, which indicates its dispersive nature. Echinacea is stimulating in nature.

Skin. Can help remedy chronic deep cystic acne and a tendency toward boils. Use for a month or so in a formula with other alteratives or blood cleansers.

At-Risk Status
Echinacea pallida, *E. tennesseensis*, and *E. angustifolia* are at risk at the time of this writing, and *E. laevagata* has been threatened for a long time. I prefer

E. angustifolia for venomous bites and serious infection, but its numbers have been threatened due to overharvesting and habitat loss. Thus, I work mostly with *E. purpurea* and save *E. angustifolia* for serious bites and conditions.

Habitat & Harvest

E. purpurea is quite adaptable but prefers full sun and sandy, rich soil. Harvest the leaves before the plant flowers, harvest seeds as they mature, and dig roots in late fall in the third year of growth. To know if the roots are mature enough, chew on a small piece of root and see whether your tongue tingles. If so, it is ready to harvest.

Preparations

Infusion: Leaf and flower—steep for an hour; drink 2 to 3 cups a day for immune support. Root—decoction; drink no more than 2 cups a day.

Tincture: Fresh root, leaf, flower (1:2, 75% alcohol); dried root, leaf, flower (1:5, 60% alcohol); seed (1:5, 80% alcohol). For acute conditions take 1 teaspoon three to four times a day until infection has subsided, then continue another ten days with ½ teaspoon three times a day.

Contraindications

Since use of echinacea increases white blood cell counts, it should not be used too soon after surgery because the increase in white blood cell count due to echinacea could be mistaken as a sign of infection. Also be cautious about offering echinacea to organ-transplant patients who are on immuno-suppressive drugs.

Those with allergies to Asteraceae or Compositae family plants may also have an allergic reaction to echinacea. There are no known serious side effects to taking echinacea.

The German *Commission E Monographs* (considered by many to be the gold standard for herbal safety standards) says that "in principle" echinacea should not be used in chronic conditions such as AIDS, HIV infection, multiple sclerosis, or other autoimmune conditions, as it would "stimulate" the immune system. In *Principles and Practice of Phytotherapy*, authors Kerry Bones and Simon Mills state, "There is now a large body of clinical observations, including those of the authors, that long term Echinacea is at least not harmful in autoimmunity and is probably beneficial." These writers go on to say, "The *British Herbal Compendium* offer no contraindications for Echinacea. In fact, the indications in the compendium for prophylaxis of colds and influenza and chronic viral and bacterial infections suggests long term useage."[20] I have used both species very safely with acute infection for those that have autoimmune conditions when it was the best remedy for the condition.

Elder

Sambucus nigra, S. canadensis
Lady Elder, Rob Elder, Pipe tree

Family	Adoxaceae (formerly Caprifoliaceae)
Part Used	flower, berry
Energetics	flower—cooling, drying; berry—cooling, nutritive
Tissue States	flower—heat, tension, cold/depression; berry—heat, tension, atrophy
Taste	flower—sweet, acrid, aromatic; berry—sour
Actions	flower—expectorant, anticatarrhal, diaphoretic, antispasmodic, circulatory stimulant, external anti-inflammatory, very mild sedative; berry—antiviral, nutritive, antioxidant, anti-inflammatory, diuretic, laxative, immunomodulator

A veritable apothecary in itself, the uses of elder are as rich and varied as the myths and folklore surrounding this revered tree. The word *elder* comes from the Anglo-Saxon word *aeld*, which meant "fire." This may refer to the use of the hollow stem after the inner pith is removed, as a pipe, possibly for smoking or to help ignite fires; hence, it also has the common name of *pipe tree*.

   In Nature, the presence of a hollow tube has always been associated with a journey medicine or a way to travel to the underworld. Even on the leaf stems of elder, there is a hollow ridge, which is one feature that helps to identify this shrub when it is not in flower.[21] Early customs associated this tree with the magic of the underworld. In most countries, most notably Denmark, it was thought that Hylde-Moer, the Elder Mother, dwelt in the leaves; she was the guardian of the underworld. It was common knowledge for hundreds of years that permission was required to cut down an elder and use its wood, or foul events would befall the trespasser. This custom continues to this day with wise lovers of plant medicine. "Old girl, give me some of thy wood and I will give thee some of mine when I grow into a tree," was a Scandinavian woodsman's plea.[22] Another Danish tradition was that if you stood under the elder on Midsummer Night's Eve, you would see the Fairy King and all his entourage. It was said if you slept under an elder, you would have visions, and not all would be pleasant.

There is toxicity associated with this magical medicine, but when prepared properly it is extremely safe. The presence of cyanide, or more precisely a cyanogenic glycoside, creates more nausea and purgative effects than fatalities, although they have occurred. According to Finnish herbalist Henriette Kress: "Cyanoglycosides are found in most if not all rose family plants, and they're the taste behind bitter almonds and amaretto. There's not all that much in elder: the irritation of elder is more due to the resin than the sambunigrin."[23] I cook (or tincture) fresh and dried berries before using them because the seeds, which constitute 50 percent of the small berry, are the source of the plant's potential toxicity.

Elder prefers moist, low-lying places and can be quite abundant in wild stands. Beautiful creamy white flowers, less than a quarter-inch wide, form large saucer-shaped umbels up to nine inches across. In late summer, these flowers become draping clusters of deep purple/black berries. The whole plant has been used medicinally, and modern authors write of using leaves, bark, and stems. I use only the flowers and berries.

There are many elders worldwide but only a few native species in North America. Black elderberry, *Sambucus nigra*, is the European variety that is the subject of much of the lore and medicinal use. Of the North American species, *S. canadensis* is the preferred species and has the greatest similarities to *S. nigra*. On the West Coast, from Oregon south to Baja, blue elderberry, *S. nigra* ssp. *caerulea* is found, which is also known as Mexican elderberry or Tapiro. The common red elderberry (*S. racemosa*) is said to be best left for wildlife as it is a major source of food for birds. Canadian First Nation peoples were known to boil the berries overnight and make the preserves into cakes, and to this day Alaskan herbalists enjoy red elder medicine, but there have been more accounts of toxicity from the red berries of this species.

Uses

Rich, purple elderberries have deservedly become a familiar elixir. The proanthocyanins found in elderberry are some of the highest-rated antioxidants. Many of the anti-inflammatory effects of elderberry are due to the nutrient-rich, cooling properties of these bioflavonoids. Herbal medicine knows of few plants who exceed the virtues of the berry of the elder tree.

While not as strong as some potent antivirals, elderberry can be offered to a diverse audience, from children to the elderly, all with great safety.

The berries seem to be most effective when taken right at the onset of a flu and continued throughout the course of the illness. A virus is a masterful creature with a very simple structure, which makes it quite adaptable but unable to replicate on its own. Viruses are equipped with an enzyme that can destroy cell membranes and commandeer a cell's genetic material. It then replicates times a thousand and sails off to do the same to neighboring cells. Elder works by preventing the virus from entering the cells, which is why early and frequent doses are the best way to shorten duration of illness.[24] According to Paul Bergner: "Viruses have the ability to alter their genetics and create new strains. This makes a problem for creating vaccines against viral diseases, such as flu or AIDS, because the vaccine can only be developed against known strains. Elder may thus be able to literally save lives, because most strains of the virus use the same enzyme mechanism to penetrate cells."[25]

Elderberry upregulates chemicals called cytokines, whose role is to signal molecules to participate in the healthy immune response.[26] There was great misinformation during the 2020 outbreak of COVID-19 that elderberry was causing the massive cytokine storms that were seen in the late stages of the disease. This was purely conjecture, based on older studies, and there are no studies reporting an increased risk of respiratory distress, cytokine storm, or ARDS (acute respiratory distress syndrome) due to use of elderberry. In fact, elderberry was attributed in shortening duration of COVID-19 infection.[27]

My favorite part of the plant is the flower, which I love to offer my students during a proving session. The taste is sweet, yet with a bit of acrid (relaxing) in the background. It is immediately warming but ever so gently. It then literally moves from the center outward. The subtle warming of the body and sharpening of the mind is remarkable. I feel it brings clarity to cognition because it softly relaxes the system. Our senses come alive with greater precision when we are relaxed and alert.

Indications
Heat/Excitation (Cooling)
Eyes. Cool elderflower tea is soothing for inflammation of the eyes.
Skin. Excellent internally and topically for eruptive skin diseases such as measles and chicken pox.

Cold/Depression (Stimulating)

Fevers. Taken hot, elderflowers are diaphoretic.

Respiratory system. Try a hot infusion of flowers for asthma, bronchitis, and irritated coughs.

General health. The berries are nutritive and are used for blood building.

Damp/Stagnation (Aromatic/Alterative)

Mouth/throat. Prepare as a mouthwash/gargle for ulcers, sore throats, and tonsillitis.

Immune system. Flowers and berries resolve damp heat and are helpful for colds, flu, and ear infections.

Endocrine system. The tea is an underutilized alterative or blood cleanser. It has great value with diabetes because it is a gentle blood sugar stabilizer and enhances the metabolic functions that rid the body of wastes.

Kidneys. As a cool infusion, the flowers enhance the kidney's ability to act as a decongestant, relieving excess fluid from the body and eliminating toxins.

Tension/Constriction (Relaxant)

Nervous system. There is a long history of using elderflowers as a relaxant for allaying anxiety, lifting spirits, and promoting restful sleep. Specific for restless children at the onset of an infection.

Habitat & Harvest

Elderberry spreads through root suckers, so if you do not want it to expand through your garden it is best to prune in late winter. Pruning every couple of years to eliminate older branches will encourage new production of flowers and fruit. If shrubs are not producing, you can prune all the way to the ground. This will delay fruit production but, in the end, will yield healthier trees. If left exposed too long to the sun before gathering, the flowers assume an undesirable brownish color when dried. Berries within a cluster may not all ripen at the same time, so discard unripe and green berries after harvesting clusters.

Elder makes excellent hedgerows and can easily be propagated through cuttings. Simply cut a healthy branch in early spring and place in the ground. Remember to stake it and water it but literally you will have a full thriving bush the next year. The magic of elder.

Preparations

Infusion: Warm flower infusion is helpful for fevers, flus, and respiratory conditions; cool infusions for kidney cleansing and as an endocrine alterative. Drink 2 to 3 cups a day for immune support.

Tincture: Fresh flowers (1:2, 75% alcohol) or dried flowers (1:5, 50% alcohol). Use ½ to 1 teaspoon three times a day for acute flus and colds.

Syrup: This is the most common preparation for berries. See Elderberry Syrup on page 193.

Wash: Make a strong infusion of the flowers to apply as a wash.

Contraindications

The bark and leaves are laxative and can be toxic. As stated above, *S. racemosa* or species with red berries have potential toxicity.

It is important to remove all stem pieces when preparing the berries. Many elixirs and cordials are made without cooking the berry. Use dried flowers for making tea.

Goldenrod

Solidago canadensis, S. odora, S. vigaurea
Woundwort, Aaron's rod, Solidago

Family	Asteraceae
Parts Used	flower, leaf
Energetics	warming, stimulating, drying
Tissue States	lax, cold
Taste	aromatic, sweet, bitter, astringent
Actions	diuretic, anticatarrhal, anti-inflammatory, antimicrobial, astringent, carminative, vulnerary, diaphoretic, stimulant

During late summer and early fall, graceful sprays of goldenrod fill meadows and woodland edges with brilliant color. The showy golden flowers are often blamed for fall allergies, but it is the inconspicuous green flowers of ragweed (*Ambrosia* spp.) that causes allergies. Ragweed has light pollen that is easily spread by wind, while goldenrod pollen is heavy and requires pollinators to spread it. Goldenrod is actually a specific medicine for fall allergies. Dark amber goldenrod honey is also an excellent medium for homeopathic dosing of this medicine.

With over one hundred species, this resilient perennial offers an array of subtle flavors, yet most species can be used interchangeably for medicine. While most are native to North America, some are native to Eurasia and Europe, such as *Solidago vigaurea*. There are lookalike plants, such as golden ragwort (*Senecio aureus*), in the Aster family that can be toxic, so before you intimately familiarize yourself with a goldenrod plant's scents and tastes, be sure you have keyed it properly. I find most goldenrods have an aromatic, resinous smell, which tells me it is stimulating, astringing, and antimicrobial. *Solidago odora*, as the species name implies, is subtly sweet smelling and tasting. All species play an important role as pollinator plants. Goldenrod is recommended for butterfly gardens, as it hosts over one hundred species of butterflies, including the beautiful monarch.[28]

Uses

Solidago means "to make whole," and this native beauty has earned her name. Goldenrod is one of our most soothing and healing medicines specific for mucous membranes and clearing inflammation. This is one of the first herbs to consider when there is congestion and inflammation in the respiratory tract, especially the sinuses. For those prone to recurrent bronchitis in the fall, I often recommend this as the primary herb in a blend. *S. odora* is especially useful for this time of year because this aromatic species is more warming than others and can work as a stimulant for seasonal depression, which often pairs with chronic bronchitis.

For those challenged with allergies from ragweed, I recommend a strong infusion of nettle and goldenrod in August to begin to tighten the weave of tissues, as well as to boost immunity. It is said that the levels of the bioflavonoid rutin are higher in goldenrod than in green tea. As mentioned earlier, bioflavonoids used to be called vitamin P (for permeability) because, as antioxidants, they add to the integrity of blood vessels as well as mucous membranes. You can see why they are so helpful for leaky, runny allergies. This is a specific indication for the red eyes, profuse secretions, and fatigue related to allergies to cat dander. This use was taught by Matthew Wood at our school years ago, and I have seen it work successfully on numerous occasions.

First Nations peoples have a long history of using this plant as a wash for wounds, burns, and infections. Again, its aromatic nature is useful in cleansing wounds especially when dealing with thrush or fungal infections.

Few herbs can compare with goldenrod as a urinary tract remedy due to its combination of potency and safety of use. Of course, any time there are kidney infections or serious pathology, it is important to work with a health care professional. However, goldenrod can bring much relief to bladder infections, cystitis, and prostatitis due to its antimicrobial and anti-inflammatory properties. Dr. John Bastyr recommended it for low urine output with back pain. German herbalist and physician Rudolf Weiss lauds *Solidago*'s potency and reliability as a diuretic.[29] Specific for sluggish kidneys, it serves well in blends to prevent formation of kidney stones. It is also a wonderful tea to drink after a long illness when the kidneys are "tired," which can manifest as heaviness or pain in lower extremities.

As if the above were not enough, this common wayside wonder is an effective digestive tonic. As an astringent, goldenrod is helpful for diarrhea. If there is fullness after eating, *S. odora* works beautifully as a carminative.

The oil of the flowers can be made into an amazing remedy for sprained and strained muscles. I have used it often with older injuries— its warming qualities penetrate deeply into bruised tissue that needs moving and clearing.

Indications
Heat/Excitation (Astringent)
Allergies. Cooling to red eyes and inflamed tissues. Works very well with hyperimmune/allergic responses from bee stings or toxic spider bites.

Bladder. Astringing remedy for hot urinary tract issues.

Digestive system. The Iroquois have used a variety of goldenrod species for intestinal bleeding and diarrhea.[30]

Damp/Stagnation (Warming/Stimulating)
Digestive system. Aromatics in this plant help to move stagnation after eating; works as a warming carminative.

Sinuses/throat. Outstanding remedy to clear sinus congestion as well as the upper respiratory tract.

Kidney. As a diuretic, goldenrod is excellent at moving suppressed urine and scant output. Safe for all ages and constitutions, especially when there is weakness or low-grade backaches. Wonderful to add to blends as a preventative for kidney stones.

Musculoskeletal system. Goldenrod oil is phenomenal at relaxing spasms, cramping, and tightness due to sprains. Works equally well on old injuries. Herbalist Kiva Rose has reported goldenrod's effectiveness when used topically for uterine and ovarian pain and cramping.

Skin. The Miwok have traditionally used California goldenrod leaf powder (*S. californica*) on sores as well as a strong infusion held in the mouth for toothaches.[31]

Habitat & Harvest

Goldenrod is a prolific plant that makes its home in open fields, savannahs, and prairies. Depending on the species, it is best to harvest leaves before the plants flower so as to avoid excess bitterness. Harvest flowers before they fully open to avoid the inconvenience of having to deal with "fluff" when processing. Goldenrod is very easy to dry as there is not a lot of moisture in this plant, as long as you do not harvest a day or two after rain.

Preparations

Infusion: Use 2 to 3 cups a day for allergies and to support kidney function.
Tincture: Fresh plant (1:2, 95% alcohol) or dry plant (1:4, 60% alcohol). Excellent in drop doses as a specific for cat allergies.
Oil: Apply often and early for relief of muscle strains, sprains, and spasms. Needs to be applied often to get relief early on, and then taper off applications over time.

Contraindications

As noted above, there are toxic lookalikes to goldenrod, so always make sure to identify *Solidago* species accurately. Allergies have been associated with *Solidago* in rare instances. Not recommended during pregnancy. Can be drying, so use caution with long-term consumption.

Goldenseal

Hydrastis canadensis
Eye balm, Yellow pucoon, Jaundice root

Family	Ranunculaceae
Parts Used	leaf, root
Energetics	cooling, drying, astringing
Tissue States	atrophy, damp/stagnation, laxity
Taste	bitter
Actions	alterative, cholagogue, lymphatic, hepatic, antiseptic

Goldenseal is one of the few plants on the UpS At-Risk List that I include in this materia medica, and I do so because I have seen it grow and flourish with relative ease in many different environs. Yet even in 1898, its survival in the wild was described as precarious in *King's American Dispensatory*:

> *With hydrastis . . . the plant disappears as soon as the ground is disturbed by the settler. Once plentiful along the Ohio riverbanks, it is now found only in isolated spots, having suffered extermination as fast as the woodland yielded to the pioneer's axe. At present the geographical center of the plant is around Cincinnati. But four states now grow sufficient* Hydrastis *to make it profitable for gathering for commercial use. These are Ohio, Indiana, Kentucky, and West Virginia.*[32]

In the Sacred Plant Traditions sanctuary garden, we have planted goldenseal in all conditions just to demonstrate its ease of cultivation. Give this plant some shade and moisture and it will move rapidly through your garden as it spreads both by rhizomes and by seed. The beautiful white flowers become clusters of ruby red berries that follow not long afterward. We have given away countless roots to students and friends, and it is a delight when they send me photos of gardens laden with spreading *Hydrastis*.

The irony of the threatened status of goldenseal is that this plant is one of the most misused herbal supplements on the market. It is touted as an "herbal antibiotic," which misleads people into immediately using it when they develop a cold, flu, or infection. Once we look at this plant's energetics, however, we see that not only is this not the appropriate use, but that goldenseal can be detrimental in these situations. Herbalist Paul Bergner said, "In my experience both selling herbs at retail, and seeing patients in the clinic, not even 10% of the goldenseal use in the U.S. is clinically appropriate. When someone pops large amounts of goldenseal 'for a cold', especially in its early stages, they are wasting both their money and an endangered plant."[33]

While all parts of goldenseal are medicinal, the root is the most highly acclaimed, yet traditional use also includes the leaves. Using the leaves is a more sustainable practice, and I have appreciated the leaf medicine especially applied topically for wounds and inflammation.

Uses

The energetics of goldenseal are bitter, cooling, drying, and astringing. While these might seem applicable in hot infections, goldenseal is the classic example where tending the terrain of the tissue will lead to greater strength and immunity. According to Herbalist Rosalee de la Floret, "Herbalists sometimes refer to goldenseal as a mucous membrane trophorestorative because it balances the mucous membranes. It can both increase mucosal secretions and inhibit mucosal secretions, depending on the need of the individual."[34] This quality is key to understanding why goldenseal is not the first herb to reach for as an acute illness comes on. There are valuable immune components in the mucus lining our membranes. The body's response with excess catarrh or phlegm is an immune response in which immunoglobulins and other vital compounds are mounting an appropriate defense. When we dry out membranes prematurely, we prevent the body's healthy response, thus allowing microbes to proliferate. If the secretions continue and our vitality is such that we cannot recuperate, then goldenseal is an appropriate astringing tonic.

The writings of Eclectic physician Harvey Felter also reinforce the use of goldenseal in deficient and lax tissue states: "*Hydrastis* preparations are among the most successful remedies in catarrhs of the nose and throat." The specific indications that he listed are as follows: "Catarrhal states of the mucous membranes unaccompanied by acute inflammation, relaxed tissues, with profuse secretion of thick and tenacious yellowish or greenish-yellow muco-pus; relaxation and ulceration of tissues of mouth and throat . . . ; atonic gastric irritability; irritation of mucous surfaces."[35]

Especially in cases of chronic sinus infections, when the tissues are boggy and have lost tone, low doses of goldenseal can help tonify and astringe this important first line of defense for the respiratory system. Goldenseal has a specificity for treating fungal growth, which attributes to the consistent success of this plant in treating sinus infections. While most infections may start out as viral or bacterial, rarely are sinus infections properly cleared with antibiotics. This leads to low-grade, asymptomatic infections lingering, which present a perfect system for fungal infections to take root. I also carry goldenseal powder with me when I am in damp tropical climates that give rise to fungal infections easily.

Goldenseal is incredibly successful with gastric ulcers and is my favorite remedy for this condition. This was one of the main ways it was used by the Eclectics.[36] Eclectic physician Harvey Felter wrote: "Without question it is our best single drug for chronic gastric catarrh, or so-called chronic gastritis. . . . For gastric ulcer no treatment should be considered without a fair and generous trial of hydrastis. . . . In the treatment of stomach disorders with hydrastis or its derivatives, the fact must be kept prominently in mind that it is only in conditions of atony, with gastric irritability."[37]

In reference to its excellent use in matters of the eye, Eclectic writers describe a clear liquid formulation that would avoid the staining that goldenseal is infamous for. Just be mindful when applying a compress that this plant imparts a dramatic yellow coloring to skin and fabrics, and to my knowledge modern-day herbalists have not come up with such a superior, non-staining remedy as that of the Eclectics.

Berberine is a bitter alkaloid found in goldenseal and other medicinal plants. The berberine-containing plants are specific for the treatment of wounds, abscesses, infections, respiratory diseases, inflammation, and pathologies of the eye. Because goldenseal is listed as an endangered plant, there is a move to use more leaf material from *Hydrastis* as well as its many analogs. Barberry (*Berberis vulgaris*), Oregon grape (*B. aquifolium*), and coptis root (*Coptis chinensis*) are the most common. Goldthread (*C. trifolia*) is the native Southern medicine that was as popular as goldenseal but was overharvested during the time of the Eclectics. While goldthread did have time to recover from overharvesting, it has now returned to the UpS At-Risk List.

What makes these three berberine-containing plants so effective is that, energetically, they are drying and clear damp heat. As we have seen, boggy, cold tissues provide a perfect host for bacterial infections. These in turn create heat and inflammation. Aside from astringing inflamed tissue, these herbs are excellent liver tonics. Berberine is a yellow alkaloid, which indicates its role as a flavonoid as well. The antioxidant effect of berberine is said to be comparable to that of vitamin C.[38]

Clinical trials for those with insulin-resistant diabetes have shown significant reductions in blood glucose through the use of berberine supplements.

These studies have shown enhancement of metabolic functions, which in turn improve insulin response and lead to much more stable levels of blood sugars.[39] Again, our traditional alteratives are at play here.

In the Berberidaceae family, the genus *Berberis* comprises 450 to 500 species, which represent the main natural source of berberine. Yet berberine is not confined to this family. Aside from goldenseal, the buttercup family, or Ranunculaceae family, has the valuable *Coptis* genus within its ranks. Our native goldthread, *C. trifolia*, was used by Native Americans for infections and so much more. Chinese goldthread, *C. chinensis*, is one of the Fifty Fundamental Herbs of the Chinese materia medica.

Unless otherwise noted, all indications do best with low doses, 5 to 10 drops as needed.

Indications

Heat/Excitation
Eye. Excellent eye wash for conjunctivitis.

General health. As a remedy goldenseal clears heat from tissues. However, there are so many other effective heat-clearing herbs that are not endangered. Save goldenseal for use where it has its greatest value.

Cold/Depression

General health. Matthew Wood wrote: "By increasing nutrition and through its own direct stimulating powers, *Hydrastis* improves the general nervous and muscular tonus of the organism, especially the respiration and circulation."[40]

Mouth. Useful for ulcers (internal and external) that are slow to heal. Tightens boggy gums that are prone to bleeding.

Damp/Stagnation (Stimulant)

Sinuses. Excellent at resolving chronic boggy conditions with excessive secretions of yellow-green mucus.

Skin. Excellent wash for indolent sores or infections that are hard to treat. Do not leave goldenseal powder on wounds that may be infected below the surface.

Digestive system. Useful for gastric ulcers, liver stagnation or constipation from lack of bile excretion, gallbladder weakness or prevalence of gallstones, colitis, gastritis.

Bladder. Useful for recurrent infections, cloudy urine, and cystitis.

Lax/Atony
Digestive system. Lack of appetite, mucus in the stools, gastritis.

At-Risk Status

Goldenseal is currently on the IUCN's (The International Union for Conservation of Nature) Red List of Threatened Species. It is also on the UpS At-Risk List. If you purchase commercially, please check veracity of sustainable harvest.

Habitat & Harvest

H. canadensis loves the moist, rich loamy soils on shaded slopes in the Appalachian Mountains. Since goldenseal does not tolerate "wet feet" very well, plant in a well-drained area or on a slight incline. At Sacred Plant Traditions, we have planted it in a variety of locations and it has even done well in partial sun (though toward the end of the season the leaves look a bit burnt). Many growers have set up areas with shade cloth and have grown beautiful healthy plants this way.

If you harvest the root of a mature plant, cut a piece closest to the stem (the oldest part) then replant the rest of the root. The approximate age of the plant in years can be determined by counting the "seals" (stem scars) on the plant.

Preparations

Infusion: Extremely bitter so other methods are preferred, such as capsules or tincture, though the leaf tea is quite effective and not as bitter as the root.

Powder: I have used powdered root and leaf to sprinkle onto superficial wounds. It will cause skin to close so make sure the wound has been thoroughly cleaned before applying. I have worked with midwives who apply powdered root to a newborn's umbilical cord to dry the tissue and prevent infection.

Tincture: Fresh root or leaf (1:2, 75% alcohol); dried root or leaf (1:5, 50% alcohol). This is one herb that needs to be taken in low doses so as to not aggravate lax or weakened tissues. Use 5 to 15 drops three times a day, or depending on need.

Contraindications

Not to be used during pregnancy or while breastfeeding.

Hawthorn

Crataegus laevigata, C. monogyna, C. pinnatifida
May flower, May tree, Thornapple

Family	Rosaceae
Parts Used	leaf, flower, berry
Energetics	leaf/flower—cooling, drying; berry—slightly warming
Tissue States	atrophy, excitation, tension, laxity
Taste	sour, sweet, astringent
Actions	cardiotonic, cardioprotective, astringent, antioxidant, relaxant, digestive, diuretic

Along the ridges of the Appalachian Mountains, the windswept and craggy outlines of hawthorns are a reminder of the ancient folklore surrounding these small trees. The trunks and branches are covered in one-inch thorns and the wood is hard as steel. The botanical name *Crataegus* defines these characteristics: *kratos*, strength; *akis*, sharp. Yet come spring, when the white five-petaled flowers bloom, you can almost feel the otherworld open. Sprigs of the tree were placed in infants' cribs as a means of protection; and it is said fairies and spirits held their gatherings under the hawthorn. A visit to the apothecary and pollinator sanctuary at Avena Botanicals in Rockport, Maine, gives one the immense pleasure of experiencing a mature hedgerow of these magnificent medicines. Owner Deb Soule keeps the small trees pruned to make for easy harvest of spring flowers and fall berries. Of course, the pollinators are in heaven. This is one of the sacred herbs of Bealtaine, symbolizing fertility and love. You can imagine the wreaths of this May Day flower adorning young girls and strewn through the fields.

Author and photographer Steven Foster wrote: "The plant group embodies the concept of endless variation with numerous hybrids and other variants that in the late nineteenth century led to the naming of upwards of 1000 species of hawthorn for North America alone!"[41] While most species can be used interchangeably, it is interesting to note the incredible variations that are found in the wild. Most apothecaries work with *C. laevigata* (also known as *C. oxyacantha*) or English hawthorn. In Europe this species is used along with *C. monogyna*, one-seeded hawthorn.

Uses

Perhaps no other medicinal plant has such an extensive and profound medicinal effect on the heart and circulation as does hawthorn. All plant parts are tonic for the heart muscle as well the walls of all blood vessels. Greater vessel tone increases blood flow, especially where there is arteriosclerosis. One of the stellar actions of hawthorn is strengthening the contraction of the heart, or positive inotropism. Flavonoids and proanthocyanidins in hawthorn help to optimize energy production, strengthen contractions, and assist in a more efficient output of blood.[42] The stronger cardiac glycosides such as lily of the valley (*Convallaria majalis*) work directly with the heart's sodium–potassium pump to increase contractility. This is a very delicate balance and use of these plants needs to be under the supervision of a trained medical professional. Hawthorn, on the other hand, directly nourishes tissue.[43] This is a gentler action, and thus hawthorn should be taken for at least three months in order to feel its full effect. It is ideal for all heart imbalances, such as arrythmias, palpitations, and enlargement of the heart, as well as congestive heart failure (CHF). There have been numerous studies of its effectiveness with CHF, a condition that can tire the heart significantly.[44]

There is extensive evidence of First Nations as well as folkloric use of hawthorn berry over a period of hundreds of years. Hawthorn berry did not enter established medical practice until the nineteenth century. In the late 1800s there was a well-known Irish physician who built his reputation on his successful treatments of heart conditions, yet he kept his remedy a secret. Upon his death his daughter revealed that his famous elixir was a tincture of fresh, ripe berries of hawthorn.

This story is one of the reasons why the berries are most popular with herbalists. It is only recently that the leaves and flowers have regained their rightful place of importance. I prefer using a tea of leaves and flowers rather than one brewed from berries mostly because the aerial parts are easier to prepare. The berries are very hard and need a good amount of heat in order to extract sufficient medicine. The flowers contain higher levels of flavonoids, and the leaves are higher in procyanidins, which are a type of proanthocyanidin.[45]

A little known but impressive use of leaf and flower is stabilizing collagen matrix. This is an excellent herb for strains and sprains and conditions in which there is a breakdown in collagen-based tissues. I have used a flower and berry combination to repair the glomerular filters in a client with kidney disease. This vital aspect of the kidney is composed of collagen and a network of delicate blood vessels.

The energetics of all parts of hawthorn make it an effective support for emotional healing and protection. Hawthorn is in the rose family, and like roses, this magnificent flower opens the physical as well as spiritual heart. The protection of sharp thorns allows vulnerability to be experienced with a sense of safety. Added to other formulas, hawthorn can bring out the heart needed for any kind of transformational work.

Indications
Heat/Excitation (Cooling)

Mental health. Cooling for irritability and anxiety related to emotional stress. Excellent for attention-deficit/hyperactivity disorder in children as well as adults.

Cardiovascular system. Useful for palpitations from anxiety (heat), especially in autoimmune conditions, and for rapid pulse, tachycardia (rapid heartbeat), and hypertension.

Dry/Atrophy (Nutritive)

Cardiovascular system. Nourishes heart tissue and builds collagen through proanthocyanins. The berries help with congestive heart failure, which manifests as difficulty breathing and fatigue, by strengthening the muscle to move stagnation. Increases blood flow and enhances warmth through circulation.

Damp/Stagnation (Warming)

Digestive system. Chinese practitioners use the berries of *C. pinnatifida* (a species native to China) for bloating and stagnation, especially after greasy food. We have used this species as well and it works remarkably quickly, though *C. laevigata* can also be used. *C. pinnatifida* is more sour.

Tension/Constriction (Relaxant)

Blood vessels. Works as a vasodilator. The Cherokee traditionally eat bitter hawthorn fruits for better circulation and relief of cramps.

Heart muscle. Decreases excessive heart rate.

Nervous system. Use as a relaxant for times of grief from broken heartedness.

Lax/Relaxation (Astringent)

Sinuses/throat. Astringency of flowers and berries help with swelling from inflammation.

Digestive system. Ojibwe tribes use the root of one species for dysentery and diarrhea.

Bladder. The Meskwaki nation of Iowa use the berry as an astringent and bladder tonic.

Habitat & Harvest

Because there are many closely related species of hawthorn, it is difficult even for pros to key out trees in this genus. Since most species are interchangeable, harvest of all plant parts from the wild is generally safe. Depending on your bioregion, harvest leaves before flowering, flowers in May or June, and berries in the fall.

Preparations of Leaf and Flower

Infusion: 2 to 3 cups a day.
Tincture: Fresh (1:2, 75% alcohol) or dried (1:5, 50% alcohol).

Preparations of Berry

Decoction: 2 cups a day.
Tincture: Best to grind berries before tincturing (1:5, 50% alcohol). Fresh berries not recommended due to high pectin content. Hawthorn berries make delicious and beautiful cordials and elixirs.
Solid extract: 1 teaspoon one to three times a day.

Contraindications

Since hawthorn is so successful for lowering blood pressure and having positive effects on cardiac function, anyone who is taking prescription medications to reduce high blood pressure should work with a qualified practitioner to ensure blood pressure does not drop too low when taking hawthorn. Dr. Bastyr cautioned not to discontinue the dose abruptly.[46] Contraindicated with hypotension.

Lobelia

Lobelia inflata

Indian tobacco, Pukeweed, Asthma weed

Family	Campanulaceae
Parts Used	aerial parts, seed pod
Energetics	relaxing, slightly warming, drying
Tissue States	tension, cold/depression, damp/stagnation
Taste	acrid
Actions	antispasmodic, emetic, expectorant, vasodilator

A delicate-looking annual (sometimes biennial) plant, lobelia grows two to three feet tall. The sweet, small flowers are mostly blue, with occasional white petals. Blooms first appear in midsummer and continue for at least a month. The ovary, or seed pod, becomes inflated just below the flower. This balloon-shaped seed pod gives the plant its name of *inflata*. Inside each bladder are hundreds of tiny seeds. The active constituent is called lobeline and its highest concentration is in the seeds. Not as showy as other native lobelias, such as cardinal flower (*Lobelia cardinalis*) and greater lobelia (*L. syphilitica*), *L. inflata* is still quite striking, especially when given best possible conditions. One would never suspect the battles waged over this plant that many hikers probably never even notice growing at trailside.

Uses

L. inflata was an indispensable remedy for Native Americans long before European colonists arrived. Cherokees use lobelia extensively, especially for croup and other bronchial spasms.[47] Early American root doctor Samuel Thomson is attributed with bringing this plant to the attention of established medicine in the late nineteenth century, but lay herbalists and midwives had also been working with this powerful plant many years before. Lobelia might be one of the most misunderstood and feared remedies because of unsubstantiated claims made by regular physicians in the mid-nineteenth century, as Paul Bergner noted in an article in *Medical Herbalism*:

> Lobelia inflata . . . *was used by all schools of medicine, but by none more so than the Thomsonian herbalists in North America . . . and by their physician successors of the Physiomedicalist school. During the*

warfare between the medical sects in that century, lobelia became a symbol. To the herbalists it was a harmless herb, one of their greatest healers. . . . Unsubstantiated and unreferenced claims of lobelia toxicity entered the medical literature of the Regulars in 1810, on the basis of selective testimony in the trial of Samuel Thomson for allegedly causing the death of Ezra Lovett the year before. Those claims have been copied and cited uncritically ever since, and remain in segments of the medical literature today as proof of prejudice and poor scholarship by their authors.[48]

High doses were given without producing emesis, the action that gives the plant its common name of pukeweed. William Cook, a wonderful Physiomedicalist physician wrote, "I have myself many times used an ounce of the herb within a few hours, and had it all retained; have given a child of five years four ounces of the seeds inside seven hours, and had it retained; and in doing so have broken up most alarming attacks of disease, and promptly restored health from spasmodic conditions that otherwise would have been fatal."[49]

The alkaloid lobeline is attributed as the source of the herb's relaxant attributes. Lobeline stimulates deeper breathing. It relaxes tense and spasming muscles from bronchitis, asthma, or pneumonia, and it is specific for musculature along the spinal column. I used to live near Front Royal, Virginia, where an Environmental Protection Agency Superfund toxic site was located along the Shenandoah River. That town was plagued with asthma and bronchitis. Our clinic was extremely successful in helping both adults and children because of the medicine of lobelia. It stimulates and releases mucus while relaxing bronchioles and surrounding musculature.

I find lobelia to be a plant of power. My understanding of the battles and alarm raised over this native species is that it is a plant of vision and voice. If you simply chew a leaf, the acridity is so intense that a wave of nausea comes over you. Once this passes, though, there is a subtle yet deep shift in consciousness; you are more present, relaxed yet incredibly alert. When I have gone on solo retreats in nature, lobelia is my ally to help clear my sight and allow me to remain in my body while engaging deeply with the environment. The alkaloid lobeline is very similar to nicotine in tobacco, *Nicotiana* spp., which has been the most sacred of plants among Indigenous Amazonians for thousands of years and continues to be so. I was taught that we offer tobacco because it is a plant that carries our prayers to Creator. Alkaloids are the language of spirit in plant form. Lobelia and tobacco are very different plants, but they share the quality of creation of disturbance (nausea) then the settling into a place of vision and peace. Many entheogens (psychotropic preparations) induce vomiting or nausea. Interestingly, lobelia is a great ally in breaking the nicotine addiction.

In thirty years of learning from lobelia, I have never induced emesis to achieve desired results. It has not been my teaching, but that is the beauty of relationships; they are satisfying in their differences. For all of the indications below I have used drop doses, or for muscular adults up to 10 to 15 drops as needed. One area where lobelia shines, aside from asthma, is to help in passing of gallstones, as described below.

Indications

All of the recommendations for *Lobelia* are low dose only, except as noted otherwise.

Cold/Depression (Stimulant)

General health. As a general relaxant, it warms tissues through enhancement of blood flow.

Musculoskeletal system. Excellent for inflammation of joints or muscle spasms. Apply poultice or prepare tincture/vinegar added to oil to rub into muscles.

Lungs. Clears phlegm and is a specific for asthma.

Damp/Stagnation (Emetic)

Digestive system. If used as an emetic, lobelia can clear obstructions in the stomach as was indicated in Thomsonian medicine.

Tense/Constriction/Wind (Relaxant)

General health. Relaxant to all parts of the body. Especially useful for wind or tension that comes and goes, such as with intermittency.

Fevers. Drop doses can relax the tension experienced during fevers.

Ears. For intense pain of earaches, drops applied in the ear canal give great relief. If tympanic membrane is not intact, place tincture on skin below ear lobe and around outside of ear.

Digestive system. Drop doses for heartburn or reflux.

Cardiovascular system. Calms rapid heartbeat (tachycardia).

Nervous system. Excellent for relaxation of nervous tics, spasms, and anxiety. Well-known remedy as an aid to help quit tobacco habit.

Respiratory system. Supreme relaxant for bronchial spasms from asthma, bronchitis, pneumonia, and spastic cough.

Throat. Helpful for people who are constantly clearing their throat when nothing is there.

Musculoskeletal system. Wonderful relaxant either internally or externally.

Gallbladder. For assistance in passing gallstones, use a tincture of equal parts lobelia and wild yam (*Dioscorea villosa*). Give 10 to 15 drops every twenty minutes until the spasms stop or the stones pass.

At-Risk Status

Lobelia species are listed on the UpS At-Risk List, and this has been an ongoing discussion among UpS members for quite some time as to whether lobelia is actually at risk. Further research is needed to affirm this status. According to NatureServe, a US nonprofit comprised of biodiversity scientists, as well as other sources, *L. inflata*'s status is not endangered. As an annual, it produces thousands of seeds every year. The beauty with this medicine is that a small amount will go a long way. We need to be watchful as to any changes in its status.

Habitat & Harvest

Lobelia loves good soil and drainage. I have seen the most beautiful species in edge habitats such as along fire roads and in transitioning meadows. If you harvest lobelia when the plant is in seed, you can open the pods and scatter the seeds in areas close to the plant. Why some annuals grow for two years is a mystery, but I have noticed that lobelia sometimes remains in the Sacred Plant Traditions garden for more than one year. If you want a gentler medicine, gather leaves before the seeds mature. We have made tinctures specifically with seeds only when desiring a strong medicine.

Preparations

Tincture: Fresh plant (1:3, 75% alcohol) or freshly dried (1:5, 50% alcohol).

Vinegar: Prefers vinegar, and this is often true of medicines high in alkaloids. Richo Cech covers this topic thoroughly in his book *Making Plant Medicine*.[50]

Contraindications

Not safe during pregnancy. For those who are sensitive or if the dose is too high, ingesting lobelia can cause nausea, vomiting, dizziness, and sometimes excess relaxation. Not to be taken by those who are weak or debilitated.

Marshmallow

Althaea officinalis
Common marshmallow, Mauve blanche, Sweet weed

Family	Malvaceae
Parts Used	leaf, root, flower
Energetics	moistening, cooling, nutritive
Tissue States	heat, atrophy
Taste	sweet, salty
Actions	demulcent, emollient, nutritive, vulnerary, immunostimulant, diuretic

The flowers, leaves, and root of *Althaea officinalis* have been used as nourishing food for over two thousand years; Romans considered this food a delicacy. Native to the salt marshes of the European coasts, as well as Africa, this member of the mallow family is named for those wetlands where it thrives. It has naturalized to many parts of the world but still prefers waterways and ditches. Its genus name originates in the Greek word *altheo*, to heal or cure.

As a hearty perennial, marshmallow can grow up to five feet with the tall stalk adorned by heart-shaped, velvety leaves. The family name Malvaceae is derived from the Latin word *mollis*, meaning soft. The familiar hollyhock (*Alcea rosea*), rose of Sharon (*Hibiscus syricus*), and other hibiscuses are all part of this family. Okra, the edible fruit of another hibiscus, is the classic demulcent food.[51] These have been used as substitutes for marshmallow as they are often more readily available.

Uses

Marshmallow is the quintessential mucilaginous herb. In my early practice I favored the use of the indominable slippery elm (*Ulmus rubra*), but as the status of this tree has shifted to endangered, I have refocused to work more with the mallows. Over the years, I have seen remarkable results from the multitude of talents this whole plant possesses.

All parts of the marshmallow plant are demulcent, with the root predominant. This superb mucilaginous medicine coats and soothes red, hot, inflamed tissue from the mouth to the anus. While not curative, this root medicine will surely relieve heartburn, gastric discomfort, and any "itis" (inflammation) along the alimentary canal. The root tea is best as a cold infusion, as cool water extracts the mucopolysaccharides. I had always wondered how this gooey, viscous healing matter could make it all the way through the fire and brimstone that is digestion. I found the answer during a class with British herbalist and author Simon Mills, who explained the reflexive response of the digestive system: Research suggests that the mechanism of action is related to embryonic development and the developmental relationships of tissues. He explained the physiology in detail, but to me, it is purely magical.

This same action is indispensable when working with dry, hacking coughs, and in this application, the leaves have a gentle yet consistent action. In my experience, marshmallow root has so much power that it can trigger too much mucus in the lungs, so it is important to track the status of the lungs. Root or leaf medicine is especially useful for coughs that persist at night. Marshmallow syrup is easily administered and can be wonderfully effective for soothing such coughs.

Marshmallow prefers salty marshes. This can be seen as a doctrine of signatures when you realize how much of the plant's medicine is the salty aspect of the root. The maxim that water follows salt is invaluable when you want to bring fluid to an area and loosen what has concretized. This mineral-rich plant has a wonderful emollient action—an ability to loosen hardened material. For example, over time, mucus in the lungs will harden and cut off oxygen exchange, leading to dyspnea or difficulty breathing. I have observed marshmallow's influence on breaking up tough mucous plugs, which are often found in the lower lobes of a smoker's lungs or the lungs of those who have had chronic bronchitis. *Althaea* also softens hardened lymph nodes.

Marshmallow is the most demulcent of the diuretics, deserving a place at the top of the list when blending recipes to ease the pain of kidney stones, urinary tract infections, and other hot, irritating conditions, especially interstitial cystitis. This debilitating and very painful chronic disease (also known as bladder pain syndrome) occurs five times more frequently in women than men. Women describe the pain of sitting down as if their bladders had "hardened." This syndrome is of unknown etiology, and treatments often yield little success. Marshmallow root, taken for an extended period of time, lessens the heat and discomfort that comes from inflammation. Marshmallow is also a key ingredient in the urinary tract infection formula I offer clients: two parts uva ursi (*Arctostaphylos uva ursi*), one part corn silk (*Zea mays*), and one part marshmallow.

Indications

Heat/Excitation (Cooling)

Eyes. Cool leaf or root compress for red, hot eyes.

Digestive system. A specific for heartburn, gastritis, and heat/pain from ulcers in the digestive system. Naturopath Bill Mitchell combined this root with ½ teaspoon deglycyrrhizinated licorice root (*Glycyrrhiza glabra*) (DGL is a form of licorice where the glycyrrhizin has been removed, as this constituent can cause complications), three times a day and found it nearly always curative.[52]

Bladder. Effective for urinary tract infection, dysuria, burning urination, and interstitial cystitis.

Dry/Atrophy (Moistening)

General health. Considered a yin tonic in TCM, *Althaea* can have a moistening effect on all systems.

Mouth. Cool infusion as a gargle for atrophic heat—canker sores, mouth ulcers.

Throat. Chew on the root for chronic dry mouth or throat. Excellent tea for sore throat, tonsillitis.

Lungs. Leaf, root, and flower tea for dry hacking cough. Good tea to begin drinking at start of the winter season to counteract drying effects of indoor heat or woodstoves. Also helpful for bronchitis, asthma, and emphysema.

Digestive system. Useful for leaky gut syndrome to heal intestinal lining, as well as supply mucopolysaccharides and prebiotics for support of beneficial bacteria.

Skin. Wash or compress of infusion of leaves and flower can be healing for dry skin conditions such as psoriasis and eczema.

Cancer. Powerful reliever of mouth ulcers and atrophic heat resulting from chemotherapy and radiation. Cool infusion is best.

Tension/Constriction (Relaxant)

General health. When the body is lubricated, there is less tension and friction, allowing the body to let go and relax.

Habitat & Harvest

A stunning presence in any garden, marshmallow is mostly harvested from cultivated plants rather than from the wild. *Althaea* prefers moist soil and full sun. Harvest the leaves before the plant flowers and the flowers just as they come into full bloom. For best results, wait to harvest the root of a plant until it is at least two years old.

Preparations

Infusion: To make cold infusion, steep 4 tablespoons dried root in 1 quart of water and let sit at least four hours or overnight. Leaves and flowers can be made as a hot infusion, but do not use boiling water. Drink ½ cup as needed throughout the day to counter dry, hot conditions.

Tincture: Whether using fresh or dried plant material, the alcohol should not be above 20 percent. Since marshmallow is mostly water soluble, I do not use tincture very often, but it is excellent for urinary tract infections and digestive conditions presenting with excess heat.

Syrup: Marshmallow leaves and flowers can be made into a syrup or used as a fomentation. Can be added to other syrup formulas, such as elderberry, for help with dry coughs.

Contraindications

Best to take prescription medicines an hour before or several hours after drinking marshmallow tea, because marshmallow may slow absorption of drugs by the digestive system.

Milk Thistle

Silybum marianum
Variegated thistle, St. Mary's thistle, Marian thistle

Family	Asteraceae
Parts Used	seed (fruit), leaf
Energetics	neutral, moistening, stimulating
Tissue States	atrophy, stagnation
Taste	sweet, bitter
Actions	hepatoprotectant, choleretic, cholagogue, anti-inflammatory, nutritive, antioxidant, galactagogue

Milk thistle is native to the Mediterranean region and notably Iran and Afghanistan. It spreads extremely easily and is considered invasive in some parts of North America. It is an annual or biennial and grows up to eight feet tall. *Silybum marianum* (previously called *Carduus marianus*) starts out as a beautiful basal rosette, but the leaves, which have prominent white veins, are so prickly it is best to admire from afar. The milky white veins are a signature that this herb, which is also referred to as Mary's milk, is excellent for increasing breast milk or as a galactagogue. The seeds, which are actually fruits, mature after the classic purple thistle flower finishes its bloom. Outside my kitchen window it is amazing to see yellow finches swaying as they balance on a huge stem while eating the seeds. This is a favorite food of other species of birds as well.

Uses

Milk thistle is the most studied of all the hepatoprotective plants.[53] It has been used for liver health for over a thousand years. In this era of environmental pollution, our livers have an onslaught of chemicals to process, and this plant deserves a place in all apothecaries. Milk thistle is regarded as an antidote to serious toxicity, ranging from imbibing too much alcohol to suffering the effects of ingesting poisonous mushrooms. In Europe, a study with over two thousand patients exposed to the deadly mushroom *Amanita* reported that intravenous silybin proved the most successful therapy against the poison amatoxin.[54] Silybin is considered the most potent antioxidant and anti-inflammatory within the flavonoid complex of milk thistle.

I saw this plant's remarkable detoxifying powers firsthand when a young mother called me late at night. After trying homeopathic remedies and herbs to no avail, she took her feverish infant to the emergency room. The ER dispensed acetaminophen, and when she returned home, her baby's temperature had dropped to 93°F. His pulse was very slow and he was extremely lethargic. I went over to the house and we gave him powdered milk thistle extract mixed with breast milk by the dropperful. In a short while he vomited and immediately came "back" to himself. While still groggy, he began nursing. It's my view that he was adversely affected by the acetaminophen, which can cause hepatotoxic effects, especially in very young infants. *Silybum* moved his body to purge itself of the offending toxin.

Silymarin is a term for a group of related flavolignans that make up its profile, which the above mentioned silybin is among. These are powerful antioxidants that protect against free radicals and oxidative stress and assist in lowering insulin resistance and normalizing blood sugar and cholesterol. The mechanism of action for *Silybum*'s detoxifying power is that silymarin acts to rearrange the outer membrane of hepatocytes (liver cells) so that poison can't enter. By increasing protein synthesis, the liver is stimulated to regenerate and make new liver cells.[55] This plant has had incredible healing and lasting effects for those suffering from hepatitis and fatty liver disease as well as cirrhosis. It has been shown to inhibit deposition in collagen fibers, which is thought to contribute to cirrhosis.[56]

It is now coming to light how this "invasive" wonder plant has a profound effect on most metabolic processes. *Silybum* increases production of glutathione, an antioxidant produced in the liver.[57] Combined with the plant alkaloid berberine, milk thistle has been shown to be effective in lowering cholesterol and reducing vascular damage from inflammation.[58]

As described in chapter 3, liver energy governs flow and this relates to my approach to menstrual cycle irregularities. According to Eclectic physician, H.W. Felter, "Amenorrhea . . . and uterine hemorrhage have all been successfully treated with it."[59] I have seen *Silybum* help those dealing with lack of menses as well as flooding (too much bleeding). By enhancing liver function, the herb helps the body to break down hormones more efficiently so rhythm and cycles are brought into balance. This may take a cycle or two to reinstate but I believe this approach of opening the body's channels to allow endogenous hormones to do their work is preferable to supplying plant hormone substitutes such as *Vitex* or black cohosh (*Actaea racemosa*). (There are times when these herbs are needed, but self-correction should be the goal first.)

As mentioned above, milk thistle is a supreme galactagogue for increasing milk production. One study found that silymarin increased production by at least 85 percent with no adverse side effects.[60]

Milk thistle has been used for hundreds of years for the treatment of melancholy. This old-time diagnostic term is related to spleen and liver congestion and presents with low appetite, sallow complexion, and malaise. Melancholy is not exactly the same as depression, but I have had good success with milk thistle taken for at least a month or two to move metabolic stagnation and lighten the temperament. In Five Phase Theory, Liver governs vision, and when this is clouded, as in melancholic moods, it is hard to see the way forward.

Indications
Dry/Atrophy
Liver. As a hepatic, milk thistle stimulates hepatic function, helping to improve metabolic processes.

Breasts. Increases production of milk.

Digestive system. As a cholagogue, bile is released, moistening the bowels and relieving constipation.

Skin. Moistens skin through increasing metabolic functions as well as enhancing circulation. Deeply nutritive with high quantities of antioxidants.

Damp/Stagnation (Stimulant)

General. From *King's American Dispensatory*, "Congestion of the liver, spleen and kidneys is relieved by its use."[61] Great for enhancing metabolic functions, especially when chronic disease has been present, most notably in diabetes.

Circulatory system. Decreases cholesterol and congestion due to impaired circulation.

Uterine health. This is a reliable remedy for excessive pelvic pain during menses. Needs to be taken for a couple of months but effects will be long lasting. Also decreases excessive clotting during cycle.

Habitat & Harvest

Milk thistle is very easy to grow. It prefers sunny and well-drained locations but can grow just about anywhere. The leaves are very nutritious when steamed but wear gloves to trim off the sharp edges when harvesting. Harvest seeds before seed tufts form or they will be blown around like dandelion seeds. We clip the flower stems, cover the seed heads with brown paper bags, and then hang the stems upside down. The seeds will fall down into the bags. Harvesting is definitely a prickly job, and once you have harvested milk thistle seed, you won't grimace at the price of organic seeds. It is a labor that deserves just compensation.

Preparations

Decoction: The outer layer of the seed is hard to penetrate. If you want to make a tea, it is best to powder seeds first (you can grind them in a coffee mill) and make a decoction.

Food: Powdered seeds can be sprinkled on food or used in baking or smoothies. Grind in a coffee mill and use up to 2 tablespoons a day. Once ground, seeds can go rancid quickly, so store seeds whole and grind as needed.

Standardized extract: For medicinal doses, I prefer this form to all others in most cases because the tincture requires a high percentage alcohol and that is not optimum for liver health. Standardized to 50 to 80 percent silymarin. Take 150 to 300 milligrams of the extract, once or twice a day depending on situation.

Tincture: Dried seed (1:3, 95% alcohol). It is good to have milk thistle tincture on hand for treating poisonings.

Contraindications

Milk thistle is extremely safe for all constitutions, but those on medications need to start slowly. Also, dosage of other medications may need to be adjusted because milk thistle will improve overall metabolic functioning, thus requiring lower doses of medication to produce the desired effect. For diabetics it is best to monitor blood sugar often as milk thistle will improve metabolism and possibly necessitate less medication.

Motherwort

Leonurus cardiaca
Lion's ear, Throw-wort, Heartwort

Family	Laminaceae
Parts Used	leaf, flower
Energetics	bitter, cooling, moving
Tissue States	heat, tension, stagnation
Taste	bitter, acrid, astringent
Actions	nervine, relaxant, bitter, antispasmodic

Leonurus cardiaca means lion-hearted. This plant teaches us that courage rises from our core when we relax and allow our authentic self to shine through. It creates the sense that you are being held in a safe embrace. In many ways this herb is the quintessential Mother. The energy of the Earth Mother is nourishing, calming yet fierce. Motherwort's lovely pink and lilac flowers are encased in a spiky structure that becomes the seed in late summer. This signature is why I have used motherwort as spirit medicine for someone who is vulnerable and needs to stay centered and calm yet protected. As a hardy perennial, it is most resilient.

The stems are square as is usual with mints, but motherwort has an exceptionally sturdy structure and can grow up to six feet tall. The pattern of leaf growth is striking; the palm-shaped leaves are borne in pairs along the stems, but the placement of the leaves alternates along the length of a stem. This gives the impression of rhythm, control, and balance yet with an energy of movement. These signatures of the plant play out beautifully in that it helps regulate the cardiac muscle, slowing down rapid heartbeat and regulating rhythm. As a blood mover, it resolves congestion in uterine tissue to help alleviate stagnation as well as tension. It also regulates the rhythm of the moon/menstrual cycle.

Uses

As you can imagine, any plant named motherwort must bear medicine that can influence women's health and cardiovascular strength. For centuries it has been employed for palpitations, arrhythmia, and tension. As a uterine tonic and blood mover, it is exceptional in helping delayed or suppressed menstruation and is incomparable for PMS symptoms. From *King's American Dispensatory*: "It is adapted to cases of nervous debility with irritation, nervous unrest, tendency to choreic or spasmodic movements, pelvic and lumbar uneasiness or pain, bearing down pains."[62] "Bearing down pains" refer to the stagnation and pressure felt often with painful menses. As a blood mover, motherwort excels at relieving this pressure. Used the world over for the heat of menopausal symptoms, it also aids menopausal women with insomnia.

Indications
Heat/Excitation (Cooling)
Thyroid. Specific for heat from hyperthyroid conditions, especially when blended with bugleweed (*Lycopus virginicus*) and lemon balm. Eases anxiety, palpitations, insomnia, and other heat symptoms.

Liver/gallbladder. As a bitter, motherwort is cooling and releases liver tension and "Liver heat rising." *Leonurus cardiaca* calms anxiety, palpitations, irritability, increased sensitivity, red face, and night sweats.

Menopause. As a bitter herb, motherwort cools hot flashes through its effect on the liver as well as through its relaxation of blood vessels.[63]

Tension/Constriction (Relaxant)
Head. Relieves tension headaches, especially those located in the temples. Oftentimes pressure headaches at the temples can indicate issues with Liver/Gallbladder.

Digestive system. Relieves heartburn and indigestion due to tension. Excellent digestive bitter.

Nervous system. Motherwort is a reliable remedy for palpitations, anxiety, and fear of the unknown, which is often what provokes panic attacks. For relaxation and cooling, use 10 to 30 drops three times a day or as needed. I find it also works very effectively in drop doses.

Cardiovascular system. Useful addition to high blood pressure formulas because it encourages vasodilation, opening vessels and allowing greater flow. Used with great success for angina by the Eclectic physicians.

Uterine health. *L. cardiaca* is used extensively to bring on delayed menses. For PMS, 10 drops once a day, from ovulation to beginning menses. When the goal is to shift the patterns of menses, it takes at least three months to establish a new rhythm. Taking a low dose as suggested can also shift pain, depression, and anxiety. Increased bleeding may occur initially as motherwort is a blood mover as well as a vasodilator. This helps relieve pain that arises from stagnation.

Thyroid. For palpitations due to hyperthyroidism.

Damp/Stagnation (Bitter/Stimulant)

Uterine health. In Chinese medicine, motherwort is used to "invigorate blood," which resolves masses such as fibroids and cysts. Most pain is some form of stagnation, whether from inflammation or cold depression, and blood-moving plants like motherwort reduce pain from stagnation. Clots in the cycle often indicate stagnation, especially clots with older, darker blood.

Mental health. The repetitive patterns and loops in thinking that can plague sufferers of obsessive-compulsive disorder have been helped by motherwort's ability to move stagnation.

Habitat & Harvest

Motherwort grows in all conditions and needs no soil amendments. Motherwort prefers full sun but will also do well in partial shade. When gathering to dry as well as to tincture, collect the top two-thirds of the plant just as the flowers are beginning to bloom.

Preparations

Infusion: Dried or fresh, 1 to 2 cups a day, but this is a very bitter brew so best to include it in a blend.

Tincture: Fresh plant (1:2, 95% alcohol) or dried (1:5, 40–60% alcohol). Low dose is often all that is needed. Take 7 to 10 drops three times a day or as part of a larger formula.

Contraindications

Since *Leonurus* is a blood mover, it is not to be used during pregnancy. Some midwives do use it to bring on labor as well to ease postpartum pain. Motherwort increases blood flow, so caution must be exercised with fibroids or conditions that create menstrual flooding. While motherwort can act as a tonic, it is not recommended to use it for atrophy (vata) unless given along with sweet, building, tonic herbs. Use with care in cardiovascular conditions as it will relax tension and may lower blood pressure.

Mullein

Verbascum thapsus
Jupiter's staff, Velvet mullein, Quaker's rouge

Family	Scrophulariaceae
Parts Used	flower, leaf, root
Energetics	flower and leaf—cooling, moistening; root—warming
Tissue States	flower and leaf—dry/atrophy, tension; root—laxity
Taste	leaf—sweet, salty; flower—astringent, sweet; root—astringent, sweet, bitter
Actions	relaxing expectorant, demulcent, nervine, diuretic, anodyne, antispasmodic.

Mullein is one of the most majestic plants in the Sacred Plant Traditions garden. *Verbascum* is usually reported to grow between three and five feet tall, but I have seen her reach up to seven feet. While our small urban garden is full of plants, it is said that mullein grows best in spots where its large basal leaves can grow wide and long, hence it prefers bare soils. Mullein loves disturbed soils, too, and will appear in abundance in recently cleared areas. It is also one of the first plants to take up residence after a fire, so this lung medicine heals burned land to prevent erosion, but also brings comforting medicine to dry, irritated lungs.

Native to Europe and west Asia, mullein has naturalized with ease in North America. As a biennial, mullein presents as a beautiful basal rosette of lanceolate leaves in its first year of growth. The leaves are very hairy, which is a signature that the plant can act to help the cilia in the lungs remove particulates or phlegm. Take care when harvesting mullein, because those hairy leaves can prove irritating to those who have sensitive skin. The common name of Quaker's rouge references how Quaker women would rub mullein leaf on the cheeks to "irritate" and enhance their skin color. I have never understood the many references I've come across proclaiming mullein as Nature's toilet paper.

Beginning in the second year, a stalk emerges from the rosette. As the stalk elongates, it is adorned with a multitude of golden yellow flowers, which open in an upward spiral around the lance-shaped stalk. Each flower stalk can produce 80,000 to 100,000 seeds, which will self-sow quite easily. Mullein seeds remain viable in the soil for hundreds of years.

Uses

No other plant tells so much of its use through its many signatures. The beautiful basal rosette reflects how grounding this plant is and its relationship to the pelvic region of the body. The soft, flannel-like leaves are soothing, yet the hairs are irritating, which reflects its medicinal action of clearing debris (phlegm) while also soothing mucous membranes. The yellow flowers bring warmth to many formulas, and the stalk appears to be a staff of light in the meadow or garden and also within us. Although it is not a well-known use, mullein is one of the best plants when working with depression—when the light seems to have left the personality. The medicinal effect feels like a return or rising of energy: like the light of the flowers on the rising stalk.

Mullein is one of those herbs that has seemingly contradictory attributes but presents a complete healing picture. The most popular use of mullein leaf is for working with respiratory ailments. Mullein is the perfect remedy for dry, hoarse coughs that occur mostly at night. Its slightly irritating quality triggers release of the cough reflex, yet its cooling, soothing, demulcent qualities help the lungs expel the irritants. The volatile oils also have a cleansing action. Less well-known are mullein's nervine and relaxant qualities. This is an invaluable asset for a cough remedy. Mullein can ease spasms and tension held in the body due to wracking pain of pneumonia or severe bronchitis.

This relaxant quality is also helpful for musculoskeletal issues, including prevention of sore muscles after strenuous exercise. A miraculous use I learned from Matthew Wood is to help in the resetting of bones, a task I usually leave to allopathic practitioners. If a client has a rib out of place or broken toes, the pain can be excruciating, and it is a watch and wait situation—there is no quick fix through conventional medicine. Simply applying dried mullein leaf to the affected area has brought startling relief. This does not work in every case, but when it does, it is very impressive.

Mullein flowers are legendary for easing pain from earaches, primarily in children. In infants the eustachian tube runs horizontally from the ear to the nose. As we age and our facial structure changes, the canal then drains downward to the nose. Most earaches are not due to ear infections, but rather to mucous buildup in the sinuses that pushes against the very sensitive tympanic membrane. It is the relaxant and demulcent effect of mullein flower oil, rather than its antimicrobial qualities, that eases the discomfort.

The root is warming and relaxing; it lowers pain from cystitis or urinary tract infections.

Indications for Leaf and Flower
Dry/Atrophy (Moistening/Nutritive)
Sinuses/throat. Mullein has the same lubricating effect on the throat and sinus as it does in the lungs.

Ears. Oil of flowers eases pain of earache. Apply to both ears even if only one presents with pain. Eclectic physicians would administer drops 3 to 4 times a day to restore uncomplicated hearing loss.[64]

Lungs. Particularly useful in cases of dry, nocturnal dyspnea (difficulty breathing), chronic bronchitis, asthma, recurring pneumonia, or blood in sputum due to excessive irritation and dryness.

Musculoskeletal system. Eases pain of arthritic joints due to dryness and atrophy and of broken bones with damage and pain to the nerves.

Tension/Constriction (Relaxant)
Sinuses/throat/ear. Relieves pain from spasm or tension.

Lungs. Eases tension from painful, racking coughs. Relaxes bronchioles in asthma.

Musculoskeletal system. Excellent muscle relaxant in the relief of pain resulting from overuse of muscles, joints, tendons. Specific for low-back pain.

Mental health. Offered for depression described as a heavy, dark cloud. Relaxation allows this rising energy or brightness to be perceived.

Indications for Root
Relaxation/Atony (Astringent)
Bladder. Very useful for bed-wetting and incontinence due to aging, pregnancy, or stress. Enhances muscular tone and improves tissue integrity, especially after repeated infections or inflammation. Also helps to ease pain from interstitial cystitis.[65]

Prostate. Excellent herb for reducing swelling and pain of an enlarged prostate or in cases of benign prostatic hypertrophy.

Habitat & Harvest

Verbascum thapsus is the most frequently used species, but the stunning Greek mullein (*V. olympicum*) is appreciated for its proliferation of flowers. Harvest leaves as well as the root at the end of the first year of growth or before the stalk rises on the second-year plant. Since individual flowers remain open only for one day, one method of harvest is to cut the stalk and place it in a vase of water indoors. This makes it easy to harvest flowers daily as they open and add them to an oil or dry them.

Preparations

Infusion: For leaf and flower, 2 to 3 cups per day. Infusion is my preferred method.

Decoction: Root best extracted in a decoction, 1 cup a day.

Tincture: Fresh leaf and flower (1:2, 50% alcohol); dried leaf (1:5, 40% alcohol); dried root (1:5, 50% alcohol).

Oil: See the Warm Oil Infusion instructions, page 213, for preparing medicinal oils and simply use mullein flowers.

Contraindications

Mullein is nontoxic, but the wooly hairs on the leaves can be irritating to the skin and may cause a rash.

Nettle

Urtica dioica, U. urens
Common nettle, Stinging nettle, Wood nettle

Family	Urticaceae
Parts Used	leaf, seed, root
Energetics	cooling, drying (yet also moistening through minerals and salt)
Tissue States	depression, atrophy, heat, relaxation
Taste	bitter, sweet, salty
Actions	diuretic, astringent, nutritive, kidney/adrenal trophorestorative

Echinacea might be the gateway plant that introduces many people to herbalism, but once through the herbal portal, it is nettle that becomes the herbalist's most beloved remedy. Nettle is one of the most useful plants to grow because it is a perennial food and medicine of great nutritional value. Nettles even make an appearance in the funeral song of a Scottish mermaid: *If they would eat nettles in March, and drink mugwort in May, so many fine maidens would not go to the clay.*

Many meet nettle for the first time inadvertently by brushing up against the leaves and getting "nettled" or stung. The sting from this herbaceous perennial is due to the hollow hairs called *trichomes* on leaf surfaces. Plants inject formic acid through the hairs into the skin of the lucky person who has intentionally applied the leaves or the one who has inadvertently brushed up against the patch. Urtification, from the genus name *Urtica* (*uro* means to burn), is the word given to the act of brushing nettle against skin in order to stimulate blood flow to areas of pain and decreased function. Interestingly, nettle is used to treat urticaria, which is hives or an allergic reaction that produces welts.

Nettle grows three to six feet tall and the square stems have been used as fiber for clothing as well as paper. The heart-shaped leaves are deeply serrated. Inconspicuous flowers grow from the base of the leaf and these become the green fruit or seeds that are harvested later in the season. Woodland nettle (*Urtica urens*) is an annual that is abundant is eastern US woodlands and is found along streams. Another common name is burning nettle, but I do not find this plant as topically stimulating as *U. dioica*. Both species prefer to grow by water or at least in moist conditions, which is a signature for its work with kidneys, both as a tonic and as a diuretic. Nettle also loves nitrogen-rich soil. Analysis of nettle powder shows it is three times richer in protein than rice, barley, and wheat.[66] The concentration of available amino acids in nettle make this an excellent herbal brew for vegans and vegetarians.

Uses

Pain is oftentimes due to stagnation, and the stimulation and circulatory enhancement (kindly put) that this plant induces has been a treatment for centuries.[67] I have used nettle topically, fresh sting, for over twenty years to aid in the restoration of sensation for those suffering from neuropathy, as well as joint pain from overuse such as carpal tunnel syndrome. I will give a client a plant from my patch in the clinic garden to transplant into their home garden for use for their own urtification needs. While this certainly does not sound inviting, this application of nettle increases circulation and over a short period of time can greatly affect chronic pain.

There is simply no other nourishing, mineral-packed remedy in our apothecary that can reach so deeply into an exhausted system nor provide such an abundant food source as nettle. For years, Sacred Plant Traditions hosted an annual women's conference, and we were able to feed over a hundred women a delicious nettle soup made from the harvest from our humble six square-foot patch. After the conference, we would gather an additional two harvests. This tonic brew is supreme for mineralizing the body, balancing blood sugar, calming allergies, lifting low blood pressure, and, as if that were not enough, restoring lost kidney function. Nettle is a supreme alterative as well as blood builder. It is high in chlorophyll as well as iron and a host of other minerals. Author and clinical herbalist David Hoffmann is famously quoted for wisely stating, "When in doubt, choose nettles."

More recently the seed has come into use through the teachings of herbalist David Winston, who has made a great contribution by highlighting the seed as a kidney trophorestorative. The root is effective in decreasing inflammation of benign prostatic hypertrophy (BPH) when combined with other herbs.[68]

Indications for Leaf
Heat/Excitation (Cooling)
Allergies. A natural astringent, it is thought that nettle also relieves allergies by decreasing histaminic reaction set off by contact with pollens. If using the infusion for prevention, it is best to start drinking 1 quart per day at least a month before allergy season.

Cold/Depression (Nutritive)
General vitality. Truly a nutritional powerhouse. It is a wonderful source of calcium, magnesium, potassium, zinc, copper, iron, phosphorus, chromium, amino acids, B complex vitamins, and carotenes measured as vitamin A.

Joints. Nettle is useful for inflammatory joint pain, and in this instance, the tincture may be most appropriate.[69] Consistent use of nettle infusion is excellent for remineralization and nutrition. Nettle may also be effective for arthritis because it is an excellent alterative.

Bones. Due to high calcium and magnesium content, regular use of nettle is indicated for osteoporosis or bone injuries.

Kidneys/adrenals. While adaptogens have become popular for kidney support, nettle leaf cannot be underestimated for reliable nutritional support for fatigue and exhaustion. I have used this tea successfully to decrease organ rejection in clients with kidney transplants. This therapy should be initiated a few months after the surgery; the results have been near miraculous in easing the transition.

Iron. Especially useful during pregnancy to increase iron levels. Makes an excellent blood-building syrup.

Indications for Root
Laxity/Atrophy (Astringing)
Prostate. Successfully used to decrease inflammation and hypertrophy from BPH.[70] While nettle can be successful as a simple, I have used it with great success in a formula blend with saw palmetto (*Serenoa serulata*), sage leaf (*Salvia officinalis*), and mullein root.

Indications for Seed
Kidneys. Trophorestorative for the kidneys. As mentioned in chapter 4, many varieties of seeds are the medicine of the kidneys, for our essence originates here and seeds hold the essence of many plants. This medicine is very supportive for adrenal exhaustion.

Mental health. Helps with mental clarity and increasing alertness.

Habitat & Harvest
I encourage my local community to grow stinging nettles in their yards because this is the epitome of sustainable harvest. All parts of the plants have great merit. Nettle loves to grow by water but I have successfully grown it in almost all settings and soil conditions. The first spring greens are the tastiest and most medicinal, but here in the mid-Atlantic region, we can enjoy three bountiful harvests of leaves every year. The seeds are worth all the time and effort it takes to harvest them. It is best to harvest when the seeds have become heavy enough to make the stalk bend over, but be sure to pick while they are green and before they turn grey or black. It's best to wear gloves when harvesting because contact with the seeds can also cause itching.

Preparations
Infusion: Dried leaves are most nutritive, but fresh leaves, handled with care or gloves, can also be used. Best to drink 1 quart a day for maximum nutritional value.

Tincture: Fresh plant (1:2, 75% alcohol) or dried (1:5, 50% alcohol). Tincture of leaves is the best form for allergies and arthritis. Fresh root tincture is specific for BPH. For seeds, prepare a tincture with freshly dried seeds (1:5, 50% alcohol); this tincture can be deeply nourishing to adrenals, using small doses of 10 to 20 drops.

Food: Fresh plants need to be steamed or cooked to remove sting from leaves, unless blending in a blender at high speeds to make nettle pesto.

Decoction: Use dried root; drink 1 cup a day.

Nettle seed: Freshly dried—start low to see sensitivities, ½ teaspoon up to 1 tablespoon two times a day mixed or sprinkled on a small amount of food.

Contraindications

Dried plants can still have the power to sting, so be careful when handling freshly dried leaves. Some people report that the seeds are energizing and stimulating, so if you are starting out, take them in the morning so you can see your individual response.

Plantain

Plantago major
Broadleaf plantain, Snakeweed, Cart track plant

Family	Plantaginaceae
Parts Used	leaf, seed
Energetics	leaf—moistening, cooling, softening, drying; seed—moistening
Tissue States	atrophy, heat, relaxation
Taste	sweet, salty, astringent
Actions	demulcent, vulnerary, astringent, antimicrobial; seeds—bulking agent

Ubiquitous to lawns and roadsides around the globe, plantain has the dubious distinction of being called "white man's footprint." Pollinated by wind and producing thousands of seeds per plant, plantain can make its home any place the soil has been disturbed. It actually has a beneficial influence in compacted soil because plantain roots penetrate and loosen dry, clay soils. This is seen as the plant's signature—it has profound drawing qualities, and it draws what it needs from any soil, even the most deficient.

There are over two hundred species, making it important to identify which types of plantain grows in your area. Ribwort plantain (*P. lanceolata*) is narrow leafed and bears its seed head on a stalk. The seeds of *P. psyllium* are used as the bulk fiber sold in health food stores as an intestinal cleanse as well as an ingredient in the laxative medication Metamucil. The seed is hydrophilic, which means it attracts water and hence swells in the presence of moisture.

P. major is low growing, with a basal rosette of leaves. *Plantago* is derived from the Latin *plantaris*, meaning sole of the foot. It has broad oval leaves, with distinct veins or ribs running the length of the leaf.

Were I ever exiled to the moon and had to choose five herbs to take, plantain would definitely be one. And I would not be surprised if *Plantago* wasn't already there!

Uses

Most children raised in a family that practices natural medicine know plantain as the "band-aid plant." Early on they are taught how to properly identify it, then how to make a spit poultice from the leaves: First wash the plant, chew the leaf to mix it well with saliva, then place the plant paste right on a bee sting, insect bite, or other red-hot inflammation. Holding the poultice on the area cools the tissue and draws the venom from the bite.

Plantain is most beloved for its ability to draw out toxins, both internally and externally. When I try to assign an energetic action for this property, it is hard to pinpoint. Astringents have an ability to draw tissue together and reduce inflammation (which plantain does), but this herb almost seems to send its demulcent quality or sugars into the tissue to loosen the object that it is removing from the skin or the cell membrane. This is how it can soothe and astringe simultaneously.

Many of my early herbal teachers were midwives. One day, the son of one of the local midwives had accidently stepped on a large sewing needle. An X-ray revealed it had migrated above his ankle, and surgery was recommended. His mother and I began thrice daily plantain soaks of her son's foot and ankle and applied slippery elm poultices between soaks. She also gave him homeopathic silica, because silica (horsetail) helps the body get rid of what it does not want. After two weeks, on the morning of his return visit to the doctor to schedule the surgery, we all heard the metal ting of the large needle dropping into the enameled soaking bin after his one last soak. A number of healing agents played a role in the remarkable process, but plantain was definitely the major player.

My other plantain story concerns the worst case of food poisoning I have ever had. I awoke in the night in distress. I picked up an herb book (this was at the beginning of my herbal career) to research what to take, but I was so ill that I ended up just holding the book and asking that it open to the right remedy. It opened to plantain. I performed this adept clinical research method twice more, and twice more plantain looked up from the page. I first discarded this offer of advice from spirit, because in my amateur's superficial understanding, I had pigeonholed this remedy as being only for topical applications to draw out poisons. Finally, light dawned. Of course, if plantain drew toxins externally, it would do the same internally. After making and drinking just one cup of plantain tea, I felt miraculously better. More tea the next day completed the adventure.

Indications

Heat/Excitation (Cooling)
Plantain has a specificity for diseases of the head, throat, teeth, and gums.

Head. Compress for clearing pink eye.

Teeth/gums. Very effective for clearing heat and infection from an abscessed tooth.

Digestive system. Counteracts food poisoning and inflammatory bowel conditions due to heat; wonderful as a poultice for hemorrhoids.

Skin. Any irritation that is red, hot, and itchy will find relief from this herb. Highly effective when made as a bath for poison ivy.

Bladder. Clears heat and is soothing to bladder irritation caused by a urinary tract infection as well as pain from interstitial cystitis.

Venomous bites. Combined with slippery elm powder, plantain is cooling and assists in drawing of toxins. Copperhead, recluse spider, and other venomous bites are greatly relieved with plantain poultice as well as infusions taken internally.

Damp/Stagnation (Alterative)
Lungs. Helpful for sore throat, laryngitis, and bronchitis and has a special affinity for clearing fluid from lungs due to pneumonia or chronic bronchitis.

Skin. Excellent for boils and skin abscesses to clear heat from stagnant conditions; this is facilitated as it softens skin to pull deep infections.

Lax/Atony (Astringent)

Mouth. As an astringent, plantain is helpful for mouth ulcers and tooth abscesses when applied as a poultice or a mouthwash.

Digestive system. Specific remedy for leaky gut syndrome, diarrhea, excessive water in stool, or internal bleeding.

Uterine health. Underutilized tonic for uterus with lack of tone and excessive bleeding.

Dry/Atrophy (Moistening/Nutritive)

While seemingly counterintuitive, plantain is soothing and moistening to the same tissues it astringes because it is so nutritive.

General health. Plantain is highly nutritious and has high levels of vitamin C. It also contains flavonoids, beta-carotene, and vitamins A, B_1, B_2, B_3, C, and K. Also rich in minerals.

Tissue regeneration. With high levels of allantoin, plantain can be used for internal healing. *P. major* has been used effectively to rebuild irritated tissues that could lead to internal bleeding. Extremely useful in atrophy of tissues especially in the gut.

Habitat & Harvest

Plantain grows in disturbed soils in well-drained areas. While it prefers sunny locations, it can also tolerate shade. The leaves are harvested in spring or early summer before they become too large, bitter, and fibrous.

Preparations

Infusion: For food poisoning, 2 to 3 cups as needed, sipped throughout the day.
Tincture: Fresh plant (1:3, 95% alcohol) or dried (1:4, 50% alcohol).
Poultice/compress: For external wounds.
Oil/salve: Apply oil via a roll-on dispenser (the type used for deodorant or perfume).

Contraindications

I know of no contraindications for *P. major*, but care needs to be exercised when harvesting, especially from lawns that may have been "sprayed"—by local dogs or lawn care companies.

Prickly Ash

Zanthoxylum americanum, Z. clava-herculus

Northern prickly ash, Toothache bark, Pepper wood, Yellow wood

Family	Rutaceae
Parts Used	root bark, bark, twig, berry
Energetics	warming, stimulating, diffusive
Tissue States	cold/depression, stagnation
Taste	pungent, acrid, aromatic
Actions	circulatory stimulant, diffusive, antirheumatic, carminative, sialagogue, anodyne, astringent, antispasmodic, tonic

Most guide books simply refer to the "prickles" on the bark and branches of *Zanthoxylum*. But when you meet this profound medicine in person you immediately know you are in the presence of a remedy that has something to do with movement and pain. The bark is covered with small protruding mounds that have painful-looking thorns jutting out. There are thorns at each leaf node as well as at other random spots. But when you bruise the leaves, you'll notice an aromatic, citrusy scent that is sweet and almost narcotic. Chewing on a small twig results in an intense awakening and tingling of the nerves of the tongue and mouth. The sensation is warming and pleasant, but if the twig is left in the mouth too long, the feeling can be overpowering.

Prickly ash is the northernmost member of the Rutaceae family, which also includes citrus fruits. It is found as far north as Ontario, in the Midwest, and as far south as Louisiana and Florida. Another common name for *Zanthoxylum* is yellow wood, and *zanthos* is the Greek word for yellow. The berries are green early in summer, ripen to a vibrant red in autumn, then turn shiny black in November. These are the infamous Sichuan peppers that are a foundation flavor in Asian cooking as a five-spice powder. The culinary red peppers are harvested from *Z. bungeanum*, and green peppers are from *Z. armatum*. I have used *Z. americanum* for many years and of late have been seeing more consistent results with *Z. clava-herculis*; some practitioners feel this is the stronger of the two.

Uses

First Nation peoples have extensive experience with this plant. The Chippewa have a tradition of bathing the legs and feet of elders or children who have weakness or even paralysis in a strong decoction of the bark. Delaware have used an infusion for weak hearts. Many First Nations such as the Ojibwe, Meskwaki, and Menominee have been known to make prickly ash into a cough syrup for many respiratory complaints.[71] The heating, pungent action certainly would have been most effective.

Prickly ash bark stimulates circulation, the lymphatic system, and mucous membranes. It is excellent for cold arthritic and painful rheumatic conditions. This supreme stimulant is ideal for sluggish peripheral circulation where there is general lack of tone, including chronic conditions where there is blood stasis and congestion. This tonic improves function in chronic fatigue, diabetes, and metabolic syndrome. It is effective in treating chilblains (painful constriction of small arteries), leg cramps, varicose veins, ulcers, and other painful problems resulting from blood congestion and cold. I have used it for years with Raynaud's syndrome, an autoimmune condition in which the fingers turn icy white and numb. Eclectic physician Finley Ellingwood described this bark perfectly: "This agent is a stimulant to the nerve centers, and through these centers it increases the tonicity and functional activity of the different organs. It is diffusive, producing a warm glow throughout the system and nervous tingling, as if a mild current of electricity was being administered."[72] The same chemical that gives echinacea its characteristic numbing tingle is found in prickly ash bark as well; hence, it also has the common name toothache tree.

I often use this herb as an activator in a formula: something that will promote distribution of the other herbs throughout the body. This has been very useful for people whose thyroid function has all but lost its fire. Remarkably, many clients state that after they started to take this plant, their foggy thinking and depression lifted. I have since been blending it in formulas for stagnant depression where symptoms of cold predominate. Something about this plant and how it awakens our vitality entrances me. Small doses are all that are required.

Author and acupuncturist Alan Tillotson reports that doctors in various parts of Africa use a relative of prickly ash, fagara (*F. zanthosyloides*), for sickle cell anemia.[73] This genetic blood disorder affects people of African descent and is often very difficult to treat. The red blood cells, which are normally round, are shaped like sickles or crescent moons. These become rigid, sticky cells lodged in small blood vessels, which creates excruciating pain. Tillotson reports a number of case studies in which he used prickly ash with *Ginkgo biloba* and was very successful in helping patients regain their quality of life and dramatically reduce the severity of attacks. While this is an extreme clinical presentation, the power of this plant cannot be underestimated.

Indications
Cold/Depression (Warming Stimulant)

Cardiovascular and circulatory systems. Strengthens function of the heart muscle and is specific for peripheral circulatory insufficiency, especially intermittent claudication and edema. Has been used for numbness in poststroke recovery.

Joints. Increases circulation in arthritis, especially brought on by cold.

Nervous system. Works admirably with healing nerve trauma or postsurgical nerve pain where nerves have been damaged. Matthew Wood writes of its homeopathic indications specific for paralysis, Bell's palsy, nerve weakness, and one-sided nerve pain.[74]

Respiratory system. Excellent in cough syrups or added to cough formulas for loosening constricted musculature. Effective for whooping cough and nighttime coughs.

Wounds. Improves wounds and ulcers that are slow in healing.

Digestive system. Superb tonic for increasing activity of digestion and helping pancreas and liver act more efficiently. Increases saliva and gastric fluids to aid digestion.

Skin. Fomentation or compress moves stagnant bruises very quickly. I have also applied tinctures directly to bruises with good results.

Damp/Stagnation (Warming)

Sinuses/lungs. Strong astringent action; moves damp stagnation or mucus.

Uterine health. Relives sharp, intense pain from ovarian cysts, stagnation, and endometriosis.

Laxity/Atony (Astringent)

Digestive system. Tonifies mucous membranes and enhances appetite and gastric secretions after chemotherapy treatments.

Circulatory system. Astringing for vasculature internally as well as topically for varicose veins.

Habitat & Harvest

Prickly ash prefers full sun; it can grow in most soil conditions but it prefers moist areas. Harvest the inner bark in early spring as the vital force is returning and before buds and leaves emerge or after berries have turned dark and the energy is descending to the root. Berries are usually harvested after they turn red.

Preparations

Decoction: Use as a low-dose botanical. Only a small amount of decoction may be needed throughout the day—¼ cup every four hours.
Tincture: Fresh bark (1:3, 75% alcohol) or dried bark (1:5, 50% alcohol).

Contraindications

Not to be used with blood-thinning medications or where there is excess heat such as ulcers or inflammation. Since it is a blood mover, *Zanthoxylum* is unsafe for use during pregnancy.

Self-heal

Prunella vulgaris
All heal, Heal-all, Woundwort

Family	Lamiaceae
Parts Used	aerial parts
Energetics	moistening, cooling, nutritive
Tissue States	heat/excitation, atrophy, stagnation
Taste	bitter, slightly acrid, sweet
Actions	demulcent, astringent, diuretic, hemostatic, lymphatic, immunomodulator, vulnerary

I have always held the highest regard for this plant. As a mint, self-heal is ubiquitous to most landscapes. Preferring cool, damp places, *Prunella vulgaris* will grow in most sunny locations and once established will spread quite happily. I have seen this low-growing mint reach up to nine inches tall in spots where it had been established for a while.

The doctrine of signatures is perfectly expressed in this plant. The purple flowers are lipped shape, opening to form a mouth and throat. It is a first-rate remedy for tonsillitis and sore throats. Oftentimes the color purple indicates sepsis or infection. The origin of the name *Prunella* is actually a German word (*Brunella*) for quinsy, which is a severe (abscessed) sore throat.

Uses

Prunella vulgaris is aptly named heal-all and self-heal. There are a multitude of uses for this humble mint. Many years ago, I had the honor of participating in a five-hour class with Michigan Anishinaabe medicine elder Keewaydinoquay, all on the uses of self-heal. She described the many applications of this heat-clearing herb with fever, infections, diarrhea, and of course sore throats. Her people, along with the Cree and Iroquois nations, use this plant almost as a panacea.[75] In Chinese medicine, this herb is used to clear Liver heat and to enhance vision. Similarly, Ojibwe peoples would make a tea to drink before going hunting to sharpen their powers of observation. Keewaydinoquay told us story after story of the plant's ability to open hearts to choose the path of self-care. To this day, I often add small doses to formulas where someone is struggling with tending themselves.

As the name woundwort implies, it is a supreme healer of wounds. Sixteenth-century botanist and author John Gerard stated in *The Herbal*, "There is not a better Wound herbe in the world than that of Self Heale is, the very name importing it to be very admirable upon this account."[76] And according to fifteenth-century herbalist Nicholas Culpeper, "It is an especial remedy for all green wounds, to close the lips of them, and to keep the place from any further inconveniencies."[77] Research studies have shown that *P. vulgaris* can disrupt biofilms.[78] When microorganisms attach to a surface, mostly a wet one, they secrete a glue-like substance that sets the scene for chronic infections. While biofilms were unknown to fifteenth-century herbalists, I am certain this capability is what earned heal-all its rank among the most revered of plants.

A plethora of recent studies have shown that heal-all has antiviral properties.[79] *P. vulgaris* is most notably successful against herpes simplex virus, human papillomavirus, and even HIV.[80] Research reveals that it inhibits viral binding activity, making it effective at prevention of new outbreaks.

Indications

Heat/Excitation (Cooling)

Eyes. Chinese medicine specifically uses self-heal for signs of "Liver fire rising" and "Liver constraint." Headaches and painful eyes that are worse at night are indications for self-heal. Self-heal is recommended for many types of eye complaints, including red eyes, conjunctivitis, and eye-tearing.

Mouth. As an antiviral, useful for herpes and cold sores.

Skin. Very useful as a wash for sunburn or kitchen burns as well as red, eruptive rashes, abscesses, and septic (pustulent) wounds.

Fevers. Especially useful for pediatric fevers, as it is gentle and nutritive.

Damp/Stagnation (Stimulant)

Skin. As noted above, few herbs compare with heal-all when it comes to wound healing.

Lymphatic system. As a lymphagogue, self-heal clears swollen glands, especially in the neck and groin area.

Dry/Atrophy (Demulcent)

General health. Wild food with nutritive value as a source of antioxidants.

Digestive system. As a gentle demulcent, self-heal is a wonderful addition to anti-inflammatory teas for colitis and irritable bowel.

Kidneys. Matthew Wood relates how renowned herbalist William LeSassier used self-heal when there was dental decay due to Kidney deficiency.[81] In TCM, Kidney governs bone formation.

Lax/Atony (Astringent)

Digestive system. An astringent, self-heal is useful for diarrhea. Effective in blends for colitis and IBS.

Habitat & Harvest

As an edge dweller, self-heal prefers moist, nutrient-rich woodland edges and meadows but will tolerate most soil and site conditions. The herb that is common in lawns is thought to be the shorter Eurasian variety but all can be used interchangeably. Best to harvest the leaves before the plant flowers, and each flower harvest will stimulate more growth.

Preparations

Infusion: Fresh or dried plant matter makes an excellent tea.

Tincture: Fresh plant (1:2, 75% alcohol) or dried plant (1:5, 50% alcohol).

Oil: The oil of self-heal leaves and flowers makes a wonderful healing salve.

Contraindications

Best to avoid if there is extreme cold and damp in the system, but other than that, it is an extremely safe herb.

Skullcap

Scutellaria lateriflora
Mad-dog scullcap, Madweed

Family	Lamiaceae
Parts Used	aerial parts
Energetics	cooling, relaxing
Tissue States	heat, tension, atrophy
Taste	bitter, slightly acrid
Actions	anodyne, antispasmodic, nervine, sedative, trophorestorative, tonic

Coming upon skullcap in the woods is like finding a treasure. At home in moist areas and streambeds, this North American native is not that easy to spot in the wild. Skullcap is a small, slender-stalked mint with light blue flowers. The color blue is a signature for the nervous system, and indeed this is one of our superior nervine tonics. The genus name comes from the Latin word *scutella*, meaning small dish. Using one's imagination, you can see that the shape of the calyx (the sepals or the protective layer around a flower in bud) is like a dish. The common name refers to a resemblance to helmets worn in medieval times.

Uses

I love the name *skullcap* not for the visual image but because it evokes this plant's gentle energetic presence above our heads, "capping" incessant thoughts and worries. This cooling mint has a special affinity for mental patterns of excess heat and excitation characteristic of the vata-pitta dosha. For those that ruminate and can't find their way out of circular thinking, this is the herb of choice, and it excels for those with insomnia. As a trophorestorative, skullcap can be taken for long periods of time. It contains monoterpenes and flavonoids that are nourishing to nerve tissue. The active constituent, scutellarin, is similar to quercetin, which decreases mast cell activity or inflammation.[82] This is one way it works to cool and sedate pain. It is not the strongest pain reliever in the apothecary, but it has a specificity for pain with muscle tension, spasms, and (in the past) epilepsy. The names mad-dog skullcap and madweed refer to its purported use in treating rabies. Many historical accounts claim great success with treating this dreaded disease, but it seems there are an equal number of stories countering the veracity of those claims. Either way, it is an excellent sedative, yet does not compromise cognition. Skullcap taught me that calming the mind has a way of making you more in touch with where you are. For insomnia, it is often our minds that provide the energy that prevents us from sleeping. When that energy is calmed, we align with the truth that, indeed, we really are tired.

Indications

Heat/Excitation (Cooling)

Fevers. It is always important to add a nervine to fever formulas to relax the tension that accompanies a fever. This is the perfect cooling relaxant because it also acts as a febrifuge.

Mental health. Calms and cools heated, agitated thoughts. Good for restlessness, anxiety, and fearful states.

Dry/Atrophy (Tonic)

Nervous system. Excellent trophorestorative, tonifying for exhausted system due to pain or stress. Works differently than adaptogens in that it specifically feeds the nerves. Takes the jagged edge off stress. Specific for people who are easily overstimulated by noise, lights, and other environmental changes.

Tension/Constriction/Wind (Relaxant)

Mental health. For tension headaches, skullcap pairs beautifully with wood betony (*Stachys officinalis*) and St. John's wort.

Insomnia. The late naturopath William Mitchell said, "I have used as much as 180 drops [a generous teaspoon] of *Scutellaria* tincture at night to aid sleep. Although this dose seems high, it is not. In fact, I have used as much as 300 drops [1.7 teaspoons] for patients with insomnia."[83] (Note that 1 teaspoon is about equal to 175 drops.)

Musculoskeletal system. Specific for anxiety accompanied by tremors, spasms, twitchy muscles, especially during sleep.

Addiction. Because of its effects on the musculoskeletal system and mental states, skullcap is extremely helpful in delirium tremens with withdrawal, as well as lesser symptoms. Larger doses may be required, such as 5 milliliters (1 teaspoon) every hour, alone or in combination with other antispasmodic herbs. Fresh milky oats (*Avena sativa*) tincture is also a specific for this challenge.

Habitat & Harvest

Skullcap grows easily from seed. As a member of the mint family, when conditions are right, it will spread with ease, yet it has never taken over in the Sacred Plant Traditions garden (much to my chagrin). It prefers shade and moist soils but has been known to occupy sunny conditions especially in cooler northern climes. All aerial parts are harvested just as flowers are beginning to bloom.

Preparations

Infusion: Use 2 to 3 cups a day. Many herbalists feel dried skullcap has no medicinal value, but my twenty-five years of clinical practice have proven otherwise.

Tincture: Fresh plant (1:2, 75% alcohol); I have only made fresh-plant tincture because skullcap is most effective when made this way. If you use dried, make sure it is very freshly dried (1:5, 50% alcohol).

Contraindications

Skullcap is one of the most adulterated herbs in the marketplace, so if you do not grow it for your own use, make sure your source is reputable.

St. John's Wort

Hypericum perforatum
Klamath weed, Goatweed

Family	Hypericaceae
Parts Used	flower bud, flower, leaf
Energetics	warming, drying
Tissue States	tension, stagnation, depression,
Taste	sweet, bitter
Actions	vulnerary, trophorestorative (nervous system), hepatic, antiviral, relaxing nervine

St. John's wort is a plant that embodies the light. Herbalist and author Maude Grieves stated: "Its name *Hypericum* is derived from the Greek and means 'over an apparition,' a reference to the belief that the herb was so obnoxious to evil spirits that a whiff of it would cause them to fly."[84] This refers to the sacred place this herb held in protection against evil forces. Dried bundles were hung on doorways during Midsummer's Eve, the Summer Solstice, in efforts to bring light and good graces upon the family. The five-petaled bright yellow flowers begin blooming near this day of longest light, which Christian churches later called St. John's Day. The species name, *perforatum*, describes the holes or perforations seen when the leaf is held up to the light. These are oil glands, and when you bruise the leaf (rub it between your fingers), a small amount of dark red oil is secreted. This oil was also said to represent the blood of St. John the Baptist, but for me this is the plant's signature, an indication that it performs beautifully as an alterative or blood cleanser as it enhances the liver's ability in the breakdown of chemicals. Cleansing can be a challenging undertaking that sometimes triggers old issues and stirs up toxins held in the body, which may result in severe headaches. I've found that formulas that include this light-filled nervine have yielded dramatic results in facilitating what can be a dark and difficult process of release.

Uses

This is one of the supreme nervines of our apothecaries. *Hypericum* has a specificity for nerve pain, and in homeopathy it is referred to as the arnica of the nerves, meaning it is a must-have remedy when there is injury and nerve pain.[85] Whole-plant medicine works equally well as does the oil made from the flowers.

According to *King's American Dispensatory*: "Hypericum has undoubted power over the nervous system, and particularly the spinal cord. It is used in injuries of the spine and in lacerated and punctured wounds of the limbs to prevent tetanic complications and to relieve the excruciating pains of such injuries."[86]

In my decades of practice, St. John's wort has been one of the most reliable remedies I have found for sciatica, nerve pain from trauma or surgery, and post-concussion challenges. Through the use of St. John's wort, I have seen nerves come back online that were once thought lost. I am hesitant to say this trophorestorative can actually regenerate nerves, but its ability in restoring nerve function is unparalleled.

This plant has gained notoriety for treatment of depression, which makes sense in the framework of the plant's relationship with light. Depression has a myriad of causes, so it is important to differentiate the cause for each individual. St. John's wort is a wonderful remedy for seasonal affective disorder, which is a response to diminished light. My sense is that the spirit of this medicine works directly on the solar plexus. In the East Indian chakra or energy system, this third chakra is our sense of self and reflects the liver, gallbladder, and digestive system. In chapter 4, I described how in Five Phase Theory the Liver/Gallbladder processes anger and aids in decision-making. These are two vital functions when working with depression because many times depression results when a person's inner fire has gone out and they feel disempowered. Herbalist David Winston wrote: "In ancient Greek medicine, the word melancholia described a state in which a person had an excess of the black (melan) bile (choler). This humoral imbalance led to symptoms including irritability, depression (often with anxiety), angry thoughts, loss of appetite, insomnia, nausea and biliousness. This symptom picture is indicative of *hepatic depression*,"[87] the feeling that the lens of life has soured. St. John's wort is a wonderful remedy here, especially blended with wood betony.

My deep love for and devotion to this plant began in the mid-eighties while I was working with folks in the HIV community. Spurred by a very specific dream, I began harvesting large quantities of fresh St. John's wort flowers and leaves, and spent hours listening to its medicine. I was not aware of this herb's antiviral capabilities at the time, but it has been shown to inhibit the ability of viruses to fuse with host cells.[88] I was working in a large metropolitan clinic at the time, and we used it primarily for its restorative effect on the nervous system. After a while, we noted a marked decrease in the secondary herpetic outbreaks that often accompany HIV among those taking St. John's wort. There is now substantial research for the use of St. John's wort in mitigating intensity and duration of viral infections, most notably herpes.[89] The pain from herpetic lesions, whether due to shingles, cold sores, or trigeminal neuralgia of the face, can be extreme. I am not certain how I could address these conditions without this remedy.

Indications

Heat/Excitation (Nervine/Sedative)

Skin. Helpful to ease pain from radiation burns, herpetic lesions (shingles, cold sores), and red, inflamed tissues with pain.

Musculoskeletal system. Decreases nerve pain from trauma, and is especially beneficial for sciatica.

Bladder. Calms excessive urination from high levels of stress. Also indicated for dark yellow urine (too much heat) with high anxiety.

Cold/Depression (Tonic)

Liver. Useful for sluggish liver metabolism.

Digestive system. Builds and tones digestive tract.

Nervous system. As a trophorestorative, *Hypericum* can be used with almost any disorder of the nerves, from multiple sclerosis to damage caused by injury or surgery. Specific for sharp, shooting pains, especially in regions that are highly enervated such as eyes and extremities.

PMS. Eases PMS, cramping, and irregular bleeding. A specific for those who suffer from melancholic thoughts and moods during their cycle.

Tension/Constriction (Relaxation)

Head. Excellent remedy for tension headaches. Combines well with skullcap.

Eyes. Specific for sharp eye pain resulting from injury or infection.

Musculoskeletal system. Helps ease any type of pain associated with spinal injuries or tension. As stated above, it is specific for sciatic pain—use both tincture and topical oil. Might need high doses for acute injuries, such as 1 teaspoon every three to four hours until pain subsides.

Bladder. Calms when excessive anxiety or stress causes urinary symptoms such as bed-wetting and increased frequency.

Habitat & Harvest

St. John's wort prefers open, well-drained fields and meadows. It is best to harvest when the sun is most radiant and all parts are dry (especially if making an oil). Fresh-plant tincture and oil is preferred. The bud is excellent, and the best medicines are a combination of bud, flower, and leaves taken from the upper branches. While many herbalists focus on the flower alone, the flavonoids in the leaves enhance the effect of hypericin, one of the principal constituents of St. John's wort, which is found in the flowers.[90]

While some growers and gardeners cultivate this healing medicine successfully, many small growers I have talked with agree that this plant is peripatetic—it likes to move and change locations—and this is my observation as well. For this reason, I continue to harvest in wild lands blessed with St. John's wort.

Preparations

Infusion: Best used fresh or freshly dried.

Tincture: Fresh plant (1:2, 95% alcohol) or recently dried (1:5, 60% alcohol).

Oil: Apply frequently for nerve pain. If fair-skinned, best to cover (with clothing) areas on which oil has been applied if you go outdoors in the sun.

Contraindications

Photosensitivity of eyes and skin can occur with high doses or certain forms of preparations, especially standardized extracts.

Clinical research has shown that St. John's wort speeds up a metabolic process in the liver. The CYP450 enzyme metabolism pathway in the liver is responsible for clearing the liver of toxins or excess hormones. This detoxification is a positive use of *Hypericum*, but when combined with some pharmaceuticals, this enhanced metabolism can decrease blood levels of medications or render them ineffective. Those on certain medications should avoid the use of this plant or consult a qualified botanical or medical practitioner.

Violet

Viola sororia, V. odorata

Sweet violet, Pansy, Heart's ease

Family	Violaceae
Parts Used	flower, leaf, root
Energetics	moistening, cooling, nutritive
Tissue States	heat, dry/atrophy, stagnation
Taste	sweet, salty, sour
Actions	antimicrobial, nutritive, expectorant, vulnerary, demulcent, lymphagogue, alterative, antineoplastic

Over the years, violet has been a great teacher for me. Ubiquitous in gardens, woodlands, forests, and those famous "waste places" some authors of guidebooks love to describe, the profound medicine of *Viola* is at almost every herbalists' disposal. While violet prefers moist, shady places (as her medicine is moistening), she is adaptable to a variety of conditions. Violet appears soft and sweet and yet has a ferocity of spirit that moves deeply with serious illnesses, including cancer and stubborn lymphatic congestion. The ability of violet to soften hard edges, mentally and physically, is most impressive. I love the truth of the words of Tennessee Williams from *Camino Real*: "The violets in the mountains have broken the rocks." *Viola* has taught me that there is great power in gentle ways.

According to Thomas Elpel, author of *Botany in a Day*, there are 16 genera and 850 species in the *Violaceae* family. While the European native *V. odorata* is the "official" violet, there are many species native to North America.

The common blue violet, *V. sororia*, a white flower with blue stripes, is said to be interchangeable with species that bear white or violet flowers when it comes to food and medicine. Heart's ease (*V. tricolor*) has three colors combined in one flower. The shiny, heart shaped leaves have scalloped edges, and the blossom is irregular and exquisite, like that of an orchid. The true flowers of violets—the ones that produce viable seed—are green, remaining hidden under the leaves, and do not emerge until fall. This is a signature for violet as a medicine for shyness, for someone who is the quintessential shrinking violet. Although it keeps its flowers hidden, violet produces seed capsules described as exploding, which is why it is so prolific.

There are actually a number of woodland violets that are endangered, so it is best to identify common ones in your area and work with those species.

Uses

First and foremost, violets are nutritious. The early spring leaves or new fall growth are the sweetest and most tender. As summer comes on, the leaves become tough, and teas with those leaves will be more bitter. Violet is rich in minerals and vitamins, especially vitamins A and C. Herbalist Susun Weed writes that 100 grams (approximately 1 cup) of fresh herb yields 264 milligrams of ascorbic acid and 20,000 IU of vitamin A.[91] Many plant lovers drink daily infusions of nettle for its nutritional value, but as a diuretic, nettle can be drying. Substitute violet tea for nettle tea, or add violets to a nettle brew to moisten the formula. This herb is undervalued in our vata-prone culture, as violets are helpful for tension and irritability.

Violet's uncanny ability to soften hard edges manifests in its ability to move lymphatic fluid and soften cysts and growths. There is also some other hidden essence of this low-growing, high-achieving plant that softens our edges, mentally and physically.

Indications

Heat/Excitation
Head. Cools throbbing headache, especially presenting at the temples, which can indicate Liver/Gallbladder tension or sinus congestion.

Respiratory system. Excellent tea for clearing damp heat from respiratory tract. The leaves are high in saponins, which are useful for expectoration.

Skin. A simple poultice of the leaves and roots clears rash from eczema, eruptions, and boils, and is a great addition to a drawing plantain poultice.

Breasts. Excellent internally as well as externally for heat and swelling from mastitis or breast inflammation/infection from blocked ducts.

Bladder. Clears heat from a urinary tract infection and can be a great pain reliever for interstitial cystitis.

Dry/Atrophy (Moistening)

Respiratory system. Violet is excellent to treat dry mucosa, which can cause hacking, unproductive coughs.

Joints. As a lubricant, it can ease pain and stiffness from arthritis, especially when there are accompanying dry, hot tissues. The leaves also contain natural salicylates, the anti-inflammatory compounds used in aspirin.

Skin. Used in a salve or cream, violet restores moisture and tone to dry, cracked skin. Take internally for atopic dermatitis and other skin eruptions.

Stagnation

Throat. As a lymphagogue, violet is excellent for swollen, sore throats.

Breasts. Violet has a specificity for moving congested lymph material in breast tissue. Massaging violet oil into breast tissue will have a profound clearing effect for fibrocystic breasts. If this treatment does not yield the desired results, adding a few drops of poke oil to the blend will move the medicine deeper. Excellent remedy for mastitis.

Liver. Useful when there are signs of congested Liver heat, such as persistent anger, irritability, and indigestion.

Cancer. Violet has a traditional role in treating cancer, both topically and internally, especially working with breast health. According to an NIH study, "*Viola odorata* extract exerted anti-cancerous activity on both breast cancer cell lines. . . . *Viola odorata* extract mostly targets cancerous cells, not normal cells with high exception in high concentration."[92]

At-Risk Status

There are a number of violet species that are endangered. Identify those in your local area to ensure harvest of the more common variety. *V. sororia* is the common blue violet and can be used interchangeably.

Habitat & Harvest

Although it prefers rich, moist, shaded areas, violet can be found in most locales. I harvest violet leaves like chickweed, gathering a bundle of leaves at the base, close to the ground, then use scissors to snip the handful. The plants spread widely by seed and rhizome (to many a gardener's frustration). Harvesting leaves encourages rapid regrowth, allowing for a few harvests per plant. You want to accomplish this before the summer heat makes the leaves tough and fibrous.

Preparations

Infusion: Fresh plants yield more mucilage, and dried plants yield more nutrition; 2 to 3 cups a day.

Tincture: I usually use violet as an infusion, but I prefer fresh-plant tincture to stimulate lymphatic movement (1:3, 95% alcohol).

Oil: Fresh-plant as well as dried-plant oil is very effective for breast tissue.

Contraindications

Many writers say that ingestion of violet roots causes emesis (vomiting), so care must be taken. According to author and herbalist Juliet Blankespoor, "Avoid internal use with individuals who have the rare inherited disorder G6PD (glucose-6-phosphate dehydrogenase) deficiency, because it can aggravate hemolytic anemia."[93]

Yarrow

Achillea millefolium

Soldier's woundwort, Knight's milfoil, Thousand weed, Staunchweed

Family	Asteraceae
Parts Used	leaf, flower
Energetics	cooling, warming,
Tissue States	stagnation, heat, depression
Taste	acrid, aromatic, pungent, bitter
Actions	aromatic, anodyne, circulatory stimulant, vulnerary, astringent, stimulating diaphoretic, antiseptic, diuretic

Even after thirty years of wildcrafting this herb, I still find myself deeply moved when I come upon a new stand of yarrow. *Achillea* stalks are strong and upright. Perhaps this is why yarrow stalks were traditionally used when throwing the I Ching.

Medicinal yarrow is the white-flowered yarrow; the flower heads often have tinges of pink. The brilliantly colored yarrows are best used for arrangements and ornamental garden design. A yarrow flower head is actually a grouping of 15 to 30 disk florets shaped like a dome or shield. (This flower structure is what botanists describe as a corymb.) The leaves are deeply segmented, finely cut two to three times along the stem, giving them a feathery appearance. These divisions are also what garners the plant its name of *millefolium*, or thousand-leaved. While yarrow is described as invasive, I have never found that to be true in my garden. It does spread by seed, so if you want to keep a stand of yarrow under better control, deadhead the flowers before they go to seed.

Revered the world over, yarrow is mentioned in the ancient texts of Ayurveda and Chinese medicine. So great was yarrow's healing prowess, it was said that no one would travel without yarrow seeds because they did not want to face settling in a new place without this medicine. And indeed, a Neanderthal skull found in Spain and reported to be over 50,000 years old had seeds of yarrow in the teeth.[94]

Uses

Legends abound about yarrow. One well-known story is that Achilles's mother Thetis, who was the goddess of water, dipped him in a brew of yarrow tea. As she had to hold him by the ankle while doing so, the protective elixir did not touch his heel. Hence our most vulnerable aspect, our Achilles's heel. It is also said that Achilles would never go into battle without this plant. It is aptly called soldier's woundwort, knight's milfoil, and militaris.

The power of this plant came home to me one hot summer day. I was blending a mass of jewelweed stems in a food processor for a friend who had a serious case of poison ivy. I was moving quickly (to aid my poor friend) and as I reached in to scoop out the plant material, I caught my finger on the blade. I immediately knew that this cut had probably gone close to the bone and stitches would be required. Not wanting to take the time for that (lesson still not learned) I quickly went out to my "lawn," gave great thanks for having a hearty stand of yarrow, chewed up a wad of leaves and applied it to my finger. The bleeding stopped immediately and not only did the pain lessen but the finger began to tingle, then was delightfully numb. Later that afternoon I went to change the bandage and saw a very clean wound with edges nearly meeting and no redness from inflammation. A few years later, I heard Matthew Wood say that yarrow was for times when you feel "cut to the bone," and I knew that was true. I do not carry yarrow seeds like the traders of old, but dried yarrow leaves are a must in my traveling first-aid kit, as I have seen dried yarrow work the same miracles with bleeding wounds.

The effectiveness of this plant in healing wounds is not simply that it stanches bleeding. Its aromatic oils are antimicrobial, and there is the numbing effect. Ayurvedic texts note that yarrow was used for anesthesia for surgery. I'm not certain what the physiological mechanism is, but if you chew a leaf and leave it wadded against your gum for a minute or two, you will experience this sensation.

Just as powerfully as it stanches blood, yarrow also moves stagnant blood. I once had a client with an old wound—a deep cut incurred from contact with a coral reef. These injuries can be dangerous for many reasons, but mostly from concern of microscopic crystals, which are full of bacteria, lodging in the skin. The site of the cut was still deep purple and swollen after almost a year. Applying yarrow salve daily for a couple of weeks completely cleared the area, but left quite a scar. We followed up with calendula salve, and now there is only a small scar left to remind my client of the wonders of herbal medicine.

Matthew Wood wrote that yarrow "is both cooling and warming, fluid generating and controlling. Remedies with contradictory but complementary properties are often of great utility since they are able to normalize opposing conditions. This is true for yarrow."[95]

With this plant in your apothecary, you really need no other diaphoretic. Yarrow brings blood to the surface, opens the pores, and circulates heat so it can move out of our systems in times of fever. And if we make a cold infusion, it moves our waters through our kidneys, releasing toxins. Warm tea moves energy up and outward and cool infusions move down and outward. At the first sign of a cold or flu, a simple hot tea of yarrow can be the perfect remedy.

In Chinese medicine there are extra meridians that are called the "sea of blood" and are responsible for healthy menstruation and moon cycles. Also, wounding from sexual trauma is often played out in menstrual history, and yarrow offers the ability to heal physical as well as emotional wounding. Again, it seems odd to use such a blood mover when a woman is experiencing a heavy cycle. But if offered in low doses, yarrow has a way of harmonizing the flow and healing of psychic wounds. With the use of yarrow, the disempowerment women, as well as men, feel from such trauma gives way to a sense that they can go to battle for themselves in ways they may never have imagined. Also, loss of blood leads to anemia and without sufficient iron to steel their way forward, women can feel disheartened and fatigued. Yarrow protects on so many levels.

Indications

Heat

Fevers. The quintessential fever remedy. Hot infusions bring on diaphoresis or sweating to help break a fever and dispel pathogens.

Digestive system. As a digestive bitter, yarrow is cooling. It can also help resolve diarrhea caused by heat and infection.

Uterine health. Menstrual flooding can be a sign of heat. Adding yarrow to other astringing and tonifying herbs can cool and normalize menstrual flow.

Mouth/gums. Chewing the root clears heat from dental infections as well as relieving the pain from swelling.

Night sweats. Clears atrophic heat—the heat that arises when the body does not have enough fluids to cool itself.

Cold/Depression (Move Stagnation)

Skin. As a blood mover, yarrow can resolve old bruises and injuries.

Head. Aromatic oils in yarrow help relieve tension headaches caused by cold conditions. The Chippewa used the leaves in a steam inhalant for headaches. They also chewed the roots and applied the saliva to their appendages as a stimulant.

Cardiovascular system. Yarrow is one of the few herbs that safely invigorates blood.

Uterine health. Cold conditions create more menstrual pain through constriction. Yarrow can warm uterine muscle by increasing blood flow.

Trauma. Excellent in drop doses after concussion or head injury.

Damp/Stagnation (Stimulant)

Respiratory system. Yarrow's volatile oils help promote the healthy flow and elimination of mucus (anticatarrhal), especially from the sinuses.

General health. As a warming diaphoretic, yarrow can be used for an at-home sauna: Drinking a cup or two of the hot infusion and soaking in a bath with water as hot as is tolerable is an effective way to detoxify.

Digestive system. Yarrow's bitter aromatic qualities make it an excellent digestive tonic where there is stagnation and bloating.

Uterine health. Fibroids are a form of stagnation, so adding yarrow to uterine formulas can help resolve these benign tumors.

Tension (Relaxant)
Uterine health. Relieves cramping from blood stagnation or tension due to emotionally related trauma: This can be from abuse or traumatic birth experiences.

Laxity (Astringent)
Digestive system. Excellent for diarrhea, especially from food poisoning.
Wounds. As a styptic, yarrow astringes and stops excess bleeding.
Nosebleeds. Very reliable remedy for nosebleeds. Make a poultice of leaves and apply directly into nostril.

Habitat & Harvest
Yarrow has two lookalikes to familiarize yourself with before harvesting. One is wild carrot (*Daucus carota*), an edible and medicinal plant also known as Queen Anne's lace. The other is poison hemlock (*Conium maculatum*), which causes central nervous system depression and respiratory failure that has led to fatalities. Unless you are well versed at recognizing yarrow in the wild, it is best to harvest only from garden plants.

If wildcrafting, be mindful of the health of the soil as yarrow is a soil remediator and can pull out heavy metals from the soil.[96] Harvest leaves before plants flower and harvest flowers at their peak flowering stage. If you plan to harvest the root, deadhead the flowers so that the plant's energy does not go into making the seed but instead returns to the root.

Preparations
Infusion: Cold infusion is best for diuresis. A hot infusion serves as a diaphoretic and most other applications.
Tincture: Fresh plant (preferred: 1:2, 95% alcohol) or dried (1:5, 75% alcohol).
Oil/salve: Best not to apply oil or salve to a pustulant wound. Use a spray (of the infusion) or poultice to draw and dry the wound before applying oil.

Contraindications
Pregnant women should avoid yarrow as it has the ability to relax the smooth muscle of the uterus and is a blood mover.

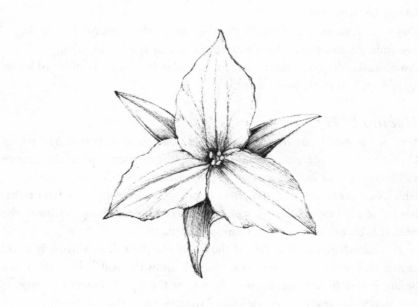

Epilogue

Before scripts, glyphs, and written language, humans shared knowledge through the art of the story. Herbalism was and remains a tradition of stories passed on by word of mouth. Whether in the context of a dream, poetic wanderings, or a long tale of healing to tide the circle through the night, we have learned the magic and pattern songs of the plants through story. I can read volumes on materia medica, plant profiles, or research, but the medicine stories are how the plant remains in my heart.

As an herbalist, instead of the requisite fifteen-minute visit, I can sit for as long as needed to hear my client's story. I listen with all my senses in order to perceive the inner and outer landscapes. So often I think providing the answer is not the solution for healing. More frequently, solutions reveal themselves when the perfect question is presented. The inquiry is the key that gently opens a place of vulnerability with someone who has come to trust you. As a practitioner, my deep listening holds space for them to hear and understand their story in a new light. The telling of the story is a most potent medicine in herbal traditions.

Over the years, I have often wondered whether I had let go of my golden thread in choosing not to join Rosemary Gladstar at the California School of Herbal Studies. As it turns out, the thread of my life did intertwine with that of Rosemary's. It was she who shone her light on me many years ago when I was a budding herbalist and she invited me to teach at her beautiful Sage Mountain Center, as well as at many of her conferences in later years. I am deeply honored to have served with her and United Plant Savers for so many years. I am certain this is exactly the place the thread intended to lead me.

The magic and medicine of our plant teachers is not simply the root or leaf or seed. It is the very song that is sung when these individual plants and their communities come into being. There are unseen forces that science cannot measure, yet are detectable to the human heart and spirit. For example, Southwestern native American peoples have a thousand-year history of using chaparral, or creosote bush (*Larrea tridentata*). This astounding desert plant grows by producing new stems underground from a crown taproot. As the new stems develop, the older central stems die back. Eventually, this appears as an expanding ring of seemingly separate plants, but all are attached belowground and all share the same genetic material. These rings grow very slowly; researchers estimate that a ring with a diameter of twenty feet can be up to three thousand years old. In the Sonoran Desert, there is an astounding specimen thought to be eighteen thousand years old. If we assume that the genetic material is the same as the original clone, then these beings are the oldest living creatures on Earth—their seeds germinated at the conclusion of the last Ice Age. Imagine planting a garden for the coming ages. . . . It begins with one dream, one seed, one garden, one sanctuary at a time.

Acknowledgments

W orking with illustrator Lara Gastinger was a dream come true. Living less than a mile away, we would meet in my garden as she would gather materials for her illustrations. How honored I was to dig roots of goldenseal and Solomon's seal and know she would not only illustrate them but replant them on her side of town. As the illustrator of *Flora of Virginia*, she knows these plants so well. To Beth Le Grand, my teacher of the heart, protector of my voice, and my Buddha in the corner. To my dear friend and wise woman Hollis Melton. Your feedback and insistence that I read every word out loud to hear it in my heart made all the difference. Suzanna Stone, you brought depth of courage and veracity to all the parts that were uncomfortable and made it all feel just right. Teresa Boardwine, your love and your cordials nourished my heart, soul, and the Dreamtime that keeps dreaming our paths together. To Mary K. Scott, whose open heart brought me the muse of the ocean. To my Light Falling Sisters of Mt. Shasta, your dreams and prayers light up these pages. To my beloved Rappahannock County community, whose magic and mountains nourished my dreams.

Very special thanks to my stellar editor, Fern Bradley, who heard me teach a number of years ago and never stopped believing. Early on I realized the co-creative process that unfolds in writing a book, and Fern's craft is with deep thought and, most importantly, much heart. Thanks also to publisher Margo Baldwin for her support. Patricia Stone brought such clarity and beauty with her production wizardry and kudos to the whole team that polished this text with professionalism and caring.

To all the students who have graced my life with your curiosity, dedication, and a desire to keep this art alive and thriving. To Heather Wetzel, who kept the clinic fires burning, and Angel Shockley; there are no words for your patience and the art you bring to details. Your warmth and humor carried me through. Heartfelt gratitude to all my teachers, named and unnamed, seen and unseen. Rosita Arvigo, Cascade Anderson-Geller, Stephen Buhner, Candis Canton, Robert Clickner, Eliot Cowan, Jim Duke,

Margi Flint, Rosemary Gladstar, David Hoffmann, Robyn Klein, Phyllis Light, Sarah Holmes, Lorna Mauney-Brodek, jim mcdonald, Rain Perrie, Karyn Sanders, Tammi Sweet, Laura Marie Thompson, Susun Weed, David Winston, Matthew Wood, and 7Song.

To those that have been there from the very beginning and kept this dream alive, well-traveled, and so well fed. I give deep thanks to my family, especially my sister Gretchen Teran and her family—Tim, Hank, Emmet. To John Bloom, many thanks for the seeds planted long ago. To Brian Rayner, whose constant love and faith in this project sustained me long into the morning hours.

To all our ancestors who hold us in their love and protection. And finally, to the Earth herself and all her relations. When I was living right, I would show up to write, light a candle, burn some wondrous wood or plant, and offer gratitude for the privilege to be in concert with the spirits of these plants.

At-Risk Assessment Tool Scoring Sheet

This scoring sheet reflects a comprehensive evaluation of a species. Plants are assigned a score in each category. Low scores reflect a plant that is less vulnerable; high scores reflect greater vulnerability. For example, a plant that requires a unique method for pollination or that takes a long time to produce mature seed would have a higher score in the seed reproduction category than a plant that is pollinated by many species and spreads easily by seed.

Appendix 1: At-Risk Assessment Tool Scoring Sheet

I. Life History
1.0 Life Span
1.1 Age at First Reproduction
1.2 Disturbance Tolerance
1.3 Vegetative Reproduction
1.4 Seed Reproduction
1.5 Interactions
Life History Total

II. Effect of Harvest on Plant
2.0 Plant Part Harvested
2.1 Post-Harvest Recovery
2.2 Harvest Interval
2.3 Length of Harvest Season
Population Total
III. Abundance and Range
3.0 Natural Abundance
3.1 Range—Current Population Size
3.2 Changes in Population Size
3.3 Habitat Specialization
Abundance Total
IV. Habitat
4.0 Habitat Vulnerability
4.1 Habitat Acreage
4.2 Habitat Fragmentation
4.3 Soil Type
4.4 List Threats to Habitat
Habitat Total
V. How Much Is Needed
5.0 Annual Demand
5.1 Yield per Acre
5.2 Alternatives
5.3 Cultivation Status
Demand Total
Overall Total

Herbal Actions Glossary

Adaptogen. In the most general of terms, this is an herb that helps the body increase resilience and adapt to stress. These plants are thought of as building herbs; they support those who have deficiencies, especially deficiencies of hormonal systems such as adrenal and endocrine weakness. Examples: reishi (*Ganoderma lucidum*), ashwagandha (*Withania somnifera*), borage (*Borago officinalis*), holy basil (*Ocimum tenuiflorum*)

Alterative. An herb that alters the body's metabolic processes so that tissues function optimally. These plants enhance detoxification through supporting elimination channels of the liver, kidneys, skin, lymphatics, and bowels. These are the beloved "blood cleansers" of traditional herbalism. They tend to be bitter, drying, and cooling, which is why they work beautifully for damp-heat conditions such as diabetes, eczema, candida, and acne. Examples: echinacea root (*Echinacea* spp.), artichoke leaves (*Cynara scolymus*), dandelion root (*Taraxacum officinale*)

Amphoteric. An herb that serves as a normalizer. These plants harmonize organs and systems, and have the ability to correct two seemingly contradictory actions; they are able to act as either an acid or a base (such as both lowering high blood pressure and raising low blood pressure). Example: garlic (*Allium sativum*)

Analgesic or **Anodyne.** An herb that reduces the sensation of pain (*ano*, meaning against; *dynia*, meaning pain). This is accomplished through cooling excess heat, relaxing spasms, moving blood stagnation, or nourishing the nervous system. Examples: Jamaican dogwood (*Piscidia erythrina*), prickly ash (*Zanthoxylum americanum*), black cohosh (*Actaea racemosa*), skullcap (*Scutellaria lateriflora*), California poppy (*Eschscholzia californica*)

Antacid. An herb that neutralizes acid. Examples: slippery elm (*Ulmus rubra*), marshmallow root (*Althaea officinalis*), chamomile (*Matricaria chamomilla*), fennel (*Foeniculum vulgare*), agrimony (*Agrimonia eupatoria*)

Antibacterial. An herb that stops or prevents the growth of bacteria. Examples: calendula (*Calendula officinalis*), elecampane (*Inula helenium*), garlic (*Allium sativum*)

Anticatarrhal. An herb that assists the body in removing excess mucus. *Catarrh* is an older term for mucus. Examples: yarrow (*Achillea millefolium*), lobelia (*Lobelia inflata*), goldenrod (*Solidago canadensis*), thyme (*Thymus vulgaris*), rosemary (*Salvia rosmarinus*)

Antiemetic. An herb that relieves nausea and helps to prevent vomiting. Examples: chamomile (*Matricaria chamomilla*), peppermint (*Mentha × piperita*), ginger (*Zingiber officinale*)

Antifungal. An herb that inhibits the growth or spread of fungal infections. Usually, such herbs contain high levels of essential oils and the aromatic compounds. Examples: black walnut hulls (*Juglans nigra*), rosemary (*Salvia rosmarinus*), oregano (*Origanum vulgare*), pau d'arco (*Tabebuia impetiginosa*), calendula (*Calendula officinalis*)

Anti-inflammatory. An herb that acts to soothe inflammation or acts directly to reduce tissue inflammation. Examples: feverfew (*Tanacetum parthenium*), plantain (*Plantago* spp.), yucca root (*Yucca glauca*), kudzu (*Pueraria montana*), meadowsweet (*Filipendula ulmaria*)

Antilithic. An herb that prevents, inhibits, or diminishes the formation of calculi (stones). *Lithos* means stones. For gallbladder stones, work with the cholagogues, but for kidney stones work with antilithics as well as antispasmodics. Examples: Joe Pye weed (*Eutrochium purpureum*), hydrangea (*Hydrangea arborescens*), celery seed (*Apium graveolens*)

Antimicrobial. Many herbs are referred to as antimicrobial but that does not help in knowing which plants to use for which types of microbes. It is much more useful to break this category into more specific categories such as antifungal, antibacterial, antiseptic, and antiviral.

Antiseptic. An herb that destroys or prevents bacterial growth; these are often pungent aromatics. Examples: yarrow (*Achillea millefolium*), rosemary (*Salvia rosmarinus*), thyme (*Thymus vulgaris*)

Antispasmodic. An herb that prevents or reduces muscular tension or spasm. Most antispasmodic herbs are acrid or high in volatile oils. Examples: respiratory—wild lettuce (*Lactuca virosa*), lobelia (*Lobelia inflata*), cramp bark (*Viburnum opulus*); gut—chamomile (*Matricaria chamomilla*), wild yam (*Dioscorea villosa*), ginger (*Zingiber officinale*); uterine—cramp bark (*Viburnum opulus*), black haw (*Viburnum prunifolium*)

Antiviral. An herb that prevents or reduces the spread of viral infections. Examples: osha root (*Ligusticum porteri*), St. John's wort (*Hypericum perforatum*), lemon balm (*Melissa officinalis*), calendula (*Calendula officinalis*), echinacea (*Echinacea* spp.)

Anxiolytic. An herb that reduces anxiety. Examples: skullcap (*Scutellaria lateriflora*), lemon balm (*Melissa officinalis*), motherwort (*Leonurus cardiaca*), blue vervain (*Verbena hastata*)

Aperient. An herb that is a bitter or a hepatic that gently works as a laxative through stimulation of the liver. Examples: juniper berry (*Juniperis communis*), dandelion root (*Taraxacum officinale*), artichoke (*Cynara scolymus*)

Aphrodisiac. An herb that increases or stimulates sexual desire. Many aphrodisiacs are reproductive tonics. Examples: damiana (*Turnera diffusa*), muira puama (*Croton echioides*), schisandra (*Schisandra chinensis*)

Aromatic or **Carminative.** An herb that is warming, stimulating, dispersing, and used to aid digestion. Known by their strong scent, these herbs contain volatile oils. Many essential oils are high in antioxidants, and thus this group is also antimicrobial and anti-inflammatory. Examples: rosemary (*Salvia rosmarinus*), sage (*Salvia officinalis*), anise seed (*Pimpinella anisum*), peppermint (*Mentha × piperita*), cinnamon (*Cinnamonum verum*)

Astringent. An herb that tightens tissue weave and reduces secretions and discharges. Through the action of tannins, astringents decrease fluids, which makes the tissues less vulnerable to infection, and thus aids in wound healing. Examples: women's health—red raspberry (*Rubus idaeus*); bladder—uva ursi (*Arctostaphylos uva ursi*); circulatory system—horse chestnut (*Aesculus hippocastanum*); digestive system—blackberry root (*Rubus fruticosus*); skin—witch hazel (*Hamamelis virginiana*)

Bitter. An herb that stimulates the digestive system and enhances the flow of juices, acids, bile, and enzymes. The sensation/taste of bitterness directly affects the central nervous system and provokes a wide range of benefits. Relaxation, increasing appetite, greater liver detoxification, and blood sugar regulation are just a few of the healthful effects of these herbs. Examples: dandelion (*Taraxacum officinale*), yellow dock root (*Rumex crispus*), artichoke leaf (*Cynara scolymus*), Oregon grape root (*Berberis aquifolium*), chamomile (*Matricaria chamomilla*)

Cardiotonics. An herb that is supportive to heart muscle and cardiovascular functioning. These tonic herbs have a marked benefit for the cardiovascular system. Although these herbs are not as strong as cardiac glycosides, it is always best to work with a licensed practitioner if there are pharmaceuticals for blood pressure involved. Examples: hawthorn leaf, flower, and berry (*Crataegus* spp.), linden flower (*Tilia cordata*), motherwort (*Leonurus cardiaca*)

Carminative. An herb that works to increase gastric emptying and thereby aid in expelling gas and relieving cramping. This is why carminatives can be found on the digestive rack in our kitchens. Rich in volatile oils. Examples: anise (*Pimpinella anisum*), fennel (*Foeniculum vulgare*), rosemary (*Salvia rosmarinus*), cloves (*Syzygium aromaticum*), angelica (*Angelica archangelica*), dill (*Anethum graveolens*), catnip (*Nepeta cataria*), chamomile (*Matricaria chamomilla*)

Cathartic. An herb that purges the bowels and stimulates glandular secretions. These herbs are rarely needed if working with other digestive remedies. Examples: rhubarb (*Rheum rhabarbarum*), senna (*Senna alexandrina*)

Cholagogue. An herb that stimulates the release and secretion of bile from the liver. Bile moistens the digestive track and helps with constipation due to dryness. Examples: artichoke leaf (*Cynara scolymus*), Oregon grape root (*Berberis aquifolium*), yellow dock (*Rumex crispus*), fringetree bark (*Chionanthus virginicus*)

Demulcent or **Emollient.** An herb that is rich in mucilage or polysaccharides, which makes it mucilaginous (slimy). This property makes these plants cooling and soothing to mucous membranes, especially those of the intestine. Emollients are demulcents that are applied topically. Examples: violet (*Viola* spp.), comfrey (*Symphytum officinale*), marshmallow leaf and root (*Althaea officinalis*), chickweed (*Stellaria media*)

Diaphoretic. An herb that promotes sweating. These herbs are divided into two useful categories:

Relaxing Diaphoretics. The analogy for these herbs is opening a window to let the heat out. These are used when there is tension in the body and signs of heat with little sweating. Heat can be expressed as high fever, restlessness, red face, and little to no urination. Examples: blue vervain (*Verbena hastata*), elderflower (*Sambucus nigra*), boneset (*Eupatorium perfoliatum*), linden flowers (*Tilia cordata*)

Stimulating Diaphoretics. These herbs are used when vitality is low and there is clammy skin with cold and shivering. Tissue states of lax and cold stagnation are predominant. Examples: ginger (*Zingiber* *officinale*), horseradish (*Armoracia rusticana*), cayenne (*Capsicum annuum*), yarrow (*Achillea millefolium*)

Diffusive. An herb that increases movement of energy to break through congestion or stagnation. Usually given in low doses, these plants move other herbs out to the periphery of the body or they can add focus to the direction of a formula. This is why cayenne was so popular with Thomsonian physicians and other practitioners at the turn of the twentieth century. It brought heat and movement to cold/stagnant situations. Examples: prickly ash (*Zanthoxylum americanum*), cayenne (*Capsicum annuum*), ginger (*Zingiber officinale*)

Diuretic. An herb that stimulates the flow of urine. There are a few different mechanisms; not all diuretics are created equal. Examples:

Increasing Blood Flow: kola nut (*Cola vera*), green tea (*Camellia sinensis*)
Irritant: juniper berry (*Juniperus communis*) works by irritating the kidney
Mineral Balancing: dandelion leaf (*Taraxacum officinale*), nettle (*Urtica dioica*)

Emetic. An herb that promotes vomiting when taken in higher doses than normal. Example: lobelia (*Lobelia inflata*)

Emmenagogue. An herb that stimulates and normalizes the menstrual flow. Useful for menses that start light or with intermittency. Not to be used during pregnancy. Examples: mugwort (*Artemisia vulgaris*), motherwort (*Leonurus cardiaca*), ginger (*Zingiber officinale*), blue cohosh (*Caulophyllum thalictroides*)

Expectorant. An herb that helps the body remove excess mucus from the lungs. When mucus is white or clear, it usually indicates a cold condition and you would choose warming herbs. If there is yellow or green in the mucus, this indicates heat so herbs to clear infection should accompany expectorants.

Relaxing expectorants. Herbs that soothe bronchial spasm and loosen thick mucus. These are appropriate for an unproductive cough or irritation. Examples: coltsfoot (*Tussilago farfara*), marshmallow (*Althaea officinalis*), licorice (*Glycyrrhiza glabra*), violet (*Viola* spp.), plantain (*Plantago major*)

Stimulating expectorants. These herbs are generally warmer in nature and used for excessive mucus production or chronic conditions of bronchial congestion. Examples: elecampane (*Inula helenium*), lobelia (*Lobelia inflata*), hyssop (*Hyssopus officinalis*), licorice (*Glycyrrhiza glabra*)

Febrifuge. An herb that reduces fevers (*febri*, meaning fever; *fugo*, meaning to chase). If not working with diaphoresis, then herbs in this category contain salicylic acid (an aspirin-like compound) and work as an anti-inflammatory. Examples: meadowsweet (*Filipendula ulmaria*), willow (*Salix alba*), elderflower (*Sambucus nigra*), peppermint (*Mentha × piperita*), yarrow (*Achillea millefolium*)

Galactagogue. An herb that helps increase the flow of breast milk in nursing mothers. Examples: blessed thistle (*Cnicus benedictus*), borage (*Borago officinalis*), fenugreek (*Trigonella foenum-graecum*), milk thistle (*Silybum marianum*), fennel (*Foeniculum vulgare*)

Hepatic. An herb that strengthens and tones the liver and increases secretion of bile. While this may seem redundant with bitters and cholagogues, the latter are focused solely on stimulation of bile and enhancing downward energy to promote bowel movements. Examples: milk thistle (*Silybum marianum*), dandelion root (*Taraxacum officinale*), turmeric (*Curcuma longa*), licorice (*Glycyrrhiza glabra*)

Hypnotic. An herb that helps induce sleep. Often containing alkaloids, these plants are usually stronger than nervines. Examples: California poppy (*Eschscholzia californica*), Jamaican dogwood (*Piscidia erythrina*), kava kava (*Piper methysticum*), wild lettuce (*Lactuca virosa*)

Hypotensive. An herb that acts to reduce elevated blood pressure. Examples: hawthorn (*Crataegus* spp.), motherwort (*Leonurus cardiaca*), reishi (*Ganoderma lucidum*), valerian (*Valeriana officinalis*), linden (*Tilia cordata*), garlic (*Allium sativum*)

Immunomodulator. An herb that could be considered more tonifying for the immune system. These plants are to be used when there are frequent colds, allergies, and immune issues. Examples: astragalus (*Astragalus membranaceus*), reishi (*Ganoderma lucidum*), shitake (*Lentinula edodes*)

Immunostimulant. An herb that boosts the immune system; should be used only for a short duration (two weeks). Examples: echinacea (*Echinacea* spp.), usnea (*Usnea* spp.), poke root (*Phytolacca americana*)*, wild indigo (*Baptisia* spp.)

Laxative. See Aperient, Bitter, and Cathartic

Lymphatic. An herb that moves congested lymph material. These are indicated for swollen glands, sluggish recovery from colds or flus, and benign

---

* drop doses only

cysts. Examples: calendula (*Calendula officinalis*), cleavers (*Galium aparine*), red root (*Ceanothus americanus*), violet (*Viola* spp.), poke root (*Phytolacca americana*)*

Nervine. An herb that affects the nervous system. There are different types that provide a wide variety of medicinal actions:

> **Tonics.** These herbs are the trophorestoratives and one of herbal medicine's greatest contributions to strengthening and nourishing the nervous system. Wonderful for working with recovery from trauma. Examples: milky oats (*Avena sativa*), gotu kola (*Centella asiatica*), St. John's wort (*Hypericum perforatum*), borage (*Borago officinalis*), blue vervain (*Verbena hastata*)
>
> **Relaxing Nervines.** These are calming herbs that in general do not affect cognition and actually increase energy by removing tension, which can cause fatigue. Examples: skullcap (*Scutellaria lateriflora*), passionflower (*Passiflora incarnata*), St. John's wort (*Hypericum perforatum*), linden (*Tilia cordata*), lemon balm (*Melissa officinalis*)
>
> **Sedative Nervines.** See Hypnotic
>
> **Stimulating Nervines.** Herbs that stimulate the nervous system. Examples: coffee (*Coffea arabica*), green tea (*Camellia sinensis*), rosemary (*Salvia rosmarinus*), kola nut (*Cola vera*), prickly ash (*Zanthoxylum americanum*), peppermint (*Mentha* × *piperita*)

Oxytocic. An herb that stimulates labor or helps with sluggish menstruation. Oxytocin is the pituitary hormone that is responsible for uterine contractions. Examples: blue cohosh (*Caulophyllum thalictroides*), red raspberry (*Rubus idaeus*), goldenseal (*Hydrastis canadensis*)

Rubefacient. An herb that simulates circulation locally when applied to the skin. With use of these herbs, increased blood flow brings nutrients to the damaged area and enhances healing. Examples: cayenne (*Capsicum annuum*), mustard seed (*Brassica nigra*), ginger (*Zingiber officinale*), nettle (*Urtica dioica*), prickly ash (*Zanthoxylum americanum*)

Sialagogue. An herb that stimulates the secretion of saliva. Examples: prickly ash (*Zanthoxylum americanum*), ginger (*Zingiber officinale*), licorice (*Glycyrrhiza glabra*)

---

* drop doses only

Stimulant. A warming herb that quickens the physiological function of the body. Examples: cerebral function—rosemary (*Rosmarinus officinalis*), ginkgo (*Ginkgo biloba*), gotu kola (*Centella asiatica*); diffuse circulatory function—yarrow (*Achillea millefolium*), prickly ash (*Zanthoxylum americanum*)

Stomachic. An herb that promotes digestion and strengthens the stomach. Examples: catnip (*Nepeta cataria*), chamomile (*Matricaria chamomilla*), chickweed (*Stellaria media*), fennel (*Foeniculum vulgare*), ginger (*Zingiber officinale*)

Styptic. An herb that is applied topically to stop bleeding. Most often these are astringent. Examples: yarrow (*Achillea millefolium*), witch hazel (*Hamamelis virginiana*), cayenne (*Capsicum annuum*)

Tonic. This action has differing meanings in Western and Eastern practices and even within those systems there are further discerning properties. In Western herbalism these are generally herbs that can be taken over a long period of time to build vitality and strength of specific systems or overall vitality. There are shades of difference in defining tonification of different systems. In TCM there are Qi tonics, blood tonics, spleen tonics, and many more. Bitter tonics are mostly alteratives. Nutritive tonics are high in minerals and chlorophyll. Nervine tonics nourish the nerves. Immune/sweet tonics are somewhat like adaptogens.

Trophorestorative. An herb that helps to restore structure and also function. The Greek derivation of the word *trophic* relates to nourishment, food, and "to make solid." Examples: nervous system—St. John's wort (*Hypericum perforatum*), milky oats (*Avena sativa*); liver—milk thistle (*Silybum marianum*), dandelion root (*Taraxacum officinale*); kidney—nettle seed (*Urtica dioica*); endocrine—licorice (*Glycyrrhiza glabra*), American ginseng (*Panax quinquefolius*); heart—hawthorn (*Crataegus* spp.); skin—chickweed (*Stellaria media*), calendula (*Calendula officinalis*); connective tissue—hawthorn (*Crataegus* spp.), gotu kola (*Centella asiatica*)

Vermifuge, Anthelmintic, or **Parasiticide.** An herb that helps clear the body of parasites and worms (*verma*, meaning vermin; *fugo*, meaning to chase). Examples: black walnut (*Juglans nigra*), chaparral leaf (*Larrea tridentata*), garlic (*Allium sativum*), pumpkin seed (*Cucurbita* spp.), wormwood (*Artemisia annua*)

Vulnerary. An herb that heals external as well as internal wounds. Examples: calendula (*Calendula officinalis*), plantain (*Plantago* spp.), comfrey (*Symphytum officinale*)

Resources

I generally suggest working with local growers and medicine makers as a way to help support vibrant, community-based herbalism. However, if you need to search further afield, here is a short list of companies that provide excellent-quality herbs and herbal products. These companies also help with conservation and educational efforts by providing support to herbalism schools, free clinics, and United Plant Savers and other conservation organizations.

Avena Botanicals

www.avenabotanicals.com
Herbalist Deb Soule has been growing herbs organically as well as biodynamically for over thirty years in her pollinator garden in Rockport, Maine. Over 75 percent of medicines used in their products come from their certified biodynamic gardens.

Banyan Botanicals

www.banyanbotanicals.com
This is a reliable source for organic Ayurvedic herbs and oils.

Gathered Threads

www.gatheredthreadsllc.com
This is a family run Virginia farm that has some of the highest quality herbs we have seen. Along with bulk herbs, they provide CSA shares not only for vegetables and herbs but also for seasonal ferments.

Healing Spirits Herb Farm & Education Center

www.healingspiritsherbfarm.com
Andrea and Matthias Reisen run this family business with some of the most beautifully dried herbs we have seen. They also have extensive medicinal mushrooms blended in wonderful herbal formulas.

Herb Pharm
www.herb-pharm.com
This was one of the first companies to supply the herbal community with high-quality extracts. Herb Pharm has continued to uphold excellent standards.

Herbalist and Alchemist
www.herbalist-alchemist.com
Founded by herbalist and author David Winston, the formulas of these extracts are some of the finest clinical blends representing Eclectic tradition as well as Chinese and Ayurvedic formulations.

Mountain Rose Herbs
www.mountainroseherbs.com
We have worked with Mountain Rose Herbs for many years and they are incredibly supportive to students, schools, and those seeking better information, through their stellar website and medicine-making videos.

Oshala Farm
www.oshalafarm.com
This family-run farm's commitment to regenerative farming can be experienced through their herbs as well as witnessed by walking their fields.

Pacific Botanicals
www.pacificbotanicals.com
Pacific Botanicals has been supplying high-quality bulk herbs for over forty years. They excel at providing fresh herbs but these need to be ordered in advance. Harvest season is clearly listed on their website.

Red Moon Herbs
www.redmoonherbs.com
This woman-owned company specializes in making fresh Appalachian extracts from organic or wildcrafted sources. Their website is a veritable gold mine of great articles on harvest, medicine making, and women's health.

Traditional Medicinals

www.traditionalmedicinals.com

These are some of our favorite blends, and they are so accessible because they are pre-bagged. Founded by Rosemary Gladstar, Traditional Medicinals is a leader in the herbal industry on sustainable practices when working with international growers and harvesters.

Urban Moonshine

www.urbanmoonshine.com

Urban Moonshine specializes in extracts with a focus on digestive bitters. They have taken the art of formulating bitters to a new level and encourage the daily ritual of bitters as nourishing medicine.

Woodland Essence

www.woodlandessence.com

Kate Gilday and Don Babineau have been supplying the herbal community with high-quality medicine for almost thirty years. Their flower essences as well as mushroom extracts are superb. They specialize in providing extracts supporting Stephen Buhner's Lyme protocols.

Zack Woods Herb Farm

www.zackwoodsherbs.com

This is a family-run farm that is committed to providing organic fresh and dried bulk plant material while maintaining as well as teaching good stewardship and healthy land practices.

Recommended Reading

General

Bennett, Robin Rose. *The Gift of Healing Herbs: Plant Medicines and Home Remedies for a Vibrantly Healthy Life*. Berkeley, CA: North Atlantic Books, 2014.

Boericke, William. *Pocket Manual of Homeopathic Materia Medica: Comprising the Characteristic and Guiding Symptoms of All Remedies (Clinical and Pathogenetic) Including Indian Drugs*. New Delhi: Jain Publishers, 1984 [reprinted from the 1927 original].

Buhner, Stephen. *The Lost Language of Plants: The Ecological Importance of Plant Medicine to Life on Earth*. White River Junction, VT: Chelsea Green Publishing, 2002.

De La Forêt, Rosalee. *Alchemy of Herbs: Transform Everyday Ingredients into Foods & Remedies That Heal*. Carlsbad, CA: Hay House, 2017.

Gladstar, Rosemary. *Rosemary Gladstar's Medicinal Herbs: A Beginner's Guide*. North Adams, MA: Storey Publishing, 2012.

Grieve, Maude. *A Modern Herbal: The Medicinal, Culinary, Cosmetic and Economic Properties, Cultivation and Folklore of Herbs, Grasses, Fungi, Shrubs and Trees with All Their Modern Scientific Uses*, Volumes I and II. New York: Dover Publishing, 1971.

Hardin, Kiva Rose. *A Weedwife's Remedy: Folk Herbalism for the Hedgewise*. Plant Healer Press, 2019.

Iwu, Maurice M. *Handbook of African Medicinal Plants*. Boca Raton, FL: CRC Press, 2014.

Kimmerer, Robin Wall. *Braiding Sweetgrass: Indigenous Wisdom, Scientific Knowledge and the Teachings of Plants*. Minneapolis, MN: Milkweed Editions, 2015.

Kloss, Jethro. *Back to Eden: A Human Interest Story of Health and Restoration to be Found in Herb, Root, and Bark*. Loma Linda: Back to Eden Books Publishing, 1939–1992.

Levy, Juliette de Baïracli. *The Illustrated Herbal Handbook*. London: Faber & Faber, 1982.

Light, Phyllis. *Southern Folk Medicine: Healing Traditions from the Appalachian Fields and Forests*. Berkeley, CA: North Atlantic Books, 2018.

Masé, Guido. *The Wild Medicine Solution: Healing with Aromatic, Bitter, and Tonic Plants*. Rochester, VT: Healing Arts Press, 2013.

Mitchen, Stephanie Y. *African American Folk Healing*. New York: NYU Press, 2007.

Popham, Sajah. *Evolutionary Herbalism: Science, Spirituality, and Medicine from the Heart of Nature*. Berkeley, CA: North Atlantic Books, 2019.

Tierra, Michael. *The Way of Herbs*. Santa Cruz, CA: Unity Press, 1980.

Treben, Maria. *Health Through God's Pharmacy: Advice and Proven Cures with Medicinal Herbs*, trans. Steyr, Austria: Willhelm Ennsthaler, 1984.

Weed, Susun. *Healing Wise*. Woodstock, NY: Ash Tree Publishing, 1989.

Winston, David. *Herbal Therapeutics: Specific Indications for Herbs and Herbal Formulas*, 10th ed. Broadway, NJ: Herbal Therapeutics Research Library, 2013.

Winston, David, and Steven Maimes. *Adaptogens: Herbs for Strength and Stress Relief*. Rochester, VT: Healing Arts Press, 2007.

Wood, Matthew. *The Book of Herbal Wisdom: Using Plants as Medicines*. Berkeley, CA: North Atlantic Books, 1997.

Wood, Matthew. *The Earthwise Herbal: A Complete Guide to New World Medicinal Plants*. Berkeley, CA: North Atlantic Books, 2008.

Wood, Matthew. *The Earthwise Herbal: A Complete Guide to Old World Medicinal Plants*. Berkeley, CA: North Atlantic Books, 2008.

Clinical/Advanced Studies

Ellingwood, Finley. *American Materia Medica, Therapeutics, and Pharmacognosy*. Portland, OR: Eclectic Medical Publications, 1983 [reprinted from the 1919 original].

Felter, Harvey, and Lloyd, John Uri. *King's American Dispensatory*. Portland, OR: Eclectic Medical Publications, 1986 [reprinted from the 1898 original].

Flint, Margi. *The Practicing Herbalist: Meeting With Clients, Reading the Body*. Marblehead, MA: EarthSong Press, 2010.

Hoffmann, David. *Medical Herbalism: The Science and Practice of Herbal Medicine*. Rochester, VT: Healing Arts Press, 2003.

Kirschbaum, Barbara. *Atlas of Chinese Tongue Diagnosis*. Seattle: Eastland Press, 2000.

Maciocia, Giovanni. *Tongue Diagnosis in Chinese Medicine*. Seattle: Eastland Press, 1995.

Mills, Simon. *Out of the Earth: The Essential Book of Herbal Medicine.* London: Viking Press, 1991.

Mills, Simon, and Kerry Bone. *Principles and Practice of Phytotherapy: Modern Herbal Medicine.* Edinburg: Churchill Livingston, 2000.

Priest, A. W., and L. R. Priest. *Herbal Medication: A Clinical and Dispensatory Handbook.* L.N. Fowler, 1982.

Scudder, John M. *The American Eclectic Materia Medica and Therapeutics,* 11th ed. Cincinnati, OH: Author, 1891.

Stansbury, Jill. *Herbal Formularies for Health Professionals.* 5 vols. White River Junction, VT: Chelsea Green Publishing, 2018.

Tilgner, Sharol Marie. *Herbal Medicine: From the Heart of the Earth.* Pleasant Hill, OR: Wise Acres, 2009.

Weiss, Rudolf. *Herbal Medicine.* Translation of *Lehrbuch der Phytotherapie.* Translated by A. Meuss. Beaconsfield, UK: Beaconsfield Publishing, 1998.

Wood, Matthew. *The Practice of Traditional Western Herbalism: Basic Doctrine, Energetics, and Classification.* Berkeley, CA: North Atlantic Press, 2004.

Chinese/Ayurvedic/Unani Tibb

Bajracharya, Valdya Madhu Bajra, Todd Tillotson, and Todd Caldecott, eds. *Ayurveda in Nepal: Volume One: Ayurvedic Principles, Diagnosis and Treatment.* Shelbyville, KY: Wasteland Press, 2009.

Beinfield, Harriet, and Efrem Korngold. *Between Heaven and Earth: A Guide to Chinese Medicine.* New York: Ballantine Books, 1991.

Bensky, Dan, Steven Clavey, and Erich Stöger. *Chinese Herbal Medicine Materia Medica,* 3rd ed. Seattle: Eastland Press, 1993.

Chishti, G. M., and N. D. Hakim. *The Traditional Healer: A Comprehensive Guide to the Principles and Practice of Unani Herbal Medicine.* Rochester, VT: Healing Arts Press, 1988.

Connelly, Dianne M. *Traditional Acupuncture: The Law of the Five Elements.* Author, 1979.

Frawley, David. *Ayurvedic Healing: A Comprehensive Guide.* Twin Lakes, WI: Lotus Press, 2000.

Haas, Elson M. *Staying Healthy with the Seasons.* Berkeley, CA: Celestial Arts, 1981, 2003.

Kaptchuk, Ted. *The Web That Has No Weaver: Understanding Chinese Medicine.* New York: Congdon & Weed, 1983.

Lad, Vasant. *Ayurveda: The Science of Self-Healing.* Santa Fe, NM: Lotus Press, 1984.

Packard, Candis Cantin. *Pocket Guide to Ayurvedic Healing*. Freedom: Crossing Press, 1996.

Tierra, Lesley. *The Herbs of Life: Health and Healing Using Western and Chinese Techniques*. Freedom: Crossing Press, 1992.

Tierra, Michael. *Planetary Herbology: An Integration of Western Herbs into the Traditional Chinese and Ayurvedic Systems*. Twin Lakes, WI: Lotus Press, 1988.

Wiseman, Nigel, and Andrew Ellis. *Fundamentals of Chinese Medicine*. Brookline, MA: Paradigm Publications, 1996.

Medicine Making

Cech, Richo. *Making Plant Medicine*. Williams, OR: Horizon Herbals, 2000.

Easley, Thomas, and Steven Horne. *The Modern Herbal Dispensatory: A Medicine-Making Guide*. Berkeley, CA: North Atlantic Books, 2016.

Green, James. *Herbal Medicine-Maker's Handbook*. Forestville, CA: Simpler's Botanical, 1986.

Field Guides

Brill, Steve, with Evelyn Dean. *Identifying and Harvesting Edible and Medicinal Plants in Wild (and Not So Wild) Places*. New York: Quill William Morrow, 1994.

Elpel, Thomas J. *Botany in a Day: The Patterns Method of Plant Identification*. Pony, MT: HOPS Press, 1997.

Foster, Steven, and James Duke. *A Field Guide to Medicinal Plants: Eastern and Central North America*. Boston: Houghton Mifflin, 2000.

Moore, Michael. *Medicinal Plants of the Mountain West*. Santa Fe, NM: Museum of New Mexico Press, 1979.

Newcomb, Lawrence. *Newcomb's Wildflower Guide*. New York: Little and Brown, 1977.

Tallamay, Douglas W. *Nature's Best Hope: A New Approach to Conversations That Starts in Your Yard*. Portland, OR: Timber Press, 2020.

Decolonizing Herbalism / Social Justice Writings

Alexander, Michelle. *The New Jim Crow: Mass Incarceration in the Age of Colorblindness*. New York: The New Press, 2010.

Bonilla-Silva, Eduardo. *Racism without Racists: Color-Blind Racism and the Persistence of Racial Inequality in the United States*. Lanham, MD: Rowman & Littlefield, 2003.

Dunbar-Ortiz, Roxanne. *An Indigenous Peoples' History of the United States.* Boston, MA: Beacon Press, 2015.

Geniusz, Wendy Djinn. *Our Knowledge is not Primitive: Decolonizing Botanical Anishinaabe Teachings.* Syracuse: Syracuse University Press, 2009.

King, Thomas. *Inconvenient Indian: A Curious Account of Native People in North America.* Minneapolis, MN: University of Minnesota Press, 2018.

LaDuke, Winona. *Recovering the Sacred: The Power of Naming and Claiming.* Boston, MA: South End Press, 2005.

Lee, Michele Elizabeth. *Working the Roots: Over 400 Years of Traditional African American Healing.* Oakland, CA: Wadastick, 2017.

Washington, Harriet A. *Medical Apartheid: The Dark History of Medical Experimentation on Black Americans from Colonial Times to the Present.* New York: Harlem Moon, 2006.

Aromidwifery. "White Privilege 101." https://aromidwifery.wordpress .com/resources/white-privilege-101/

Aromidwifery. "Intersections of Race, Gender, Class." https://aromidwifery .wordpress.com/resources/intersections-of-race-gender-class/

Scott, Toi. *Queering Herbalism: Brown. Queer. Herbalism.* http:// queerherbalism.blogspot.com

History/Ethnobotany

Anderson, M. Kat. *Tending the Wild: Native American Knowledge and the Management of California's Natural Resources.* Oakland: University of California Press, 2013.

Deloria, Vine. *Behind the Trail of Broken Treaties: An Indian Declaration of Independence.* Austin, TX: University of Texas Press, 1985.

Fett, Sharla. *Working Cures: Healing, Healing and Power on Southern Slave Plantations.* Chapel Hill: The University of North Carolina Press, 2002.

Griggs, Barbara. *Green Pharmacy: The History and Evolution of Western Herbal Medicine.* Rochester, VT: Healing Arts Press, 1981, 1991, 1997.

Mitchell, Faith. *Hoodoo Medicine: Gullah Herbal Remedies.* Columbia, SC: Summerhouse Press, 2011.

Moerman, Daniel. *Native American Ethnobotany.* Portland, OR: Timber Press, 1998.

Turner, Nancy J. *Ancient Pathways, Ancestral Knowledge: Ethnobotany and Ecological Wisdom of Indigenous Peoples of Northwestern North America.* Montreal: McGill-Queen's University Press, 2014.

Wood, Matthew. *Vitalism: The History of Herbalism, Homeopathy, and Flower Essences*. Berkeley, CA: North Atlantic Books, 2000.

Reproductive Health

Buhner, Stephen. *The Natural Testosterone Plan: For Sexual Health and Energy*. Rochester, VT: Healing Arts Press, 2007.

Buhner, Stephen. *Vital Man: Natural Healthcare for Men at Midlife*. New York, NY: Avery, 2003.

Crawford, Amanda McQuade. *The Herbal Menopause Book*. Freedom: Crossing Press, 1996.

Erikson-Schroth, Laura, ed. *Trans Bodies, Trans Selves: A Resource for the Transgender Community*. New York: Oxford University Press, 2014.

Gladstar, Rosemary. *Herbal Healing for Women*. Englewood Cliffs, NJ: Prentice Hall, 1995.

Green, James. *The Male Herbal: Health Care for Men and Boys*. Freedom: Crossing Press, 1991.

Hobbs, Christopher, and Kathi Keville. *Women's Herbs, Women's Health*. Loveland, CO: Interweave Press, 1998.

Soule, Deb. *The Roots of Healing: A Woman's Book of Herbs*. New York: Citadel Press, 1995.

Weed, Susun. *The Wise Woman Herbal for the Menopause Years*. Woodstock, NY: Ash Tree Publishing, 1986.

Plant Spirit/Shamanic Studies

Berry, Thomas. *The Dream of the Earth*. San Francisco: Sierra Club Books, 1988.

Buhner, Stephen. *Secret Teachings of Plants: The Intelligence of the Heart in the Direct Perception of Nature*. Rochester, VT: Bear and Co, 2004.

Cowan, Eliot. *Plant Spirit Medicine: The Healing Power of Plants*. Portland, OR: Swan, Raven & Co., 1995.

McKenna, Terence. *Food of the Gods: The Search for the Original Tree of Knowledge: A Radical History of Plants, Drugs, and Human Evolution*. New York: Bantam Books, 1992.

Shultes, Richard. *Plants of the Gods: Their Sacred, Healing, and Hallucinogenic Powers*. Rochester, VT: Healing Arts Press, 2001.

Notes

Introduction: Honoring the Sacred

1. Stephen Buhner, *The Secret Teachings of Plants: The Intelligence of the Heart in the Direct Perception of Nature* (Rochester, VT: Bear & Company, 2004).
2. Thomas Berry, *The Dream of the Earth* (Berkeley, CA: Counterpoint Press, 2015).
3. Teju Cole, "The White-Savior Industrial Complex," *The Atlantic*, March 21, 2012.
4. Tyler Smith et al., "US Sales of Herbal Supplements Increase by 8.6% in 2019," *Herbal Gram*, Fall 2020, 54–69.
5. Belinda Hawkins, "Plants for Life: Medicinal Plant Conservation and Botanic Gardens," Botanic Gardens Conservation International (2008), https://www.bgci.org/files/Worldwide/Publications/PDFs/medicinal.pdf.
6. Svevo Brooks, *The Art of Good Living* (Boston: Houghton Mifflin, 1990).

Chapter 1: The Language of Energetics

1. Ted J. Kaptchuk, *The Web That Has No Weaver: Understanding Chinese Medicine* (Chicago: Congdon & Weed, Inc., 1983), 434.
2. David Winston and Alan M. Dattner, "The American System of Medicine," *Clinics in Dermatology* 17, no. 1 (1999): 53–56, https://doi.org/10.1016/S0738-081X(98)00063-7.
3. Dogwood School of Botanical Medicine, "History of Physiomedicalism," https://dogwoodbotanical.com/history-of-physiomedicalism.
4. Simon Mills and Kerry Bone, *Principles and Practice of Phytotherapy: Modern Herbal Medicine* (London: Churchill Livingstone, 2000), 13.
5. Robert Bly, trans., *Kabir: Ecstatic Poems* (Boston: Beacon Press, 2007).
6. Rosita Arvigo (founder, The Abdominal Therapy Collective) in discussion with the author, May 6, 2021.

Chapter 2: Plant Relations with All the Senses

1. Sajah Popham, *Evolutionary Herbalism: Science, Medicine, and Spirituality from the Heart of Nature* (Berkeley, CA: North Atlantic Books, 2019).

2. Buhner, *Secret Teachings of Plants*.

3. Simon Mills, *Out of the Earth: The Essential Book of Herbal Medicine* (London: Viking Arkana, 1993).

4. Brian C. Freeman and Gwyn A. Beattie, "An Overview of Plant Defenses against Pathogens and Herbivores," *The Plant Health Instructor* (2008), https://doi.org/10.1094/PHI-I-2008-0226-01.

5. C. H. Brieskorn and P. Noble, "The Terpenes of the Essential Oil of Myrrh," in vol. 7 of *Aromatic Plants. World Crops: Production, Utilization, and Description*, edited by N. Margaris, A. Koedam, and D. Vokou (Berlin: Springer, Dordrecht), https://doi.org/10.1007/978-94-009-7642-9_19.

6. "Science," Institute for the Preservation of Medical Traditions, https://medicaltraditions.org/research/science.

7. H. G. O. Blake, ed., *Winter: From the Journal of Henry David Thoreau* (Boston: Houghton, Mifflin, 1888).

8. Joseph Pearce, *The Biology of Transcendence: A Blueprint of the Humans Spirit* (Rochester, VT: Inner Traditions, 2004).

9. Henry Corbin, *Mundus Imaginalis, or The Imaginary and the Imaginal* (Brussels: Cahiers Internationaux de Symbolisme, 1964).

10. Karyn Sanders (clinical herbalist, Blue Otter School of Herbal Medicine), in email communication with the author, July 7, 2020.

11. Robin Wall Kimmerer, "Returning the Gift," Center for Humans & Nature, accessed August 19, 2021, https://www.humansandnature.org/earth-ethic-robin-kimmerer.

12. Robin Wall Kimmerer, *Braiding Sweetgrass: Indigenous Wisdom, Scientific Knowledge and the Teachings of Plants* (Minneapolis, MN: Milkweed Editions, 2013).

Chapter 3: Medicine of Place

1. Eliot Cowan, *Plant Spirit Medicine: A Journey into the Healing Wisdom of Plants* (Boulder, CO: Sounds True, 2015).

2. Often the word *dreamtime* is used to describe this cosmology, but none of the hundreds of Aboriginal languages contain a word for *time*. Aboriginal spirituality is thought to be better described by *dreaming*, as it conveys as a timeless concept where one moves from "dream" into reality. The other important language distinction to make is that the noun *Aborigine* is no longer in use as it is considered dehumanizing. The adjective *aboriginal* at least recognizes that there are a multitude

of diverse First Nation cultures. For the most part, the preference of each culture is to be referred to them as their language group.

3. Richard Bugbee, email message to the author, March 26, 2021.

4. Lindsay P. Galway et al., "Mapping the Solastalgia Literature: A Scoping Review Study," *International Journal of Environmental Research and Public Health* 16, no. 15 (2019): 2662, https://doi.org/10.3390 /ijerph16152662.

5. Kat Anderson, *Tending the Wild: Native American Knowledge and the Management of California's Natural Resources* (Berkeley: University of California Press, 2013).

6. Lyla June Johnston, "Lyla June on the Forest as Farm," the Esperanza Project, https://www.esperanzaproject.com/2019/native-american -culture/lyla-june-on-the-forest-as-farm.

7. Kudzayi Chiwanza et al., "Challenges in Preserving Indigenous Knowledge Systems: Learning from Past Experiences," *Information and Knowledge Management* 3, no. 2 (2013), https://www.iiste.org/Journals /index.php/IKM/article/view/4280.

8. Kirsten Vinyeta and Kathy Lynn, *Exploring the Role of Traditional Ecological Knowledge in Climate Change Initiatives*, Gen. Tech. Rep. PNW-GTR-879 (Portland, OR: US Department of Agriculture, Forest Service, Pacific Northwest Research Station, 2021) https:// permanent.fdlp.gov/gpo37896/pnw_gtr879.pdf.

9. Repatriation is the act or process of restoring or returning someone or something to the country of origin, allegiance, or citizenship. The Indigenous definition of *rematriation* is in reference to the reclamation of spirituality, ancestral objects, knowledge, and resources. These may be returned to Indigenous peoples, but in essence they are returned to the Mother Earth.

10. Toby Hemenway, *Gaia's Garden: A Guide to Home-Scale Permaculture* (White River Junction, VT: Chelsea Green Publishing, 2009).

11. Miriam Rose, "Miriam's Story," Miriam Rose Foundation, https:// www.miriamrosefoundation.org.au/about-miriam-rose-foundation.

12. Sharon Blackie, "Dipping Our Toes into the Mystery of Place," July 11, 2020, https://sharonblackie.net/dipping-our-toes-into-the -mystery-of-place.

13. United Plant Savers, "Our Mission at UpS," https://unitedplantsavers .org/40-our-mission-ups.

14. Stuart A. Kallen, *The War at Home* (San Diego, CA: Lucent Books, 2000).

15. Laura Schumm, "America's Patriotic Victory Gardens," *History*, May 29, 2014, updated August 31, 2018, https://www.history.com/news /americas-patriotic-victory-gardens.

16. *Merriam-Webster*, s.v. "Anthropocene (*n.*)," accessed May 19, 2021, https://www.merriam-webster.com/dictionary/Anthropocene. "The period of time during which human activities have had an environmental impact on the Earth regarded as constituting a distinct geological age."

Chapter 4: Medicine of the Seasons

1. Ilza Veith, trans., *The Yellow Emperor's Classic of Internal Medicine* (Berkeley: University of California Press, 1972).

2. Ted J. Kaptchuk, *The Web That Has No Weaver: Understanding Chinese Medicine* (Chicago: Congdon & Weed, Inc., 1983).

3. Kaptchuk, *The Web That Has No Weaver*.

4. Veith, *The Yellow Emperor's Classic of Internal Medicine*.

5. Gottfried Novacek, "Gender and Gallstone Disease," *Wiener Medizinische Wochenschrift* 156 (2006): 527–33, https://doi.org/10.1007 /s10354-006-0346-x.

6. Veith, *The Yellow Emperor's Classic of Internal Medicine*.

7. Martín Prechtel, *The Smell of Rain on Dust: Grief and Praise* (Berkeley, CA: North Atlantic Books, 2015).

Chapter 5: Our Elemental Selves

1. Vaidya Madhu Bajra Bajracharya et al. eds., *Ayurveda in Nepal: Volume 1: Ayurvedic Principles, Diagnosis and Treatment* (Shelbyville, KY: Wasteland Press, 2009).

2. Sajah Popham, *Evolutionary Herbalism: Science, Spirituality, and Medicine from the Heart of Nature* (Berkeley, CA: North Atlantic Press, 2019).

3. Vasant Lad, *Ayurveda: The Science of Self-Healing* (Sante Fe, NM: Lotus Press, 1985).

Chapter 6: Our Inner Terrain

1. Hakim G. M. Chishti, *The Traditional Healer's Handbook: A Classic Guide to the Medicine of Avicenna* (Rochester, VT: Healing Arts Press, 1991).

2. Samuel Thomson, *The Thomsonian Materia Medica* (Albany, NY: J. Munsell 1841).

3. John S. Haller, Jr., *The People's Doctors: Samuel Thomson and the American Botanical Movement, 1790–1860* (Carbondale, IL: Southern Illinois University Press, 2000), 184.

4. jim mcDonald, *Foundational Herbcraft: Actions and Energetics in Western Herbalism*, collected writings from http://www.PlantHealer Magazine.com.

5. Alugoju Phaniendra et al., "Free Radicals: Properties, Sources, Targets, and Their Implication in Various Diseases," *Indian Journal of Clinical Biochemistry* 30, no. 1 (2015): 11–26, https://doi.org/10.1007/s12291 -014-0446-0.

6. Allison L. Hopkins et al., "*Hibiscus sabdariffa* L. in the Treatment of Hypertension and Hyperlipidemia: A Comprehensive Review of Animal and Human Studies," *Fitoterapia* 85 (2013): 84–94, https:// doi.org/10.1016/j.fitote.2013.01.003.

7. Rosemary Gladstar, *Fire Cider!: 101 Zesty Recipes for Health-Boosting Remedies Made with Apple Cider Vinegar* (North Adams, MA: Storey, 2019).

8. Matthew Wood, *The Earthwise Herbal, Volume I: A Complete Guide to Old World Medicinal Plants* (Berkeley, CA: North Atlantic Books, 2008), 178.

9. T. P. J. Solomon and A. K. Blannin, "Effects of Short-Term Cinnamon Ingestion on *In Vivo* Glucose Tolerance," *Diabetes, Obesity, and Metabolism* 9, no. 6 (2007): 895–901, https://doi.org/10.1111/j.1463 -1326.2006.00694.x.

10. Robert Clickner, in discussion with the author, May 8, 2019.

Chapter 7: The Wheel of the Year

1. Sharon Blackie, *This Mythic Life*, podcast, January 6, 2020, https:// sharonblackie.net/podcast.

2. Martín Prechtel, *The Smell of Rain on Dust: Grief and Praise* (Berkeley, CA: North Atlantic Books, 2015).

3. Sharon Blackie, "Reclaiming Our Native 'Insular Celtic' Spirituality," *Celtic Studies*, February 9, 2020, https://sharonblackie.net /decolonising-and-reclaiming-our-native-insular-celtic-spirituality.

Chapter 8: Kitchen Apothecary Practices

1. Email communication with the author, May 18, 2021.

2. James Green, *The Herbal Medicine-Maker's Handbook: A Home Manual* (Freedom: Crossing Press, 2000), 114.

3. "What Are Flower Essences?," Flower Essence Services, http://www
.fesflowers.com/learn-about-flower-essences/what-are-flower-essences.

4. Thomas Easley and Steven Horne, *The Modern Herbal Dispensatory: A
Medicine-Making Guide* (Berkeley, CA: North Atlantic Books, 2016).

5. C. S. Johnston and C. A. Gaas, "Vinegar: Medicinal Uses and Antigly-
cemic Effect," *Medscape General Medicine* 8, no. 2 (2006): 61.

6. C. S. Johnston, C. M. Kim, and A. J. Buller, "Vinegar Improves Insulin
Sensitivity to a High-Carbohydrate Meal in Subjects with Insulin
Resistance or Type 2 Diabetes," *Diabetes Care* 27, no. 1 (2004): 281–2,
https://doi.org/10.2337/diacare.27.1.281.

7. J. Darzi et al., "Influence of the Tolerability of Vinegar as an Oral Source
of Short-Chain Fatty Acids on Appetite Control and Food Intake,"
International Journal of Obesity 38, no. 5 (2014): 675–81, https://doi
.org/10.1038/ijo.2013.157.

Chapter 9: The Plants: Materia Medica

1. David Winston and Alan M. Dattner, "The American System of
Medicine," *Clinics in Dermatology* 17 (1999): 53–56, http://doi.org
/10.1016/s0738-081x(98)00063-7.

2. Herbal Education Services, *2018 Medicines from the Earth Symposium:
Conference Book*, https://www.botanical-medicine.org/2018
-Medicines-from-the-Earth-Herb-Symposium-Conference-Book
-Download-PDF, p. 337.

3. Matthew Wood, *The Book of Herbal Wisdom: Using Plants as Medicines*
(Berkeley, CA: North Atlantic Books, 1997), 86.

4. Wood, *The Book of Herbal Wisdom*, 95.

5. N. Singh et al., "An Overview on Ashwagandha: A Rasayana (Rejuvenator)
of Ayurveda," *African Journal of Traditional, Complementary, and Alternative Medicines* 8, no. 5S (2011), https://doi.org/10.4314/ajtcam.v8i5S.9.

6. L. C. Mishra et al., "Scientific Basis for the Therapeutic Use of *Withania
somnifera* (Ashwagandha): A Review," *Alternative Medicine Review* 5,
no. 4 (2000): 334–46, https://pubmed.ncbi.nlm.nih.gov/10956379.

7. A. K. Sharma et al., "Efficacy and Safety of Ashwagandha Root Extract
in Subclinical Hypothyroid Patients: A Double-Blind, Randomized
Placebo-Controlled Trial," *Journal of Alternative and Complementary
Medicine* 24, no. 3 (2018), https://doi.org/10.1089/acm.2017.0183.

8. Richo Cech, *Making Plant Medicine* (Williams, OR: Horizon Herbs
Publications, 2000).

9. L. E. Jones and J. M. Scudder, *The American Eclectic Materia Medica and Therapeutics* (Cincinnati, OH: Moore, Wilstach, Keys, 1863).

10. Richard Whelan, "Burdock," https://www.rjwhelan.co.nz/herbs%20A-Z/burdock.html.

11. David Hoffmann, *Medical Herbalism: The Science and Practice of Herbal Medicine* (Rochester, VT: Healing Arts Press, 2003), 528.

12. Ann McIntyre, *Flower Power: Flower Remedies for Healing Body and Soul through Herbalism, Homeopathy, Aromatherapy, and Flower Essences* (New York: Henry Holt, 1996).

13. Maude Grieve, *A Modern Herbal, Volume II* (New York: Dover Publishing, 1971), 517.

14. N. De Tommasi et al., "Structure and *In Vitro* Antiviral Activity of Triterpenoid Saponins from *Calendula arvensis*," *Planta Medica* 57, no. 3 (1991): 250–53, https://doi.org/10.1055/s-2006-960084.

15. Finley Ellingwood, *American Materia Medica, Therapeutics and Pharmacognosy* (Portland, OR: Eclectic Medical Publications, 1994 [reprint of 1919 original]), 390.

16. Z. Amirghofran, M. Azadbakht, and M. H. Karimi, "Evaluation of the Immunomodulatory Effects of Five Herbal Plants," *Journal of Ethnopharmacology* 72, no. 1–2 (2000): 167–72, http://doi.org/10.1016/s0378-8741(00)00234-8.

17. V. D. Ashwlayan et al., "Therapeutic Potential of *Calendula officinalis*," *Pharmacy and Pharmacology International Journal* 6, no. 2 (2018): 149–55, http://doi.org/10.15406/ppij.2018.06.00171.

18. William Mitchell, *Plant Medicine in Practice: Using the Teachings of John Bastyr* (St. Louis, MI: Churchill Livingstone, 2003), 391-92.

19. "Root Doctors," Gale Library of Daily Life: Slavery in America, *Encyclopedia.com*, accessed September 30, 2020, https://www.encyclopedia.com/humanities/applied-and-social-sciences-magazines/root-doctors.

20. Simon Mills and Kerry Bone, *Principles and Practice of Phytotherapy: Modern Herbal Medicine* (Edinburg: Churchill Livingston, 2000), 360.

21. jim mcdonald, "Elder," https://herbcraft.org/elder.html.

22. Charlotte Sophia Burne, *The Handbook of Folklore* (Whitefish, MT: Kessinger Publishing, 2003).

23. Henriette Kress, "Elder Toxicity," January 16, 2006, https://www.henriettes-herb.com/blog/elder-toxicity.html.

24. J. E. Vlachojannis et al., "A Systematic Review on the Sambuci Fructus Effect and Efficacy Profiles," *Phytotherapy Research* 24, no. 1 (2010): 1–8.

25. "COVID-19 Coronavirus Resources," North American Institute of Medical Herbalism, https://www.naimh.com/coronavirus.
26. Z. Zakay-Rones et al., "Randomized Study of the Efficacy and Safety of Oral Elderberry Extract in the Treatment of Influenza A and B Virus Infections," *Journal of International Medical Research* 32, no. 2, (2004): 132–40, http://doi.org/10.1177/147323000403200205.
27. Paul Bergner, "Sambucus (Elderberry), Echinacea, and Cytokine Storm in Respiratory Infection," North American Institute of Medical Herbalism, https://c1c17220-5aa6-46c5-a11f-1b9d7595d5fa.filesusr.com/ugd/ee530d_15bfda32644340b18e9dbc3bed24b93f.pdf.
28. Thomas J. Allen et al., *Caterpillars in the Field and Garden: A Field Guide to the Butterfly Caterpillars of North America* (Oxford: Oxford University Press, 2005).
29. Rudolf Weiss, *Herbal Medicine* (Beaconsfield, UK: Arcanum 1988), 241–42.
30. Daniel Moerman, *Native American Ethnobotany* (Portland, OR: Timber Press, 1998).
31. Moerman, *Native American Ethnobotany*.
32. Harvey Felter and John Uri Lloyd, *King's American Dispensatory* (1898), as found in " Hydrastis USP – Hydrastis," Henriette's Herbal Homepage, https://www.henriettes-herb.com/eclectic/kings/hydrastis.html.
33. Paul Bergner, *Medical Herbalism: A Journal for the Clinical Practitioner*, vol. 8, no. 4 (Winter 1996–1997).
34. Rosalee de la Forêt, "Benefits of Goldenseal," Herbs with Rosalee, https://www.herbalremediesadvice.org/benefits-of-goldenseal.html.
35. Harvey Wickes Felter, *The Eclectic Materia Medica: Pharmacology and Therapeutics*, (Sandy, OR: Eclectic Medical Publications, 1994) [reprinted from 1922 original], 418.
36. Felter, *The Eclectic Materia Medica*.
37. Felter, *The Eclectic Materia Medica*.
38. Annie Shirwaikar et al., "In Vitro Antioxidant Studies on the Benzyl Tetra Isoquinoline Alkaloid Berberine," *Biological and Pharmaceutical Bulletin* 29, no. 9 (2006): 1906–10, http://doi.org/10.1248/bpb.29.1906.
39. Jun Yin et al., "Efficacy of Berberine in Patients with Type 2 Diabetes Mellitus," *Metabolism* 57, no. 5 (2008), https://doi.org/10.1016/j.metabol.2008.01.01.

40. Matthew Wood, *The Earthwise Herbal: A Complete Guide to New World Medicinal Plants* (Berkeley, CA: North Atlantic Books, 2008), 194.

41. "Hawthorn," Steven Foster Group, 2009, https://www.stevenfoster .com/education/monograph/hawthorn.html.

42. J. M. Rigelsky and B. V. Sweet, "Hawthorn: Pharmacology and Therapeutic Uses," *American Journal of Health-System Pharmacy* 59, no. 5 (2002): 417–22, https://doi.org/10.1093/ajhp/59.5.417.

43. I. E. Orhan, "Phytochemical and Pharmacological Activity Profile of *Crataegus oxyacantha* L. (Hawthorn)—A Cardiotonic Herb," *Current Medical Chemistry* 25, no. 37 (2018): 4854–65, https://doi.org/10 .2174/0929867323666160919095519.

44. M. H. Pittler et al., "Hawthorn Extract for Treating Chronic Heart Failure: Meta-analysis of Randomized Trials" *The American Journal of Medicine* 114, no. 8, (2003): 665–74, https://doi.org/10.1016/s0002 -9343(03)00131-1.

45. Mills and Bone, *Principles and Practice of Phytotherapy*, 440–2.

46. Mitchell, *Plant Medicine in Practice*, 134.

47. Paul B. Hamel and Mary U. Chiltoskey, *Cherokee Plants and Their Uses—A 400 Year History* (Sylva, NC: Herald Publishing Co., 1975).

48. Paul Bergner, "Lobelia: Is Lobelia Toxic?," *Medical Herbalism: Journal for the Clinical Practitioner* 10 (1–2): 1, http://medherb.com/Materia _Medica/Lobelia_-_Is_lobelia_toxic_.htm.

49. William Cook, *The Physiomedical Dispensatory* (1869), as found in "Lobelia Inflata. Lobelia, Emetic Weed," Henriette's Herbal Homepage, https://www.henriettes-herb.com/eclectic/cook/LOBELIA _INFLATA.htm, from scan by Paul Bergner at http://medherb.com.

50. Cech, *Making Plant Medicine.*

51. Thomas Elpel, *Botany in a Day: The Patterns Method of Plant Identification* (Pony, MT: HOPS Press, 2008).

52. Mitchell, *Plant Medicine in Practice*, 164.

53. Merrily A. Kuhn and David Winston, *Winston & Kuhn's Herbal Therapy and Supplements: A Scientific and Traditional Approach* (Philadelphia: Lippincott Williams & Wilkins, 2008), 229.

54. A. B. Siegel and J. Stebbing, "Milk Thistle: Early Seeds of Potential," *Lancet Oncology* 14, no. 10 (2013): 929–30, https://doi.org/10.1016 /S1470-2045(13)70414-5.

55. Christopher Hobbs, *Milk Thistle: The Liver Herb* (Capitola, CA: Botanica Press, 1992).

56. M. Bahmani et al., "*Silybum marianum*: Beyond Hepatoprotection," *Journal of Evidence-Based Complementary & Alternative Medicine* 20, no. 4 (2015): 292–301, https://doi.org/10.1177/2156587215571116.

57. Kuhn and Winston, *Winston & Kuhn's Herbal Therapy and Supplements*, 228.

58. F. Di Pierro, "Clinical Role of a Fixed Combination of Standardized *Berberis aristata* and *Silybum marianum* Extracts in Diabetic and Hypercholesterolemic Patients Intolerant to Statins," *Diabetes, Metabolic Syndrome and Obesity: Targets and Therapy* 8, (2015): 89–96, https://doi.org/10.2147/DMSO.S78877.

59. Harvey Felter and John Uri Lloyd, *King's American Dispensatory* (1898), as found in "Carduus Marianus – St Mary's Thistle," Henriette's Herbal Homepage, https://www.henriettes-herb.com/eclectic/kings/silybum.html.

60. A. B. Forinash et al., "The Use of Galactogogues in the Breastfeeding Mother," *The Annals of Pharmacotherapy* 46, no. 10 (2012):1392–404, https://doi.org/10.1345/aph.1R167.

61. Felter and Lloyd, *King's American Dispensatory* (1898), "Carduus Marianus – St Mary's Thistle," Henriette's Herbal Homepage.

62. Harvey Felter and John Uri Lloyd, *King's American Dispensatory* (1898), as found in "Leonurus – Motherwort" Henriette's Herbal Homepage, https://www.henriettes-herb.com/eclectic/kings/leonurus.html.

63. One of the mechanisms of hot flashes is that the body is requesting more estrogen via a pituitary hormone called follicle stimulating hormone (FSH). In menopause, when estrogen is decreasing and the FSH does not get the result it is hoping for, the body sends out adrenaline to "force" production of estrogen. This surge in adrenaline is one factor producing hot flashes, which is why supplementing with estrogen or giving herbs to mimic this hormone subdue the heat from flashes.

64. Ellingwood stated: "The most direct use of this agent is in the treatment of simple uncomplicated cases of deafness, or in the early stages of progressive deafness where the cause is not apparent. In these cases, from, two to five drops in the ear, three or four times each day, will stop the progress of the disease, and will cure many simple cases."

65. Christa Sinadinos, "Medicinal Uses of Mullein Root," *Medical Herbalism* 16, no. 2 (2009): 1–15, http://medherb.com/eletter/Mullein-Sinadinos.pdf.

66. B. M. Adhikari et al., "Comparison of Nutritional Properties of Stinging Nettle (*Urtica dioica*) Flour with Wheat and Barley Flours," *Food Science and Nutrition* 4, no. 1 (2015): 119–24, https://doi.org/10.1002/fsn3.259.

67. C. Randall et al., "Randomized Controlled Trial of Nettle Sting for Treatment of Base-of-Thumb Pain," *Journal of the Royal Society of Medicine* 93, no. 6 (2000): 30, https://doi.org/10.1177/014107680009300607.

68. Cathleen Rapp, "Special Saw Palmetto and Stinging Nettle Root Combination as Effective as Pharmaceutical Drug for Prostate Symptoms," *American Botanical Council's Herbalgram* 72 (2006): 20–21.

69. R. Dhouibi et al., "Screening of Pharmacological Uses of *Urtica dioica* and Others Benefits," *Progress in Biophysic and Molecular Biology* 150 (2020): 67–77, https://doi.org/10.1016/j.pbiomolbio.2019.05.008.

70. Mills and Bone, *Principles and Practices of Phytotherapy*, 494–5.

71. Moerman, *Native American Ethnobotany*.

72. Ellingwood, *American Materia Medica, Therapeutics and Pharmacognosy*, 165–6.

73. Alan Keith Tillotson, *The One Earth Herbal Sourcebook: Everything You Need to Know about Chinese, Western, and Ayurvedic Herbal Treatments* (New York: Kensington Books 2001).

74. Wood, *The Earthwise Herbal: A Complete Guide to New World Medicinal Plants*, 363–66.

75. Moerman, *Native American Ethnobotany*.

76. M. Grieve, "Self-Heal," Botanical.com: A Modern Herbal, https://www.botanical.com/botanical/mgmh/s/selfhe40.html.

77. Grieve, "Self-Heal."

78. H. Wu et al., "Strategies for Combating Bacterial Biofilm Infections," *International Journal of Oral Science* 7, no. 1 (2015): 1–7, https://doi.org/10.1038/ijos.2014.65.

79. X. Fang et al., "Immune Modulatory Effects of *Prunella vulgaris* L. on Monocytes/Macrophages," *International Journal of Molecular Medicine* 16, no. 6 (2005): 1109–16, http://www.ncbi.nlm.nih.gov/pubmed/16273294.

80. ChoonSeok Oh et al., "Inhibition of HIV-1 Infection by Aqueous Extracts of *Prunella vulgaris* L.," *Virology Journal* 8 (2011) 188, https://doi.org/10.1186/1743-422X-8-188.

81. Wood, *The Earthwise Herbal: A Complete Guide to Old World Medicinal Plants*, 404.

82. Mitchell, *Plant Medicine in Practice*, 345.

83. Mitchell, *Plant Medicine in Practice*, 345.

84. Maude Grieve, *A Modern Herbal, Volume II,* 708.
85. *Arnica montana* is a very popular homeopathic remedy for removing congestion and swelling after injury. It prevents bruising and clears stagnation so that blood supply continues to heal the injury. There are other indications but this is the most well-known.
86. Harvey Felter and John Uri Lloyd, *King's American Dispensatory* (1898), as found in "Hypericum – St. Johns Wort," Henriette's Herbal Homepage, https://www.henriettes-herb.com/eclectic/kings/hypericum.html.
87. David Winston, "Differential Treatment of Depression and Anxiety with Botanical and Nutritional Medicines," 2014, https://www.americanherbalistsguild.com/sites/default/files/Proceedings/winston_david_-_differ_treat-depression.pdf.
88. S. Degar et al., "Inactivation of the Human Immunodeficiency Virus by Hypericin: Evidence for Photochemical Alterations of p24 and a Block in Uncoating," *AIDS Research and Human Retroviruses* 8, no. 11 (1992): 1929–36, https://doi.org/10.1089/aid.1992.8.1929.
89. Kenneth M. Klemow et al., "Medical Attributes of St. John's Wort (*Hypericum perforatum*)," in *Herbal Medicine: Biomolecular and Clinical Aspects,* 2nd edition, edited by S. Wachtel-Galor and Iris F. F. Benzie (Boca Raton, FL: CRC Press, 2011), Chapter 11.
90. Cech, *Making Plant Medicine.*
91. Susun Weed, *Healing Wise* (Woodstock, NY: Ash Tree Publishing, 2003).
92. S. Yousefnia et al., "Suppressive Role of *Viola odorata* Extract on Malignant Characters of Mammosphere-Derived Breast Cancer Stem Cells," *Clinical and Translational Oncology* 22 (2020): 1619–34, https://doi.org/10.1007/s12094-020-02307-9.
93. Juliet Blankespoor, "Violet's Edible and Medicinal Uses," Chestnut School of Herbal Medicine, https://chestnutherbs.com/violets-edible-and-medicinal-uses.
94. Colin Barras, "Neanderthal Dental Tartar Reveals Evidence of Medicine," *New Scientist,* July 18, 2012, http://www.newscientist.com/article/dn22075-neanderthal-dental-tartar-reveals-evidence-of-medicine.
95. Wood, *The Earthwise Herbal: A Complete Guide to New World Medicinal Plants,* 52.
96. Toby Heminway, *Gaia's Garden: A Guide to Home-Scale Permaculture* (White River Junction, VT: Chelsea Green Publisher, 2009).

Index

Note: Page numbers in *italics* refer to figures and illustrations. Page numbers followed by *t* refer to tables.

About the Author

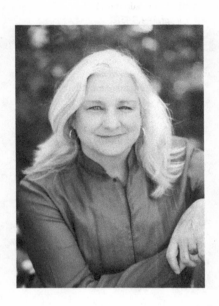

Kat Maier, RH (AHG), is the founder and director of Sacred Plant Traditions, a center for herbal studies in Charlottesville, Virginia. One of her greatest accomplishments has been to train many clinical herbalists who have gone on to begin other schools or apothecaries or to open their own practices. In clinical practice for over thirty years, Kat teaches internationally at universities, conferences, and herbal schools. She is a founding member of Botanica Mobile Clinic, a nonprofit dedicated to providing accessible herbal medicine to local communities. The Botanica clinic arose from her school's free clinic, which was one of the first on the East Coast and served as a template for other herbalism schools. She began her study of plants as a Peace Corps volunteer, and her training as a physician's assistant allows her to weave the language of biomedicine into her practice of traditional energetic herbalism. She is coauthor of *Bush Medicine of San Salvador Island, Bahamas.* As a passionate steward of the plants, Kat also served as president of United Plant Savers and was the recipient of the organization's first Medicinal Plant Conservation Award.